COMPUTATIONAL INTELLIGENCE AND PATTERN ANALYSIS IN BIOLOGICAL INFORMATICS

T0305628

Wiley Series on

Bioinformatics: Computational Techniques and Engineering

A complete list of the titles in this series appears at the end of this volume.

COMPUTATIONAL INTELLIGENCE AND PATTERN ANALYSIS IN BIOLOGICAL INFORMATICS

Edited by

UJJWAL MAULIK
Department of Computer Science and Engineering, Jadavpur University,
Kolkata, India

SANGHAMITRA BANDYOPADHYAY
Machine Intelligence Unit, Indian Statistical Institute, Kolkata, India

JASON T. L. WANG
Department of Computer Science, New Jersey Institute of Technology,
Newark, New Jersey

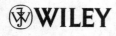

A JOHN WILEY & SONS, INC., PUBLICATION

For general information on our other products and services or for technical support, please contact our Customer Care Department within the United States at (800) 762-2974, outside the United States at (317) 572-3993 or fax (317) 572-4002.

Wiley also publishes its books in a variety of electronic formats. Some content that appears in print may not be available in electronic formats. For more information about Wiley products, visit our web site at www.wiley.com.

ISBN   978-0-470-58159-9

Library of Congress Cataloging-in-Publication Data is available.

Printed in the United States of America

10   9   8   7   6   5   4   3   2   1

To Utsav, our students and parents
—U. Maulik and
S. Bandyopadhyay

To my wife Lynn and
daughter Tiffany
—J. T. L. Wang

CONTENTS

PART III STRUCTURE ANALYSIS

PART IV MICROARRAY DATA ANALYSIS

PART V SYSTEMS BIOLOGY

PREFACE

Computational biology is an interdisciplinary field devoted to the interpretation and analysis of biological data using computational techniques. It is an area of active research involving biology, computer science, statistics, and mathematics to analyze biological sequence data, genome content and arrangement, and to predict the function and structure of macromolecules. This field is a constantly emerging one, with new techniques and results being reported every day. Advancement of data collection techniques is also throwing up novel challenges for the algorithm designers to analyze the complex and voluminous data. It has already been established that traditional computing methods are limited in their scope for application to such complex, large, multidimensional, and inherently noisy data. Computational intelligence techniques, which combine elements of learning, adaptation, evolution, and logic, are found to be particularly well suited to many of the problems arising in biology as they have flexible information processing capabilities for handling huge volume of real-life data with noise, ambiguity, missing values, and so on. Solving problems in biological informatics often involves search for some useful regularities or patterns in large amounts of data that are typically characterized by high dimensionality and low sample size. This necessitates the development of advanced pattern analysis approaches since the traditional methods often become intractable in such situations.

In this book, we attempt to bring together research articles by active practitioners reporting recent advances in integrating computational intelligence and pattern analysis techniques, either individually or in a hybridized manner, for analyzing biological data in order to extract more and more meaningful information and insights from them. Biological data to be considered for analysis include sequence, structure, and microarray data. These data types are typically complex in nature, and require advanced methods to deal with them. Characteristics of the methods and algorithms reported here include the use of domain-specific knowledge for reducing the search space, dealing with uncertainty, partial truth and imprecision, efficient linear and/or sublinear scalability, incremental approaches to knowledge discovery, and increased level and intelligence of interactivity with human experts and decision makers. The techniques can be sequential or parallel in nature.

Computational Intelligence (CI) is a successor of artificial intelligence that combines elements of learning, adaptation, evolution, and logic to create programs that are, in some sense, intelligent. Computational intelligence exhibits an ability to learn and/or to deal with new situations, such that the system is perceived to possess one or more attributes of reason, (e.g., generalization, discovery, association, and abstraction). The different methodologies in CI work synergistically and provide, in one form or another, flexible information processing capabilities. Many biological data are characterized by high dimensionality and low sample size. This poses grand challenges to the traditional pattern analysis techniques necessitating the development of sophisticated approaches.

This book has five parts. The first part contains chapters introducing the basic principles and methodologies of computational intelligence techniques along with a description of some of its important components, fundamental concepts in pattern analysis, and different issues in biological informatics, including a description of biological data and their sources. Detailed descriptions of the different applications of computational intelligence and pattern analysis techniques to biological informatics constitutes the remaining chapters of the book. These include tasks related to the analysis of sequences in the second part, structures in the third part, and microarray data in part four. Some topics in systems biology form the concluding part of this book.

In Chapter 1, Das et al. present a lucid overview of computational intelligence techniques. They introduce the fundamental aspects of the key components of modern computational intelligence. A comprehensive overview of the different tools of computational intelligence (e.g., fuzzy logic, neural network, genetic algorithm, belief network, chaos theory, computational learning theory, and artificial life) is presented. It is well known that the synergistic behavior of the above tools often far exceeds their individual performance. A description of the synergistic behaviors of neuro-fuzzy, neuro-GA, neuro-belief, and fuzzy-belief network models is also included in this chapter. It concludes with a detailed discussion on some emerging trends in computational intelligence like swarm intelligence, Type-2 fuzzy sets, rough sets, granular computing, artificial immune systems, differential evolution, bacterial foraging optimization algorithms, and the algorithms based on artificial bees foraging behavior.

Chakraborty provides an overview of the basic concepts and the fundamental techniques of pattern analysis with an emphasis on statistical methods in Chapter 2. Different approaches for designing a pattern recognition system are described. The pattern recognition tasks of feature selection, classification, and clustering are discussed in detail. The most popular statistical tools are explained. Recent approaches based on the soft computing paradigm are also introduced in this chapter, with a brief representation of the promising neural network classifiers as a new direction toward dealing with imprecise and uncertain patterns generated in newer fields.

In Chapter 3, Byron et al. deal with different aspects of biological informatics. In particular, the biological data types and their sources are mentioned, and two software tools used for analyzing the genomic data are discussed. A case study in biological informatics, focusing on locating noncoding RNAs in Drosophila genomes, is presented. The authors show how the widely used Infernal and RSmatch tools can be combined to mine roX1 genes in 12 species of Drosophila for which the entire genomic sequencing data is available.

The second part of the book, Chapters 4 and 5, deals with the applications of computational intelligence and pattern analysis techniques for biological sequence analysis. In Chapter 4, Rani et al. extract features from the genomic sequences in order to predict promoter regions. Their work is based on global signal-based methods using a neural network classifier. For this purpose, they consider two global features: n-gram features and features based on signal processing techniques by mapping the sequence into a signal. It is shown that the n-gram features extracted for $n = 2, 3, 4,$ and 5 efficiently discriminate promoters from nonpromoters.

In Chapter 5, Masulli et al. deal with the task of computational prediction of microRNA (miRNA) targets with focus on miRNAs' influence in prostate cancer. The miRNAs are capable of base-pairing with imperfect complementarity to the transcripts of animal protein-coding genes (also termed targets) generally within the 3' untranslated region (3' UTR). The existing target prediction programs typically rely on a combination of specific base-pairing rules in the miRNA and target mRNA sequences, and conservational analysis to score possible 3' UTR recognition sites and enumerate putative gene targets. These methods often produce a large number of false positive predictions. In this chapter, Masulli et al. improve the performance of an existing tool called miRanda by exploiting the updated information on biologically validated miRNA gene targets related to human prostate cancer only, and performing automatic parameter tuning using genetic algorithm.

Chapters 6–10 constitute the third part of the book dealing with structural analysis. Chapter 6 deals with the structural search in RNA motif databases. An RNA structural motif is a substructure of an RNA molecule that has a significant biological function. In this chapter, Wen and Wang present two recently developed structural search engines. These are useful to scientists and researchers who are interested in RNA secondary structure motifs. The first search engine is installed on a database, called RmotifDB, which contains secondary structures of the noncoding RNA sequences in Rfam. The second search engine is installed on a block database, which contains the 603 seed alignments, also called blocks, in Rfam. This search engine employs a novel tool, called BlockMatch, for comparing multiple sequence alignments. Some experimental results are reported to demonstrate the effectiveness of the BlockMatch tool.

In Chapter 7, Bhattacharya et al. explore the construction of neighborhood-based kernels on protein structures. Two types of neighborhoods, and two broad classes of kernels, namely, sequence and structure based, are defined. Ways of combining these kernels to get kernels on neighborhoods are discussed. Detailed experimental results are reported showing that some of the designed kernels perform competitively with the state of the art structure comparison algorithms, on the difficult task of classifying 40% sequence nonredundant proteins into SCOP superfamilies.

The use of protein blocks to characterize structural variations in enzymes is discussed in Chapter 8 using kinases as the case study. A protein block is a set of 16 local structural descriptors that has been derived using unsupervised machine learning algorithms and that can approximate the three-dimensional space of proteins. In this chapter, Agarwal et al. first apply their approach in distinguishing between conformation changes and rigid-body displacements between the structures of active and inactive forms of a kinase. Second, a comparison of the conformational patterns of active forms of a kinase with the active and inactive forms of a closely related kinase has been performed. Finally, structural differences in the active states of homologous kinases have been studied. Such studies might help in understanding the structural differences among these enzymes at a different level, as well as guide in making drug targets for a specific kinase.

In Chapter 9, Smalter and Huan address the problem of graph classification through the study of kernel functions and the application of graph classification in chemical quantitative structure–activity relationship (QSAR) study. Graphs, especially the connectivity maps, have been used for modeling chemical structures for decades. In connectivity maps, nodes represent atoms and edges represent chemical bonds between atoms. Support vector machines (SVMs) that have gained popularity in drug design and cheminformatics are used in this regard. Some graph kernel functions are explored that improve on existing methods with respect to both classification accuracy and kernel computation time. Experimental results are reported on five different biological activity data sets, in terms of the classifier prediction accuracy of the support vector machine for different feature generation methods.

Computational ligand design is one of the promising recent approaches to address the problem of drug discovery. It aims to search the chemical space to find suitable drug molecules. In Chapter 10, genetic algorithms have been applied for this combinatorial problem of ligand design. The chapter proposes a variable length genetic algorithm for *de novo* ligand design. It finds the active site of the target protein from the input protein structure and computes the bond stretching, angle bending, angle rotation, van der Waals, and electrostatic energy components using the distance dependent dielectric constant for assigning the fitness score for every individual. It uses a library of 41 fragments for constructing ligands. Ligands have been designed for two different protein targets, namely, Thrombin and HIV-1 Protease. The ligands obtained, using the proposed algorithm, were found to be similar to the real known inhibitors of these proteins. The docking energies using the proposed methodology designed were found to be lower compared to three existing approaches.

Chapters 11–13 constitute the fourth part of the book dealing with microarray data analysis. In Chapter 11, Saha and Maulik develop a differential evolution-based fuzzy clustering algorithm (DEFC) and apply it on four publicly available benchmark microarray data sets, namely, yeast sporulation, yeast cell cycle, Arabidopsis Thaliana, and human fibroblasts serum. Detailed comparative results demonstrating the superiority of the proposed approach are provided. In a part of the investigation, an interesting study integrating the proposed clustering approach with an SVM classifier has been conducted. A fraction of the data points is selected from different clusters based on their proximity to the respective centers. This is used for training an SVM.

The clustering assignments of the remaining points are thereafter determined using the trained classifier. Finally, a biological significance test has been carried out on yeast sporulation microarray data to establish that the developed integrated technique produces functionally enriched clusters.

The classification capability of SVMs is again used in Chapter 12 for identifying potential gene markers that can distinguish between malignant and benign samples in different types of cancers. The proposed scheme consists of two phases. In the first, an ensemble of SVMs using different kernel functions is used for efficient classification. Thereafter, the signal-to-noise ratio statistic is used to select a number of gene markers, which is further reduced by using a multiobjective genetic algorithm-based feature selection method. Results are demonstrated on three publicly available data sets.

In Chapter 13, Maulik and Sarker develop a parallel algorithm for clustering gene expression data that exploits the property of symmetry of the clusters. It is based on a recently developed symmetry-based distance measure. The bottleneck for the application of such an approach for microarray data analysis is the large computational time. Consequently, Maulik and Sarker develop a parallel implementation of the symmetry-based clustering algorithm. Results are demonstrated for one artificial and four benchmark microarray data sets.

The last part of the book, dealing with topics related to systems biology, consists of Chapters 14–16. Jeong and Chen deal with the problem of gene prioritization in Chapter 14, which aims at achieving a better understanding of the disease process and to find therapy targets and diagnostic biomarkers. Gene prioritization is a new approach for extending our knowledge about diseases and potentially about other biological conditions. Jeong and Chen review the existing methods of gene prioritization and attempt to identify those that were most successful. They also discuss the remaining challenges and open problems in this area.

In Chapter 15, Bagchi discusses the various aspects of protein–protein interactions (PPI) that are one of the central players in many vital biochemical processes. Emphasis has been given to the properties of the PPI. A few basic definitions have been revisited. Several computational PPI prediction methods have been reviewed. The various software tools involved have also been reviewed.

Finally, in Chapter 16, Bhattacharyya and Bandyopadhyay study PPI networks in order to investigate the system level activities of the genotypes. Several topological properties and structures have been discussed and state-of-the-art knowledge on utilizing these characteristics in a system level study is included. A novel method of mining an integrated network, obtained by combining two types of topological properties, is designed to find dense subnetworks of proteins that are functionally coherent. Some theoretical analysis on the formation of dense subnetworks in a scale-free network is also provided. The results on PPI information of *Homo Sapiens*, obtained from the Human Protein Reference Database, show promise with such an integrative approach of topological analysis.

The field of biological informatics is rapidly evolving with the availability of new methods of data collection that are not only capable of collecting huge amounts of data, but also produce new data types. In response, advanced methods of searching for useful regularities or patterns in these data sets have been developed. Computational intelligence, comprising a wide array of classification, optimization, and representation methods, have found particular favor among the researchers in biological informatics. The chapters dealing with the applications of computational intelligence and pattern analysis techniques in biological informatics provide a representative view of the available methods and their evaluation in real domains. The volume will be useful to graduate students and researchers in computer science, bioinformatics, computational and molecular biology, biochemistry, systems science, and information technology both as a text and reference book for some parts of the curriculum. The researchers and practitioners in industry, including pharmaceutical companies, and R & D laboratories will also benefit from this book.

We take this opportunity to thank all the authors for contributing chapters related to their current research work that provide the state of the art in advanced computational intelligence and pattern analysis methods in biological informatics. Thanks are due to Indrajit Saha and Malay Bhattacharyya who provided technical support in preparing this volume, as well as to our students who have provided us the necessary academic stimulus to go on. Our special thanks goes to Anirban Mukhopadhyay for his contribution to the book and Christy Michael from Aptara Inc. for her constant help. We are also grateful to Michael Christian of John Wiley & Sons for his constant support.

U. MAULIK, S. BANDYOPADHYAY, AND J. T. L. WANG

November, 2009

CONTRIBUTORS

Ajith Abraham, Machine Intelligence Research Labs (MIR Labs), Scientific Network for Innovation and Research Excellence, Auburn, Washington

G. Agarwal, Molecular Biophysics Unit, Indian Institute of Science, Bangalore, India

Angshuman Bagchi, Buck Institute for Age Research, 8001 Redwood Blvd., Novato, California

Sanghamitra Bandyopadhyay, Machine Intelligence Unit, Indian Statistical Institute, Kolkata, India

Chiranjib Bhattacharyya, Department of Computer Science and Automation, Indian Institute of Science, Bangalore, India

Malay Bhattacharyya, Machine Intelligence Unit, Indian Statistical Institute, Kolkata, India

Sourangshu Bhattacharya, Department of Computer Science and Automation, Indian Institute of Science Bangalore, India

S. Durga Bhavani, Department of Computer and Information Sciences, University of Hyderabad, Hyderabad, India

Kevin Byron, Department of Computer Science, New Jersey Institute of Technology, Newark, New Jersey

Miguel Cervantes-Cervantes, Department of Biological Sciences, Rutgers University, Newark, New Jersey

Basabi Chakraborty, Department of Software and Information Science, Iwate Prefectural University, Iwate, Japan

Nagasuma R. Chandra, Bioinformatics Center, Indian Institute of Science, Bangalore, India

Jake Y. Chen, School of Informatics, Indiana University-Purdue University, Indianapolis, Indiana

Swagatam Das, Department of Electronics and Telecommunication, Jadavpur University, Kolkata, India

Alexandre G. de Brevern, Université Paris Diderot-Paris, Institut National de Transfusion Sanguine (INTS), Paris, France

D. C. Dinesh, Molecular Biophysics Unit, Indian Institute of Science, Bangalore, India

Jun Huan, Department of Electrical Engineering and Computer Science, University of Kansas, Lawrence, Kansas

Jieun Jeong, School of Informatics, Indiana University-Purdue University, Indianapolis, Indiana

Francesco Masulli, Department of Computer and Information Sciences, University of Genova, Italy

Ujjwal Maulik, Depatment of Computer Science and Engineering, Jadavpur University, Kolkata, India

Anirban Mukhopadhyay, Department of Theoretical Bioinformatics, German Cancer Research Center, Heidelberg, Germany, on leave from Department of Computer Science and Engineering, University of Kalyani, India

B. K. Panigrahi, Department of Electrical Engineering, Indian Institute of Technology (IIT), Delhi, India

S. Bapi Raju, Department of Computer and Information Sciences, University of Hyderabad, Hyderabad, India

T. Sobha Rani, Department of Computer and Information Sciences, University of Hyderabad, Hyderabad, India

Stefano Rovetta, Department of Computer and Information Sciences, University of Genova, Italy

Giuseppe Russo, Sbarro Institute for Cancer Research and Molecular Medicine, Temple University, Philadelphia, Pennsylvania

Indrajit Saha, Interdisciplinary Centre for Mathematical and Computational Modeling, University of Warsaw, Poland

Anasua Sarkar, LaBRI, University Bordeaux 1, France

Soumi Sengupta, Machine Intelligence Unit, Indian Statistical Institute, Kolkata, India

Aaron Smalter, Department of Electrical Engineering and Computer Science, University of Kansas, Lawrence, Kansas

N. Srinivasan, Molecular Biophysics Unit, Indian Institute of Science, Bangalore, India

Jason T. L. Wang, Department of Computer Science, New Jersey Institute of Technology, Newark, New Jersey

Dongrong Wen, Department of Computer Science, New Jersey Institute of Technology, Newark, New Jersey

PART I

INTRODUCTION

1

COMPUTATIONAL INTELLIGENCE: FOUNDATIONS, PERSPECTIVES, AND RECENT TRENDS

SWAGATAM DAS, AJITH ABRAHAM, AND B. K. PANIGRAHI

The field of computational intelligence has evolved with the objective of developing machines that can think like humans. As evident, the ultimate achievement in this field would be to mimic or exceed human cognitive capabilities including reasoning, understanding, learning, and so on. Computational intelligence includes neural networks, fuzzy inference systems, global optimization algorithms, probabilistic computing, swarm intelligence, and so on. This chapter introduces the fundamental aspects of the key components of modern computational intelligence. It presents a comprehensive overview of various tools of computational intelligence (e.g., fuzzy logic, neural network, genetic algorithm, belief network, chaos theory, computational learning theory, and artificial life). The synergistic behavior of the above tools on many occasions far exceeds their individual performance. A discussion on the synergistic behavior of neuro-fuzzy, neuro-genetic algorithms (GA), neuro-belief, and fuzzy-belief network models is also included in the chapter.

1.1 WHAT IS COMPUTATIONAL INTELLIGENCE?

Machine Intelligence refers back to 1936, when Turing proposed the idea of a universal mathematics machine [1,2], a theoretical concept in the mathematical theory of computability. Turing and Post independently proved that determining the decidability of mathematical propositions is equivalent to asking what sorts of sequences of a

Computational Intelligence and Pattern Analysis in Biological Informatics, Edited by Ujjwal Maulik, Sanghamitra Bandyopadhyay, and Jason T. L. Wang
Copyright © 2010 John Wiley & Sons, Inc.

finite number of symbols can be recognized by an abstract machine with a finite set of instructions. Such a mechanism is now known as a Turing machine [3]. Turing's research paper addresses the question of machine intelligence, assessing the arguments against the possibility of creating an intelligent computing machine and suggesting answers to those arguments, proposing the Turing test as an empirical test of intelligence [4]. The Turing test, called the imitation game by Turing, measures the performance of a machine against that of a human being. The machine and a human (A) are placed in two rooms. A third person, designated the interrogator, is in a room apart from both the machine and the human (A). The interrogator cannot see or speak directly to either (A) or the machine, communicating with them solely through some text messages or even a chat window. The task of the interrogator is to distinguish between the human and the computer on the basis of questions he/she may put to both of them over the terminals. If the interrogator cannot distinguish the machine from the human then, Turing argues, the machine may be assumed to be intelligent. In the 1960s, computers failed to pass the Turing test due to the low-processing speed of the computers.

The last few decades have seen a new era of artificial intelligence focusing on the principles, theoretical aspects, and design methodology of algorithms gleaned from nature. Examples are artificial neural networks inspired by mammalian neural systems, evolutionary computation inspired by natural selection in biology, simulated annealing inspired by thermodynamics principles and swarm intelligence inspired by collective behavior of insects or micro-organisms, and so on, interacting locally with their environment causing coherent functional global patterns to emerge. These techniques have found their way in solving real-world problems in science, business, technology, and commerce.

Computational Intelligence (CI) [5–8] is a well-established paradigm, where new theories with a sound biological understanding have been evolving. The current experimental systems have many of the characteristics of biological computers (brains in other words) and are beginning to be built to perform a variety of tasks that are difficult or impossible to do with conventional computers. To name a few, we have microwave ovens, washing machines, and digital cameras that can figure out on their own what settings to use to perform their tasks optimally with reasoning capability, make intelligent decisions, and learn from the experience. As usual, defining CI is not an easy task. Bezdek defined a computationally intelligent system [5] in the following way:

"A system is **computationally intelligent** when it: deals with only numerical (low-level) data, has pattern recognition components, does not use knowledge in the AI sense; and additionally when it (begins to) exhibit i) computational adaptivity, ii) computational fault tolerance, iii) speed approaching human-like turnaround and iv) error rates that approximate human performance."

The above definition infers that a computationally intelligent system should be characterized by the capability of computational adaptation, fault tolerance, high computational speed, and be less error prone to noisy information sources. It also implies high computational speed and less error rates than human beings. It is true that a high computational speed may sometimes yield a poor accuracy in the results. Fuzzy logic and neural nets that support a high degree of parallelism usually have a fast response to input excitations. Further, unlike a conventional production (rule-based) system, where only a single rule is fired at a time, fuzzy logic allows firing of a large number of rules ensuring partial matching of the available facts with the antecedent clauses of those rules. Thus the reasoning capability of fuzzy logic is humanlike, and consequently it is less error prone. An artificial neural network (ANN) also allows firing of a number of neurons concurrently. Thus it has a high computational speed; it usually adapts its parameters by satisfying a set of constraints that minimizes the error rate. The parallel realization of GA and belief networks for the same reason have a good computational speed, and their inherent information filtering behavior maintain accuracy of their resulting outcome.

In an attempt to define CI [9], Marks clearly mentions the name of the constituent members of the family. According to him:

">... neural networks, genetic algorithms, fuzzy systems, evolutionary programming and artificial life are the building blocks of computational intelligence."

At this point, it is worth mentioning that *artificial life* is also an emerging discipline based on the assumption that physical and chemical laws are good enough to explain the intelligence of the living organisms. Langton defines artificial life [10] as:

">.... an inclusive paradigm that attempts to realize lifelike behavior by imitating the processes that occur in the development or mechanics of life."

Now, let us summarize exactly what we understand by the phrase CI. Figure 1.1 outlines the topics that share some ideas of this new discipline.

The early definitions of CI were centered around the logic of fuzzy sets, neural networks, genetic algorithms, and probabilistic reasoning along with the study of their synergism. Currently, the CI family is greatly influenced by the biologically inspired models of machine intelligence. It deals with the models of fuzzy as well as granular computing, neural computing, and evolutionary computing along with their interactions with artificial life, swarm intelligence, chaos theory, and other emerging paradigms. Belief networks and probabilistic reasoning fall in the intersection of traditional AI and the CI. Note that artificial life is shared by the CI and the physicochemical laws (not shown in Fig. 1.1).

Note that Bezdek [5], Marks [9], Pedrycz [11–12], and others have defined computational intelligence in different ways depending on the then developments of this new discipline. An intersection of these definitions will surely focus to fuzzy logic, ANN, and GA, but a union (and generalization) of all these definitions includes many other subjects (e.g., *rough set, chaos,* and *computational learning theory*). Further, CI being an emerging discipline should not be pinpointed only to a limited number of topics. Rather it should have a scope to expand in diverse directions and to merge with other existing disciplines.

In a nutshell, which becomes quite apparent in light of the current research pursuits, the area is heterogeneous as being dwelled on such technologies as neural networks,

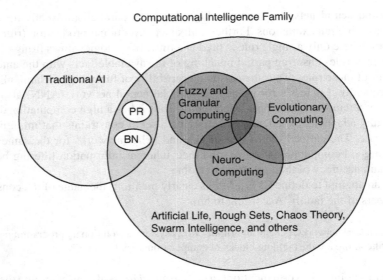

PR= Probabilistic reasoning, BN= Belief networks.

FIGURE 1.1 The building blocks of CI.

fuzzy systems, evolutionary computation, swarm intelligence, and probabilistic reasoning. The recent trend is to integrate different components to take advantage of complementary features and to develop a synergistic system. Hybrid architectures like neuro-fuzzy systems, evolutionary-fuzzy systems, evolutionary-neural networks, evolutionary neuro-fuzzy systems, and so on, are widely applied for real-world problem solving. In the following sections, the main functional components of CI are explained with their key advantages and application domains.

1.2 CLASSICAL COMPONENTS OF CI

This section will provide a conceptual overview of common CI models based on their fundamental characteristics.

1.2.1 Artificial Neural Networks

Artificial neural networks [13–15] have been developed as generalizations of mathematical models of biological nervous systems. In a simplified mathematical model of the neuron, the effects of the synapses are represented by *connection weights* that modulate the effect of the associated input signals, and the nonlinear characteristic exhibited by neurons is represented by a transfer function, which is usually the sigmoid, Gaussian, trigonometric function, and so on. The neuron impulse is then computed as the weighted sum of the input signals, transformed by the transfer function. The learning capability of an artificial neuron is achieved by adjusting the weights in

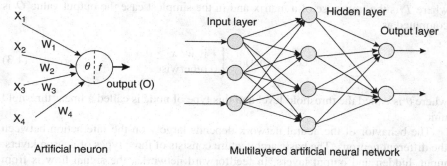

FIGURE 1.2   Architecture of an artificial neuron and a multilayered neural network.

accordance to the chosen learning algorithm. Most applications of neural networks fall into the following categories:

Prediction. Use input values to predict some output.

Classification. Use input values to determine the classification.

Data Association. Like classification, but it also recognizes data that contains errors.

Data Conceptualization. Analyze the inputs so that grouping relationships can be inferred.

A typical multilayered neural network and an artificial neuron are illustrated in Figure 1.2. Each neuron is characterized by an activity level (representing the state of polarization of a neuron), an output value (representing the firing rate of the neuron), a set of input connections, (representing synapses on the cell and its dendrite), a bias value (representing an internal resting level of the neuron), and a set of output connections (representing a neuron's axonal projections). Each of these aspects of the unit is represented mathematically by real numbers. Thus each connection has an associated weight (synaptic strength), which determines the effect of the incoming input on the activation level of the unit. The weights may be positive or negative. Referring to Figure 1.2, the signal flow from inputs $x_1 \cdots x_n$ is considered to be unidirectional indicated by arrows, as is a neuron's output signal flow (O). The neuron output signal O is given by the following relationship:

$$O = f(\text{net}) = f \left(\sum_{j=1}^{n} w_j x_j \right) \qquad (1.1)$$

where w_j is the weight vector and the function $f(\text{net})$ is referred to as an activation (transfer) function and is defined as a scalar product of the weight and input vectors

$$\text{net} = w^T x = w_1 x_1 + \cdots + w_n x_n \qquad (1.2)$$

where T is the transpose of a matrix and in the simplest case the output value O is computed as

$$O = f(\text{net}) = \begin{cases} 1 \text{ if } w^T x \geq \theta \\ 0 \text{ otherwise} \end{cases} \tag{1.3}$$

where θ is called the threshold level and this type of node is called a linear threshold unit.

The behavior of the neural network depends largely on the interaction between the different neurons. The basic architecture consists of three types of neuron layers: input, hidden and output layers. In feedforward networks, the signal flow is from input to output units strictly in a feedforward direction. The data processing can extend over multiple (layers of) units, but no feedback connections are present, that is, connections extending from outputs to inputs of units in the same or previous layers.

Recurrent networks contain feedback connections. Contrary to feedforward networks, the dynamical properties of the network are important. In some cases, the activation values of the units undergo a relaxation process such that the network will evolve to a stable state in which these activations do not change anymore. In other applications, the changes of the activation values of the output neurons are significant, such that the dynamical behavior constitutes the output of the network. There are several other neural network architectures (Elman network, adaptive resonance theory maps, competitive networks, etc.) depending on the properties and requirement of the application. The reader may refer to [16–18] for an extensive overview of the different neural network architectures and learning algorithms.

A neural network has to be configured such that the application of a set of inputs produces the desired set of outputs. Various methods to set the strengths of the connections exist. One way is to set the weights explicitly, using *a priori* knowledge. Another way is to train the neural network by feeding its teaching patterns and letting it change its weights according to some learning rule. The learning situations in neural networks may be classified into three distinct types. These are supervised, unsupervised, and reinforcement learning. In supervised learning, an input vector is presented at the inputs together with a set of desired responses, one for each node, at the output layer. A forward pass is done and the errors or discrepancies, between the desired and actual response for each node in the output layer, are found. These are then used to determine weight changes in the net according to the prevailing learning rule. The term 'supervised' originates from the fact that the desired signals on individual output nodes are provided by an external teacher. The best-known examples of this technique occur in the back-propagation algorithm, the delta rule, and perceptron rule. In unsupervised learning (or self-organization) an (output) unit is trained to respond to clusters of patterns within the input. In this paradigm, the system is supposed to discover statistically salient features of the input population [19]. Unlike the supervised learning paradigm, there is no *a priori* set of categories into which the patterns are to be classified; rather the system must develop its own representation of the input stimuli. Reinforcement learning is learning what to do—how to map situations to actions—so as to maximize a numerical reward signal. The learner is not told which actions to take, as in most forms of machine learning, but instead must discover which actions yield the most reward by trying them. In the most interesting and challenging cases, actions may affect not only the immediate reward, but also the next situation and, through that, all subsequent rewards. These two characteristics, trial-and-error search and delayed reward are the two most important distinguishing features of reinforcement learning.

1.2.2   Fuzzy Logic

Professor Zadeh [20] introduced the concept of fuzzy logic (FL) to present vagueness in linguistics, and further implement and express human knowledge and inference capability in a natural way. Fuzzy logic starts with the concept of a fuzzy set. A *fuzzy set* is a set without a crisp, clearly defined boundary. It can contain elements with only a partial degree of membership. A membership function (MF) is a curve that defines how each point in the input space is mapped to a membership value (or degree of membership) between 0 and 1. The input space is sometimes referred to as the universe of discourse.

Let X be the universe of discourse and x be a generic element of X. A classical set A is defined as a collection of elements or objects $x \epsilon X$, such that each x can either belong to or not belong to the set A, $A \sqsubseteq X$. By defining a characteristic function (or membership function) on each element x in X, a classical set A can be represented by a set of ordered pairs $(x, 0)$ or $(x, 1)$, where 1 indicates membership and 0 nonmembership. Unlike the conventional set mentioned above, the fuzzy set expresses the degree to which an element belongs to a set. Hence, the characteristic function of a fuzzy set is allowed to have a value between 0 and 1, denoting the degree of membership of an element in a given set. If X is a collection of objects denoted generically by x, then a fuzzy set A in X is defined as a set of ordered pairs:

$$A = \{(x, \mu_A(x)) | x \epsilon X\} \tag{1.4}$$

$\mu_A(x)$ is called the MF of linguistic variable x in A, which maps X to the membership space M, $M = [0,1]$, where M contains only two points 0 and 1, A is crisp and μ_A is identical to the characteristic function of a crisp set. Triangular and trapezoidal membership functions are the simplest membership functions formed using straight lines. Some of the other shapes are Gaussian, generalized bell, sigmoidal, and polynomial-based curves. Figure 1.3 illustrates the shapes of two commonly used MFs. The most important thing to realize about fuzzy logical reasoning is the fact that it is a superset of standard Boolean logic.

It is interesting to note about the correspondence between two- and multivalued logic operations for **AND**, **OR**, and **NOT**. It is possible to resolve the statement A **AND** B, where A and B are limited to the range $(0,1)$, by using the operator *minimum* (A, B). Using the same reasoning, we can replace the **OR** operation with the *maximum* operator, so that A **OR** B becomes equivalent to *maximum* (A, B). Finally, the operation **NOT** A becomes equivalent to the operation 1-A.

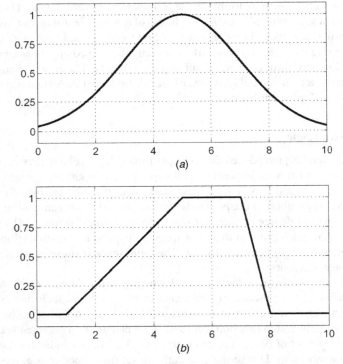

FIGURE 1.3   Examples of FM functions (*a*) Gaussian and (*b*) trapezoidal.

In FL terms, these are popularly known as fuzzy intersection or conjunction (AND), fuzzy union or disjunction (OR), and fuzzy complement (NOT). The intersection of two fuzzy sets A and B is specified in general by a binary mapping T, which aggregates two membership functions as follows:

$$\mu_{A \cap B}(x) = T(\mu_A(x), \mu_B(x)) \qquad (1.5)$$

The fuzzy intersection operator is usually referred to as a T-norm (Triangular norm) operator. The fuzzy union operator is specified in general by a binary mapping S.

$$\mu_{A \cup B}(x) = S(\mu_A(x), \mu_B(x)) \qquad (1.6)$$

This class of fuzzy union operators are often referred to as T-conorm (or S-*norm*) operators.

The fuzzy rule base is characterized in the form of *if–then* rules in which preconditions and consequents involve linguistic variables. The collection of these fuzzy rules forms the rule base for the FL system. Due to their concise form, fuzzy *if–then* rules are often employed to capture the imprecise modes of reasoning that play an essential role in the human ability to make decisions in an environment of uncertainty and imprecision. A single fuzzy *if–then* rule assumes the form

$$if\ x\ is\ A\ then\ y\ is\ B$$

where A and B are linguistic values defined by fuzzy sets on the ranges (universes of discourse) X and Y, respectively. The *if*–part of the rule "x is A" is called the *antecedent (precondition)* or premise, while the *then*–part of the rule "y is B" is called the *consequent* or conclusion. Interpreting an *if–then* rule involves evaluating the antecedent (*fuzzification of* the input and applying any necessary *fuzzy operators*) and then applying that result to the consequent (known as *implication*). For rules with multiple antecedents, all parts of the antecedent are calculated simultaneously and resolved to a single value using the logical operators. Similarly, all the consequents (rules with multiple consequents) are affected equally by the result of the antecedent. The consequent specifies a fuzzy set be assigned to the output. The *implication function* then modifies that fuzzy set to the degree specified by the antecedent. For multiple rules, the output of each rule is a fuzzy set. The output fuzzy sets for each rule are then *aggregated* into a single output fuzzy set. Finally, the resulting set is *defuzzified*, or resolved to a single number.

The defuzzification interface is a mapping from a space of fuzzy actions defined over an output universe of discourse into a space of non-fuzzy actions, because the output from the inference engine is usually a fuzzy set while for most practical applications crisp values are often required. The three commonly applied defuzzification techniques are, *max-criterion*, *center-of-gravity*, and the *mean- of- maxima*. The *max-criterion* is the simplest of these three to implement. It produces the point at which the possibility distribution of the action reaches a maximum value.

Reader, please refer to [21–24] for more information related to fuzzy systems. It is typically advantageous if the fuzzy rule base is adaptive to a certain application. The fuzzy rule base is usually constructed manually or by automatic adaptation by some learning techniques using evolutionary algorithms and/or neural network learning methods [25].

1.2.3   Genetic and Evolutionary Computing Algorithms

To tackle complex search problems, as well as many other complex computational tasks, computer-scientists have been looking to nature for years (both as a model and as a metaphor) for inspiration. Optimization is at the heart of many natural processes (e.g., Darwinian evolution itself). Through millions of years, every species had to optimize their physical structures to adapt to the environments they were in. This process of adaptation, this morphological optimization is so perfect that nowadays, the similarity between a shark, a dolphin or a submarine is striking. A keen observation of the underlying relation between optimization and biological evolution has led to the development of a new paradigm of CI (the evolutionary computing techniques [26,27]) for performing very complex search and optimization.

Evolutionary computation uses iterative progress (e.g., growth or development in a population). This population is then selected in a guided random search using parallel processing to achieve the desired end. Such processes are often inspired by biological mechanisms of evolution. The paradigm of evolutionary computing techniques dates back to the early 1950s, when the idea to use Darwinian principles for automated problem solving originated. It was not until the 1960s that three distinct interpretations of this idea started to be developed in three different places. Evolutionary programming (EP) was introduced by Lawrence J. Fogel in the United States [28], while John Henry Holland called his method a genetic algorithm (GA) [29]. In Germany Ingo Rechenberg and Hans-Paul Schwefel introduced the evolution strategies (ESs) [30,31]. These areas developed separately for 15 years. From the early 1990s on they are unified as different representatives (dialects) of one technology, called evolutionary computing. Also, in the early 1990s, a fourth stream following the general ideas had emerged—genetic programming (GP) [32]. They all share a common conceptual base of simulating the evolution of *individual* structures via processes of *selection*, *mutation*, and *reproduction*. The processes depend on the perceived performance of the individual structures as defined by the environment (problem).

The GAs deal with parameters of finite length, which are coded using a finite alphabet, rather than directly manipulating the parameters themselves. This means that the search is unconstrained by either the continuity of the function under investigation, or the existence of a derivative function. Figure 1.4 depicts the functional block diagram of a GA and the various aspects are discussed below. It is assumed that a potential solution to a problem may be represented as a set of parameters. These parameters (known as genes) are joined together to form a string of values (known as a chromosome). A gene (also referred to a feature, character, or detector) refers to a specific attribute that is encoded in the chromosome. The particular values the genes can take are called its alleles.

Encoding issues deal with representing a solution in a chromosome and unfortunately, no one technique works best for all problems. A fitness function must be devised for each problem to be solved. Given a particular chromosome, the fitness function returns a single numerical fitness or figure of merit, which will determine the ability of the individual, that chromosome represents. Reproduction is the second critical attribute of GAs where two individuals selected from the population are allowed to mate to produce offspring, which will comprise the next generation. Having selected the parents, the off springs are generated, typically using the mechanisms of crossover and mutation.

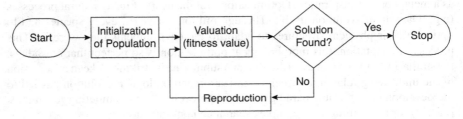

FIGURE 1.4   Flow chart of genetic algorithm iteration.

Selection is the survival of the fittest within GAs. It determines which individuals are to survive to the next generation. The selection phase consists of three parts. The first part involves determination of the individual's fitness by the fitness function. A fitness function must be devised for each problem; given a particular chromosome, the fitness function returns a single numerical fitness value, which is proportional to the ability, or utility, of the individual represented by that chromosome. The second part involves converting the fitness function into an expected value followed by the last part where the expected value is then converted to a discrete number of offspring. Some of the commonly used selection techniques are the roulette wheel and stochastic universal sampling. If the GA has been correctly implemented, the population will evolve over successive generations so that the fitness of the best and the average individual in each generation increases toward the global optimum.

Currently, evolutionary computation techniques mostly involve meta-heuristic optimization algorithms, such as:

1. Evolutionary algorithms (comprising of genetic algorithms, evolutionary programming, evolution strategy, genetic programming, learning classifier systems, and differential evolution)
2. Swarm intelligence (comprised of ant colony optimization and particle swarm optimization) [33].

And involved to a lesser extent in the following:

3. Self-organization (e.g., self-organizing maps, growing neural gas) [34].
4. Artificial life (digital organism) [10].
5. Cultural algorithms [35].
6. Harmony search algorithm [36].
7. Artificial immune systems [37].
8. Learnable evolution model [38].

1.2.4 Probabilistic Computing and Belief Networks

Probabilistic models are viewed as similar to that of a game, actions are based on expected outcomes. The center of interest moves from the deterministic to probabilistic models using statistical estimations and predictions. In the probabilistic modeling process, risk means uncertainty for which the probability distribution is known. Therefore risk assessment means a study to determine the outcomes of decisions along with their probabilities. Decision makers often face a severe lack of information. Probability assessment quantifies the information gap between what is known, and what needs to be known for an optimal decision. The probabilistic models are used for protection against adverse uncertainty, and exploitation of propitious uncertainty [39].

A good example is the probabilistic neural network (Bayesian learning) in which probability is used to represent uncertainty about the relationship being learned. Before we have seen any data, our *prior* opinions about what the true relationship might be can be expressed in a probability distribution over the network weights that define this relationship. After we look at the data, our revised opinions are captured by a *posterior* distribution over network weights. Network weights that seemed plausible before, but which donot match the data very well, will now be seen as being much less likely, while the probability for values of the weights that do fit the data well will have increased. Typically, the purpose of training is to make predictions for future cases in which only the inputs to the network are known. The result of conventional network training is a single set of weights that can be used to make such predictions.

A Bayesian belief network [40,41] is represented by a directed acyclic graph or tree, where the nodes denote the events and the arcs denote the cause–effect relationship between the parent and the child nodes. Here, each node, may assume a number of possible values. For instance, a node A may have n number of possible values, denoted by $A_1, A_2, \ldots, A_n$. For any two nodes, A and B, when there exists a dependence A→B, we assign a conditional probability matrix $[P(B/A)]$ to the directed arc from node A to B. The element at the jth row and ith column of $P(B/A)$, denoted by $P(B_j/A_i)$, represents the conditional probability of B_j assuming the prior occurrence of A_i. This is described in Figure 1.5.

Given the probability distribution of A, denoted by $[P(A_1) P(A_2) \cdots \cdot P(A_n)]$, we can compute the probability distribution of event B by using the following expression:

$$
\begin{aligned}
\mathbf{P(B)} &= [P(B_1) P(B_2) \cdots \cdot P(B_m)]_{1 \times m} \\
&= [P(A_1) P(A_2) \cdots \cdot P(A_n)]_{1 \times n} \cdot [\mathbf{P(B/A)}]_{n \times m} \\
&= [\mathbf{P(A)}]_{1 \times n} \cdot [P(B/A)]_{n \times m}
\end{aligned}
\tag{1.7}
$$

We now illustrate the computation of P(B) with an example.

Pearl [39–41] proposed a scheme for propagating beliefs of evidence in a Bayesian network. First, we demonstrate his scheme with a Bayesian tree like that in Figure 1.5. However, note that like the tree of Figure 1.5 each variable, say A, B . . . need not have only two possible values. For example, if a node in a tree denotes German measles (GM), it could have three possible values like severe-GM, little-GM, and moderate-GM.

In Pearl's scheme for evidential reasoning, he considered both the causal effect and the diagnostic effect to compute the belief function at a given node in the Bayesian belief tree. For computing belief at a node, say V, he partitioned the tree into two parts: (1) the subtree rooted at V and (2) the rest of the tree. Let us denote the subset of the evidence, residing at the subtree of V by e_v^- and the subset of the evidence

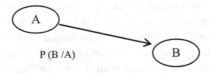

FIGURE 1.5 Assigning a conditional probability matrix in the directed arc connected from A to B.

from the rest of the tree by $e_v{}^+$. We denote the belief function of the node V by Bel(V), where it is defined as

$$Bel\ (V) = P(V/e_v{}^+, e_v{}^-)$$
$$= P(e_v{}^-/V) \cdot P(V/e_v{}^+)/\alpha$$
$$= \lambda(V)\Pi(V)/\alpha \tag{1.8}$$

where, $\lambda\ (V) = P(e_v{}^-/V)$ }

$$\Pi(V) = P(V/e_v{}^+) \tag{1.9}$$

and α is a normalizing constant, determined by

$$\alpha = \Sigma_{v \in (\text{true, false})}P(e_v{}^-/V) \cdot P(V/e_v{}^+) \tag{1.10}$$

It seems from the last expression that v could assume only two values: true and false. It is just an illustrative notation. In fact, v can have a number of possible values.

Pearl designed an interesting algorithm for belief propagation in a causal tree. He assigned *a priori* probability of one leaf node to be defective, then propagated the belief from this node to its parent, and then from the parent to the grandparent, until the root is reached. Next, he considered a downward propagation of belief from the root to its children, and from each child node to its children, and so on, until the leaves are reached. The leaf having the highest belief is then assigned *a priori* probability and the whole process described above is repeated. Pearl has shown that after a finite number of up–down traversal on the tree, a *steady-state* condition is reached following which a particular leaf node in all subsequent up–down traversal yields a maximum belief with respect to all other leaves in the tree. The leaf thus selected is considered as the defective item.

1.3   HYBRID INTELLIGENT SYSTEMS IN CI

Several adaptive hybrid intelligent systems (HIS) have in recent years been developed for model expertise, image and video segmentation techniques, process control, mechatronics, robotics and complicated automation tasks, and so on. Many of these approaches use the combination of different knowledge representation schemes, decision making models, and learning strategies to solve a computational task. This integration aims at overcoming limitations of individual techniques through hybridization or fusion of various techniques. These ideas have led to the emergence of several different kinds of intelligent system architectures. Most of the current HIS consists of three essential paradigms: artificial neural networks, fuzzy inference systems, and global optimization algorithms (e.g., evolutionary algorithms). Nevertheless, HIS is an open instead of conservative concept. That is, it is evolving those relevant

TABLE 1.1   Hybrid Intelligent System Basic Ingredients

Methodology	Advantage
Artificial neural networks	Adaptation, learning, and approximation
Fuzzy logic	Approximate reasoning
Global optimization algorithms	Derivative-free optimization of multiple parameters

techniques together with the important advances in other new computing methods. Table 1.1 lists the three principal ingredients together with their advantages [42].

Experience has shown that it is crucial for the design of HIS to primarily focus on the integration and interaction of different techniques rather than merge different methods to create ever-new techniques. Techniques already well understood, should be applied to solve specific domain problems within the system. Their weakness must be addressed by combining them with complementary methods.

Neural networks offer a highly structured architecture with learning and generalization capabilities. The generalization ability for new inputs is then based on the inherent algebraic structure of the neural network. However, it is very hard to incorporate human *a priori* knowledge into a neural network. This is mainly because the connectionist paradigm gains most of its strength from a distributed knowledge representation.

In contrast, fuzzy inference systems exhibit complementary characteristics, offering a very powerful framework for approximate reasoning as it attempts to model the human reasoning process at a cognitive level. Fuzzy systems acquire knowledge from domain experts and this is encoded within the algorithm in terms of the set of *if–then* rules. Fuzzy systems employ this rule-based approach and interpolative reasoning to respond to new inputs. The incorporation and interpretation of knowledge is straight forward, whereas learning and adaptation constitute major problems.

Global optimization is the task of finding the absolutely best set of parameters to optimize an objective function. In general, it may be possible to have solutions that are locally, but not globally, optimal. Evolutionary computing (EC) works by simulating evolution on a computer. Such techniques could be easily used to optimize neural networks, fuzzy inference systems, and other problems.

Due to the complementary features and strengths of different systems, the trend in the design of hybrid systems is to merge different techniques into a more powerful integrated system, to overcome their individual weaknesses.

The various HIS architectures could be broadly classified into four different categories based on the systems overall architecture: (1) Stand alone architectures, (2) transformational architectures, (3) hierarchical hybrid architectures, and (4) integrated hybrid architectures.

1. *Stand-Alone Architecture.* Stand-alone models of HIS applications consist of independent software components, which do not interact in anyway. Developing stand-alone systems can have several purposes. First, they provide direct means of comparing the problem solving capabilities of different techniques with reference to a certain application. Running different techniques in a

parallel environment permits a loose approximation of integration. Stand-alone models are often used to develop a quick initial prototype, while a more time-consuming application is developed. Some of the benefits are simplicity and ease of development using commercially available software packages.

2. *Transformational Hybrid Architecture.* In a transformational hybrid model, the system begins as one type of system and ends up as the other. Determining which technique is used for development and which is used for delivery is based on the desirable features that the technique offers. Expert systems and neural networks have proven to be useful transformational models. Variously, either the expert system is incapable of adequately solving the problem, or the speed, adaptability, or robustness of neural network is required. Knowledge from the expert system is used to set the initial conditions and training set for a neural network. Transformational hybrid models are often quick to develop and ultimately require maintenance on only one system. Most of the developed models are just application oriented.

3. *Hierarchical Hybrid Architectures.* The architecture is built in a hierarchical fashion, associating a different functionality with each layer. The overall functioning of the model will depend on the correct functioning of all the layers. A possible error in one of the layers will directly affect the desired output.

4. *Integrated Hybrid Architectures.* These models include systems, which combine different techniques into one single computational model. They share data structures and knowledge representations. Another approach is to put the various techniques on a side-by-side basis and focus on their interaction in the problem-solving task. This method might allow integrating alternative techniques and exploiting their mutuality. The benefits of fused architecture include robustness, improved performance, and increased problem-solving capabilities. Finally, fully integrated models can provide a full range of capabilities (e.g., adaptation, generalization, noise tolerance, and justification). Fused systems have limitations caused by the increased complexity of the intermodule interactions and specifying, designing, and building fully integrated models is complex.

1.4 EMERGING TRENDS IN CI

This section introduces a few new members of the CI family that are currently gaining importance owing to their successful applications in both science and engineering. The new members include swarm intelligence, Type-2 fuzzy sets, chaos theory, rough sets, granular computing, artificial immune systems, differential evolution (DE), bacterial foraging optimization algorithms (BFOA), and the algorithms based on artificial bees foraging behavior.

1.4.1 Swarm Intelligence

Swarm intelligence (SI) is the name given to a relatively new interdisciplinary field of research, which has gained wide popularity in recent times. Algorithms belonging to this field draw inspiration from the collective intelligence emerging from the behavior of a group of social insects (e.g., bees, termites, and wasps). These insects even with very limited individual capability can jointly (cooperatively) perform many complex tasks necessary for their survival. The expression "Swarm Intelligence" was introduced by Beni and Wang in 1989, in the context of cellular robotic systems [43].

Swarm intelligence systems are typically made up of a population of simple agents interacting locally with one another and with their environment. Although there is normally no centralized control structure dictating how individual agents should behave, local interactions between such agents often lead to the emergence of global behavior. Swarm behavior can be seen in bird flocks, fish schools, as well as in insects (e.g., mosquitoes and midges). Many animal groups (e.g., fish schools and bird flocks) clearly display structural order, with the behavior of the organisms so integrated that even though they may change shape and direction, they appear to move as a single coherent entity [44]. The main properties (traits) of collective behavior can be pointed out as follows (see Fig. 1.6):

Homogeneity. Every bird in a flock has the same behavior model. The flock moves without a leader, even though temporary leaders seem to appear.

Locality. Its nearest flock-mates only influence the motion of each bird. Vision is considered to be the most important senses for flock organization.

Collision Avoidance. Avoid colliding with nearby flock mates.

Velocity Matching. Attempt to match velocity with nearby flock mates.

Flock Centering. Attempt to stay close to nearby flock mates.

Individuals attempt to maintain a minimum distance between themselves and others at all times. This rule is given the highest priority and corresponds to a frequently

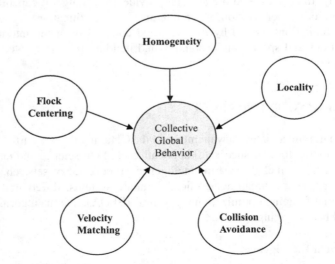

FIGURE 1.6   Main traits of collective behavior.

observed behavior of animals in nature [45]. If individuals are not performing an avoidance man oeuvre, they tend to be attracted toward other individuals (to avoid being isolated) and to align themselves with neighbors [46,47].

According to Milonas, five basic principles define swarm intelligence [48]. First is the proximity principle: The swarm should be able to carry out simple space and time computations. Second is the quality principle: The swarm should be able to respond to quality factors in the environment. Third is the principle of diverse response: The swarm should not commit its activities along excessively narrow channels. Fourth is the principle of stability: The swarm should not change its mode of behavior every time the environment changes. Fifth is the principle of adaptability: The swarm must be able to change behavior mote when it is worth the computational price. Note that principles four and five are direct opposites; opposite sides of the same coin.

Below we provide a brief outline of two most popular algorithms of SI paradigm, namely, the particle swarm optimization (PSO) algorithm and the ant colony optimization (ACO) algorithm.

1.4.1.1 The PSO Algorithm. The concept of particle swarms, although initially introduced for simulating human social behavior, has become very popular these days as an efficient means of intelligent search and optimization. The PSO [49], as it is called now, does not require any gradient information of the function to be optimized, uses only primitive mathematical operators, and is conceptually very simple. The PSO emulates swarming behavior of insects, animals, and so on, and also draws inspiration from the boid's method of Reynolds and sociocognition [49]. Particles are conceptual entities, which search through a multidimensional search space. At any particular instant, each particle has a position and velocity. The position vector of a particle with respect to the origin of the search space represents a trial solution to the search problem. The efficiency of PSO is mainly attributed to the efficient communication of information among the search agents.

The classical PSO starts with the random initialization of a population of candidate solutions (particles) over the fitness landscape. However, unlike other evolutionary computing techniques, PSO uses no direct recombination of genetic material between individuals during the search. Rather, it works depending on the social behavior of the particles in the swarm. Therefore, it finds the best global solution by simply adjusting the trajectory of each individual toward its own best position and toward the best particle of the entire swarm at each time-step (generation). In a D-dimensional search space, the position vector of the ith particle is given by $\vec{X}_i = (x_{i,1}, x_{i,2}, \ldots, x_{i,D})$ and velocity of the ith particle is given by $\vec{V}_i = (v_{i,1}, v_{i,2}, \ldots, v_{i,D})$. Positions and velocities are adjusted and the objective function to be optimized, $f(\vec{X}_i)$, is evaluated with the new coordinates at each time-step. The velocity and position update equations for the dth dimension of the ith particle in the swarm may be represented as

$$v_{i,d,t} = \omega^* v_{i,d,t-1} + C_1{}^* rand_1{}^* (pbest_{i,d} - x_{i,d,t-1}) + C_2{}^* rand_2{}^* (gbest_d - x_{i,d,t-1})$$

$$(1.11)$$

$$x_{i,d,t} = x_{i,d,t-1} + v_{i,d,t}$$

$$(1.12)$$

where $rand_1$ and $rand_2$ are random positive numbers uniformly distributed in $(0,1)$ and are drawn anew for each dimension of each particle. *pbest* is the personal best solution found so far by an individual particle while *gbest* represents the fittest particle found so far by the entire community. The first term in the velocity updating formula is referred to as the "cognitive part". The last term of the same formula is interpreted as the "social part", which represents how an individual particle is influenced by the other members of its society. The acceleration coefficients C_1 and C_2 determine the relative influences of the cognitive and social parts on the velocity of the particle. The particle's velocity is clamped to a maximum value $\vec{V}_{max} = [v_{max,1}, v_{max,2}, \ldots, v_{max,D}]^T$. If in dth dimension, $|v_{i,d}|$ exceeds $v_{max,d}$ specified by the user, then the velocity of that dimension is assigned to $sign(v_{i,d})*v_{max,d}$, where $sign(x)$ is the triple-valued signum function.

1.4.1.2 The ACO Algorithm. The main idea of ACO [50,51] is to model a problem as the search for a minimum cost path in a graph. Artificial ants as those walking on this graph, looking for cheaper paths. Each ant has a rather simple behavior capable of finding relatively costlier paths. Cheaper paths are found as the emergent result of the global cooperation among ants in the colony. The behavior of artificial ants is inspired from real ants: They lay pheromone trails (obviously in a mathematical form) on the graph edges and choose their path with respect to probabilities that depend on pheromone trails. These pheromone trails progressively decrease by evaporation. The basic idea of a real ant system is illustrated in Figure 1.7. In (*a*), the ants move in a straight line to the food. Part (*b*) illustrates the situation soon after an obstacle is inserted between the nest and the food. To avoid the obstacle, initially each ant chooses to turn left or right at random. Let us assume that ants move at the same speed depositing pheromone in the trail uniformly. However, the ants that, by chance, choose to turn left will reach the food sooner, whereas the ants that go around the obstacle turning right will follow a longer path, and so will take a longer time to circumvent the obstacle. As a result, pheromone accumulates faster in the shorter path around the obstacle. Since ants prefer to follow trails with larger amounts of

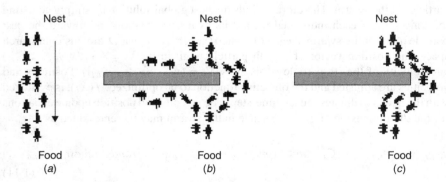

FIGURE 1.7   Illustrating the behavior of real ant movements.

pheromone, eventually all the ants converge to the shorter path around the obstacle, as shown in (c).

In addition, artificial ants have some extra features not seen in their counterpart in real ants. In particular, they live in a discrete world (a graph) and their moves consist of transitions from nodes to nodes. Pheromone placed on the edges acts like a *distributed long-term memory*. The memory, instead of being stored locally within individual ants, remains distributed on the edges of the graph. This indirectly provides a means of communication among the ants called *stigmergy* [50]. In most cases, pheromone trails are updated only after having constructed a complete path and not during the walk, and the amount of pheromone deposited is usually a function of the quality of the path. Finally, the probability for an artificial ant to choose an edge not only depends on pheromones deposited on that edge in the past, but also on some problem dependent local heuristic functions.

1.4.2   Type-2 Fuzzy Sets

The idea of types-2 fuzzy sets emerged from a 1975 paper by Zadeh [52], where he tried to address a typical problem with type-1 fuzzy sets that the membership function of type-1 fuzzy sets has no uncertainty associated with it. Thus this sometimes contradicts the word fuzzy, since that word has the connotation of lots of uncertainty. Type-2 fuzzy sets [53–55] are special kinds of fuzzy sets, the membership grades of which are themselves fuzzy (i.e., they incorporate a blurring of the type-1 membership function). The idea of type-2 fuzzy sets emerged from a 1975 paper by Zadeh [53], where he tried to address a typical problem with type-1 fuzzy sets that the membership function of a type-1 fuzzy set has no uncertainty associated with it. Thus this finding sometimes contradicts the word fuzzy, since that word has the connotation of lots of uncertainty. Now, in type-2 fuzzy sets, there is no longer a single value for the membership function for any input measurement or x value, but there are a few. This fact has been illustrated in Figure 1.8.

In order to symbolically distinguish between a type-1 fuzzy set and a type-2 fuzzy set, researchers use a tilde symbol over the symbol for the latter fuzzy set; so, if A denotes a type-1 fuzzy set, $\tilde{A}$ may denote the comparable type-2 fuzzy set. The

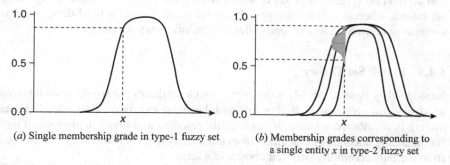

(a) Single membership grade in type-1 fuzzy set

(b) Membership grades corresponding to a single entity x in type-2 fuzzy set

FIGURE 1.8   Illustrating the membership grades in (a) type-1 and (b) type-2 fuzzy sets.

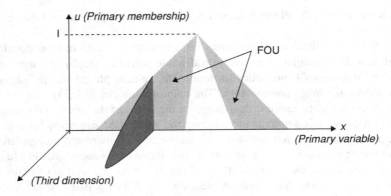

FIGURE 1.9   Illustrating the 3D membership of a general type-2 fuzzy set. A cross section of one slice of the third dimension is shown. This cross section, as well as all others, sits on the FOU.

distinguishing feature of Ã versus A is the membership function values of Ã are blurred, (i.e., they are no longer a single number from 0 to 1), but are instead a continuous range of values between 0 and 1, say [a, b]. We can either assign the same weighting or a variable weighting to the interval of membership function values [a, b]. When the former is done, the resulting type-2 fuzzy set is called either an interval type-2 fuzzy set or an interval valued fuzzy set (although different names may be used, they are the same fuzzy set). When the latter is done, the resulting type-2 fuzzy set is called a general type-2 fuzzy set (to distinguish it from the special interval type-2 fuzzy set).

The membership function of a general type-2 fuzzy set, Ã, is three-dimensional (3D) and the third dimension represents the value of the membership function at each point on its two-dimensional (2D) domain that is called its footprint of uncertainty (FOU). It is illustrated in Figure 1.9. For an interval type-2 fuzzy set that 3D value is the same (e.g., 1) everywhere, which means that no new information is contained in the third dimension of an interval type-2 fuzzy set. So, for such a set, the third dimension is ignored, and only the FOU is used to describe it. It is for this reason that an interval type-2 fuzzy set is sometimes called a first-order uncertainty fuzzy set model, whereas a general type-2 fuzzy set (with its useful third dimension) is sometimes referred to as a second-order uncertainty fuzzy set model.

1.4.3   Rough Set Theory

Introduced by Pawlak [56,57] in the 1980s, rough set theory constitutes a sound basis for discovering patterns in hidden data and thus have extensive applications in data mining in distributed systems. It has recently emerged as a major mathematical tool for managing uncertainty that arises from granularity in the domain of discourse (i.e., from the indiscernibility between objects in a set).

Rough sets can be considered sets with fuzzy boundaries: Sets that cannot be precisely characterized using the available set of attributes. The basic concept of the rough set theory (RST) is the notion of approximation space, which is an ordered pair $A = (U, R)$, where

U: Nonempty set of objects, called universe.

R: Equivalence relation on U, called indiscernibility relation. If x, y $\in U$ and xRy then x and y are indistinguishable in A.

Each equivalence class induced by R, (i.e., each element of the quotient set $\tilde{R} = U/R$), is called an elementary set in A. An approximation space can be alternatively noted by $A = (U, \tilde{R})$. It is assumed that the empty set is also elementary for every approximation space A. A definable set in A is any finite union of elementary sets in A. For x $\in U$ let $[x]_R$ denote the equivalence class of R, containing x. For each $\mathbf{X} \subseteq U$, $\mathbf{X}$ is characterized in A by a pair of sets: its lower and upper approximation in A, defined respectively as

$$A_{\text{low}}(\mathbf{X}) = \{x \in U \,|\, [x]_R \subseteq \mathbf{X}\}$$
$$A_{\text{upp}}(\mathbf{X}) = \{x \in U \,|\, [x]_R \cap \mathbf{X} \neq \emptyset\}$$

A rough set in A is the family of all subsets of U having the same lower and upper approximations. Figure 1.10 illustrates rough boundaries $A_{\text{low}}(\mathbf{X})$ [the lower approximation and $A_{\text{upp}}(\mathbf{X})$] the upper approximation of a given point set $\mathbf{X}$.

Many different problems can be addressed by RST. During the last few years, this formalism has been approached as a tool used in connection with many different areas of research. There have been investigations of the relations between RST and the Dempster–Shafer theory and between rough sets and fuzzy sets. The RST

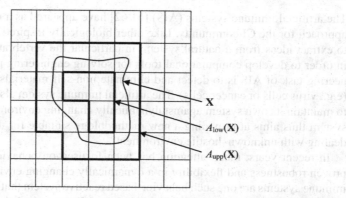

FIGURE 1.10   The rough boundaries $A_{\text{low}}(\mathbf{X})$ [the lower approximation and $A_{\text{upp}}(\mathbf{X})$] the upper approximation of a given point set $\mathbf{X} \subseteq U$-the universe of discourse.

has also provided the necessary formalism and ideas for the development of some propositional machine learning systems. It has also been used for, among many others, knowledge representation; data mining; dealing with imperfect data; reducing knowledge representation, and for analyzing attribute dependencies. The notions of rough relations and functions are based on RST and can be applied as a theoretical basis for rough controllers, among others.

1.4.4 Granular Computing

The philosophy of rough set analysis is general enough to be applicable to many problem-solving tasks. It, in fact, has a major influence on an emerging field of study known as granular computing (GrC) [58–60]. The theory of rough sets and the theory of granularity offer artificial intelligence perspectives on granular computing. Specifically, granular computing can be viewed as a study of human-inspired problem solving and information processing. Granular computing concerns the processing of complex information entities called information granules, which arise in the process of data abstraction and derivation of knowledge from information. Generally speaking, information granules are collections of entities that usually originate at the numeric level and are arranged together due to their similarity, functional or physical adjacency, indistinguishability, coherency, or the like.

Currently, granular computing is more a theoretical perspective than a coherent set of methods or principles. As a theoretical perspective, it encourages an approach to data that recognizes and exploits the knowledge present in data at various levels of resolution or scales. In this sense, it encompasses all methods that provide flexibility and adaptability in the resolution at which knowledge or information is extracted and represented.

1.4.5 Artificial Immune Systems

The artificial immune systems (AIS) [61,62] have appeared as a new computational approach for the CI community. Like other biologically inspired techniques, it tries to extract ideas from a natural system, in particular the vertebrate immune system, in order to develop computational tools for solving engineering problems. The pioneering task of AIS is to detect and eliminate non-self materials, called "antigens" (e.g., virus cells or cancer cells). The artificial immune system also plays a great role to maintain its own system against dynamically changing environment. The immune system thus aims at providing a new methodology suitable for dynamics problems dealing with unknown–hostile environment.

In recent years, much attention has been focused on behavior-based AI for its proven robustness and flexibility in a dynamically changing environment. Artificial immune systems are one such behavior-based reactive system that aims at developing a decentralized consensus making mechanism, following the behavioral characteristics of biological immune system.

The basic components of the biological immune system are macrophages, antibodies, and lymphocytes, the last one being classified into two types: B- and T-lymphocytes [63], which are the cells stemming from the bone marrow. The human blood circulatory system contains roughly 10^7 distinct types of B-lymphocytes, each of which has a distinct molecular structure and produces Y-shaped [63] antibodies from its surface. Antibodies can recognize foreign substances, called antigens, that invade a living creature. Virus, cancer cells, and so on, are typical examples of antigens. To cope with a continuously changing environment, a living system possesses an enormous repertoire of antibodies in advance. The T-lymphocytes, on the other hand, are the cells maturing in the thymus, and are used to kill infected cells and regulate the generation of antibodies from B-lymphocytes as outside circuits of B-lymphocyte networks. It is interesting to note that an antibody recognizes an antigen by part of its structure called epitope. The portion of the antibody that has the recognizing capability of an antigen is called paratope. Usually, epitope is the key portion of the antigen, and paratope is the keyhole portion of the antibody. Recent study in immunology reveals that each type of antibody has its specific antigen determinant, called idiotope.

Jerne [63–65] proposed the *idiotypic network hypothesis* to explain the biological communication among different species of antibodies. According to the hypothesis, antibodies–lyphocytes are not isolated, but they communicate to each other among their variant species.

A simple model of the immune system can be put forward in the following way: Let

$\alpha_i(t)$ be the concentration of the ith antibody

m_{ij} be the affinity between antibody j and antibody i

m_{ik} be the affinity between antibody i and the detected antigen k

k_i be the natural decay rate of antibody i

N and M, respectively, denote the number of antibodies that stimulate and suppress antibody i

The growth rate of antibody is given below:

$$\frac{d\alpha_i}{dt} = \left\{ \sum_{j=1}^{N} m_{ji} \cdot a_j(t) - \sum_{k=1}^{N} m_{ik} \cdot a_k(t) - m_i - k_i \right\} \alpha_i(t) \quad (1.13)$$

and $\alpha_i(t+1) = \dfrac{1}{1 + \exp(0.5 - \alpha_i(t))}$ \hfill (1.14)

The first and the second term on the right-hand side of Eq. (1.13), respectively, denote the stimulation and suppression by other antibodies, respectively. The third term denotes the stimulation from the antigen, and the fourth term represents the natural decay of the ith antibody. Equation (1.14) is a squashing function used to ensure the stability of the concentration.

1.4.6   Chaos Theory

In mathematics, chaos theory [66,67] describes the behavior of certain dynamical systems (i.e., systems whose states evolve with time) that may exhibit dynamics that are highly sensitive to initial conditions (popularly referred to as the butterfly effect). As a result of this sensitivity, which manifests itself as an exponential growth of perturbations in the initial conditions, the behavior of chaotic systems appears to be random. This happens even though these systems are deterministic, meaning that their future dynamics are fully defined by their initial conditions with no random elements involved. This behavior is known as deterministic chaos, or simply chaos. Chaos theory describes the behavior of certain nonlinear dynamical systems that under certain conditions exhibit a peculiar phenomenon known as chaos. One important characteristic of the chaotic systems is their sensitivity to initial conditions (popularly referred to as the butterfly effect). Because of this sensitivity, the behavior of these systems appears to be random, even though the dynamics is deterministic in the sense that it is well defined and contains no random parameters. Examples of such systems include the atmosphere, the solar system, plate tectonics, turbulent fluids, economics, and population growth.

Currently, fuzzy logic and chaos theory form two of the most intriguing and promising areas of mathematical research. Recently, fuzzy logic and chaos theory have merged to form a new discipline of knowledge, called fuzzy chaos theory [68,69]. The detailed implications of fuzzy chaotic models are beyond the scope of this chapter.

1.4.7   The Differential Evolution Algorithm

Differential evolution (DE) [70–72] is well known as a simple and efficient scheme for global optimization over continuous spaces. It has reportedly outperformed a few evolutionary algorithms (EAs) and other search heuristics like the PSO when tested over both benchmark and real-world problems. Differential evolution is a population-based global optimization algorithm that uses a floating-point (real-coded) representation. The ith individual (parameter vector or *chromosome*) of the population at generation (time) t is a D-dimensional vector containing a set of D optimization parameters:

$$\vec{Z}_i(t) = [Z_{i,1}(t), Z_{i,2}(t), \ldots, Z_{i,D}(t)] \tag{1.15}$$

Now, in each generation (or one iteration of the algorithm) to change the population members $\vec{Z}_i(t)$ (say), a *donor* vector $\vec{Y}_i(t)$ is created. It is the method of creating this donor vector that distinguishes the various DE schemes. In one of the earliest variants of DE, now called the DE–rand–1 scheme, to create $\vec{Y}_i(t)$ for each ith member, three other parameter vectors (say the r_1, r_2, and r_3th vectors such that $r_1, r_2, r_3 \in [1, NP]$ and $r_1 \neq r_2 \neq r_3$) are chosen at random from the current population. Next, the difference of any two of the three vectors is multiplied by a scalar number F and the scaled difference is added to the third one, hence we obtain the donor vector $\vec{Y}_i(t)$.

The process for the jth component of the ith vector may be expressed as,

$$Y_{i,j}(t) = Z_{r1,j}(t) + F \cdot (Z_{r2,j}(t) - Z_{r3,j}(t)) \qquad (1.16)$$

Next, a crossover operation takes place to increase the potential diversity of the population. The DE family primarily uses two kinds of crossover schemes, namely, "exponential" and "binomial" [70]. To save space here, we briefly describe the binomial crossover, which is also employed by the modified DE algorithm. The binomial crossover is performed on each of the D variables whenever a randomly picked number between 0 and 1 is within the Cr value. In this case, the number of parameters inherited from the mutant has a (nearly) binomial distribution. Thus for each target vector $\vec{Z}_i(t)$, a trial vector $\vec{R}_i(t)$ is created in the following fashion:

$$
\begin{aligned}
R_{i,j}(t) &= Y_{i,j}(t) \quad \text{if } rand_j\,(0, 1) \le Cr \text{ or } j = rn(i) \\
&= Z_{i,j}(t) \quad \text{if } rand_j\,(0, 1) > Cr \text{ or } j \ne rn(i)
\end{aligned} \qquad (1.17)
$$

for $j = 1, 2, \ldots, D$ and $rand_j\,(0, 1) \in [0, 1]$ is the jth evaluation of a uniform random number generator. The Paramiter $rn(i) \in [1, 2, \ldots, D]$ is a randomly chosen index that ensures $\vec{R}_i(t)$ gets at least one component from $\vec{Z}_i(t)$. To keep the population size constant over subsequent generations, the next step of the algorithm calls for "selection" in order to determine which one between the target and trial vector will survive in the next generation (i.e., at time $t = t + 1$). If the trial vector yields a better value of the fitness function, it replaces its target vector in the next generation; otherwise the parent is retained in the population:

$$
\begin{aligned}
\vec{Z}_i(t + 1) &= \vec{R}_i(t) \quad \text{if } f(\vec{R}_i(t)) \le f(\vec{Z}_i(t)) \\
&= \vec{Z}_i(t) \quad \text{if } f(\vec{R}_i(t)) > f(\vec{Z}_i(t))
\end{aligned} \qquad (1.18)
$$

where $f(.)$ is the function to be minimized.

The DE has successfully been applied to diverse domains of science and engineering (e.g., mechanical engineering design, signal processing, chemical engineering, machine intelligence, and pattern recognition, see [73]). It has been shown to perform better than the GA and PSO over several numerical benchmarks [74].

1.4.8   BFOA

In 2002, Passino and co-workers proposed the BFOA [75,76] based on the foraging theory of natural creatures that try to optimize (maximize) their energy intake per unit time spent for foraging, considering all the constraints presented by their own physiology (e.g., sensing and cognitive capabilities), and environment (e.g., density of prey, risks from predators, physical characteristics of the search space). Although BFOA has certain characteristics analogous to an evolutionary algorithm ([75], p. 63), it is not directly connected to Darwinian evolution and natural genetics, which formed the basis of the GA type algorithms in the early 1970s.

During foraging of the real bacteria, locomotion is achieved by a set of tensile flagella. Flagella help an *Escherechia coli* bacterium to tumble or swim, which are two basic operations performed by a bacterium at the time of foraging [70]. When they rotate the flagella in the clockwise direction, each flagellum pulls on the cell. That results in the moving of flagella independently and finally the bacterium tumbles with a lesser number of tumbling, whereas in a harmful place it tumbles frequently to find a nutrient gradient. Moving the flagella in the counterclockwise direction helps the bacterium to swim at a very fast rate. In the above-mentioned algorithm, the bacteria undergoes chemotaxis, where they like to move toward a nutrient gradient and avoid noxious environment. Generally, the bacteria move for a longer distance in a friendly environment. Figure 1.11 depicts how clockwise and counterclockwise movement of a bacterium take place in a nutrient solution.

When they get sufficient food, they increased in length, and in the presence of a suitable temperature, they break in the middle to from an exact replica of themselves. This phenomenon inspired Passino to introduce an event of reproduction in BFOA. Due to the occurrence of sudden environmental changes or attack, the chemotactic progress may be destroyed and a group of bacteria may move to some other places or something else may be introduced in the swarm of concern. This constitutes the event of elimination dispersal in the real bacterial population, where all the bacteria in a region are killed or a group is dispersed into a new part of the environment.

Now, suppose that we want to find the minimum of $J(\theta)$, where $\theta \in \Re^p$ (i.e., θ is a p-dimensional vector of real numbers), and we do not have measurements or an analytical description of the gradient $\nabla J(\theta)$. The BFOA mimics the four principal mechanisms observed in a real bacterial system: chemotaxis, swarming, reproduction, and elimination dispersal to solve this nongradient optimization problem. Below, we introduce the formal notations used in BFOA literature, and then provide the complete pseudocode of the BFO algorithm.

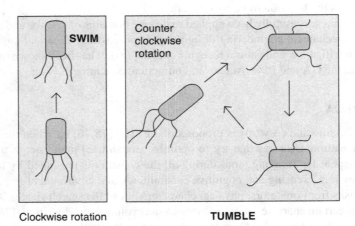

FIGURE 1.11   Swim and tumble of a bacterium.

Let us define a chemotactic step to be a tumble followed by a tumble or a tumble followed by a run. Let j be the index for the chemotactic step. Let k be the index for the reproduction step. Let l be the index of the elimination-dispersal event. Also, let

p = Dimension of the search space

S = Total number of bacteria in the population

Nc = The number of chemotactic steps

N_s = The swimming length

N_{re} = The number of reproduction steps

N_{ed} = The number of elimination-dispersal events

P_{ed} = Elimination-dispersal probability

$C(i)$ = The size of the step taken in the random direction specified by the tumble

Let $P(j, k, l) = \{\theta^i(j, k, l) | i = 1, 2, \ldots, S\}$ represent the position of each member in the population of the S bacteria at the jth chemotactic step, kth reproduction step, and lth elimination-dispersal event. Here, let $J(i, j, k, l)$ denote the cost at the location of the ith bacterium $\theta^i(j, k, l) \in \Re^p$ (sometimes we drop the indices and refer to the ith bacterium position as θ^i). *Note*: We will interchangeably refer to J as being a "cost" (using terminology from optimization theory) and as being a nutrient surface (in reference to the biological connections). For actual bacterial populations, S can be very large (e.g., $S = 109$), but $p = 3$. In our computer simulations, we will use much smaller population sizes and will keep the population size fixed. However, the BFOA, allows $p > 3$ so that we can apply the method to higher dimensional optimization problems. Below we briefly describe the four prime steps in BFOA. We also provide a pseudocode of the complete algorithm.

1. **Chemotaxis**. This process simulates the movement of an *E. coli* cell through swimming and tumbling via flagella. Suppose $\theta^i(j, k, l)$ represents ith bacterium at the jth chemotactic, kth reproductive, and lth elimination-dispersal step. The parameter $C(i)$ is a scalar and indicates the size of the step taken in the random direction specified by the tumble (run length unit). Then in computational chemotaxis, the movement of the bacterium may be represented by

$$\theta^i(j + 1, k, l) = \theta^i(j, k, l) + C(i)\frac{\Delta(i)}{\sqrt{\Delta^T(i)\Delta(i)}} \qquad (1.19)$$

where Δ indicates a unit length vector in the random direction.

2. **Swarming**. An interesting group behavior has been observed for several motile species of bacteria including *E. coli* and *Salmonella typhimurium*, where stable spatiotemporal patterns (swarms) are formed in a semisolid nutrient medium. A group of *E. coli* cells arrange themselves in a traveling ring by moving up the nutrient gradient when placed amid a semisolid matrix with a single nutrient

chemoeffecter. The cells when stimulated by a high level of *succinate*, release an attractant *aspertate*, which helps them to aggregate into groups and thus move as concentric patterns of swarms with high bacterial density. The cell-to-cell signaling in *E. coli* swarm may be represented by the following function:

$$J_{cc}(\theta, P(j, k, l)) = \sum_{i=1}^{S} J_{cc}(\theta, \theta^i(j, k, l))$$

$$= \sum_{i=1}^{S}[-d_{attractant}\exp(-w_{attractant}\sum_{m=1}^{P}(\theta_m - \theta_m^i)^2)]$$

$$+ \sum_{i=1}^{S}[h_{repellant}\exp(-w_{repellant}\sum_{m=1}^{P}(\theta_m - \theta_m^i)^2)] \qquad (1.20)$$

where $J_{cc}(\theta, P(j, k, l))$ is the objective function value to be added to the actual objective function (to be minimized) to present a time varying objective function. The coefficients $d_{attractant}$, $w_{attractant}$, $h_{repellant}$, and $w_{repellant}$ control the strength of the cell-to-cell signaling. More specifically $d_{attractant}$ is the depth of the attractant released by the cell; $w_{attractant}$ is a measure of the width of the attractant signal (a quantification of the diffusion rate of the chemical); $h_{repellant} = d_{attractant}$ is the height of the repellant effect (a bacterium cell also repels a nearby cell in the sense that it consumes nearby nutrients and it is not physically possible to have two cells at the same location); and $w_{repellant}$ is a measure of the width of the repellant. For a detailed discussion on the function J_{cc}, please see [70].

3. *Reproduction.* The least healthy bacteria eventually die while each of the healthier bacteria (those yielding lower value of the objective function) asexually split into two bacteria, which are then placed in the same location. This keeps the swarm size constant.

4. *Elimination and Dispersal.* To simulate this phenomenon in BFOA, some bacteria are liquidated at random with a very small probability while the new replacements are randomly initialized over the search space.

1.4.9   Bees Foraging Algorithm

Besides the gradually increasing popularity of BFOA, the current decade also witnessed the development of a family of computer algorithms mimicking the foraging strategies of honey bees. A colony of honey bees can extend itself over long distances (up to 14 km) and in multiple directions simultaneously to exploit a large number of food sources. A colony prospers by deploying its foragers to good fields. In principle, flower patches with plentiful amounts of nectar or pollen that can be collected with less effort should be visited by more bees, whereas patches with less nectar or pollen should receive fewer bees [77,78]. The foraging process begins in a colony by scout bees being sent to search for promising flower patches. Scout bees move randomly from one patch to another. During the harvesting season, a colony continues its exploration, keeping a percentage of the population as scout bees. When they return to the hive, those scout bees founding a patch that is rated above a certain quality threshold (measured as a combination of some constituents, e.g., sugar content) deposit their nectar or pollen and go to the "dance floor" to perform a dance known as the *Waggle Dance* [41]. The family of *Artificial Bee Foraging* algorithms try to mimic the above aspects of the foraging strategies employed by real bee colonies. The key members of the family and their applications to several different engineering optimization problems have been summarized in Table 1.2.

TABLE 1.2   A Summary of State-of-the-art Research Works on Bees Foraging Algorithm

Researchers	References	Related Algorithms	Applications
1. Yonezawa and Kikuchi (1996)	[79]		*Biological Simulations*
2. Seeley and Buhrman (1999)	[80],		
3. Schmickl et al. (2005)	[81],		
4. Lemmens (2006)	[82],		
Sato and Hagiwara (1997)	[83]	Bee System	*Genetic Algorithm Improvement*
Karaboga (2005)	[84]	Artificial Bee Colony (ABC)	*Continuous Optimization*
Yang (2005)	[85]	Virtual Bee Algorithm (VBA)	*Continuous Optimization*
Pham et al. (2006)	[86]	Bees Algorithm (BA)	*Continuous Optimization*
Lucic and Teodorovic (2001)	[87]	Bee System (BS)	*Travelling Salesman Problem (TSP)*
Lucic and Teodorovic (2002)	[88]	BS	*TSP and Stochastic Vehicle Routing Problem*
Teodorovic and Dell'Orco (2005)	[89]	Bee Colony Optimization (BCO) + Fuzzy Bee System (FBS)	*Ride-Matching Problem*
Nakrani and Tovey (2003)	[90]	A Honey Bee Algorithm	*Dynamic Allocation of Internet Service*
Wedde et al. (2004)	[91]	Bee Hive	*Telecommunication Network Routing*
Drias et al. (2005)	[92]	Bees Swarm	*Max-W-Sat Problem*
Pham et al. (2006)	[93]	BA	*LVQ-Neural Network*

Recently, Quijano et al. [94] modeled the social foraging behavior of honey bees for nectar, involving the environment representation, activities during bee expeditions (exploration and foraging), unloading nectar, dance strength decisions, explorer allocation, recruitment on the dance floor, and accounting for interactions with other hive functions [95]. They used the computational model of bee foraging to (1) solve a continuous optimization problem underlying resource allocation, and (2) provide novel strategies for multizone temperature control, an important industrial engineering application. They also established the global optimality of such algorithms for single or multiple hives theoretically on the resource allocation problem.

1.5 SUMMARY

This chapter introduced different fundamental components of CI, discussed their scope of possible synergism, and also focused on the most prominent recent topics emerging in the field. It is clear from the discussions that fuzzy logic is a fundamental tool for reasoning with approximate data and knowledge. Neural network plays a significant role in machine learning and GA has an extensive application in intelligent search and optimization problems. Belief networks are capable of propagating beliefs of an event node based on the probabilistic support of its cause and effect nodes in the causal tree–graph. The chapter also provided a list of possible synergism of two or more computational models that fall under the rubric of CI. It ends with a brief exposure to some very recently developed methodologies, which are gaining rapid importance in the realm of CI.

REFERENCES

1. A. M. Turing (1936), On Computable Numbers, with an Application to the Entscheidungs problem, Proc. London Math. Soc., 2, 42: 230–265.

2. Turing Machine: Available at http://www.turing.org.uk/turing/.

3. A. M. Turing (1950), Computing Machinery and Intelligence Available at http://abelard. org/turpap/turpap.htm.

4. A. M. Turing (1948), Machine Intelligence, in B. J. Copeland (Ed.), *The Essential Turing: The ideas that gave birth to the computer age*, Oxford University Press, Oxford, UK.

5. J. C. Bezdek (1994), What is Computational Intelligence? *Computational Intelligence Imitating Life*, J. M., Zurada, R. J. Marks, and C. J. Robinson (Eds.), IEEE Press, NY, pp. 1–12.

6. A. Konar (2005), *Computational Intelligence, Principles, Techniques, and Applications*, Springer-Verlag, Berlin, Heidelberg.

7. D. Poole, A. Mackworth, and R. Goebel (1998), *Computational Intelligence—A Logical Approach*, Oxford University Press, NY.

8. A. P. Engelbrecht (2007), *Computational Intelligence: An Introduction*, John Wiley & Sons, Inc., NY.

9. R. J., Marks (1993), Intelligence: Computational versus Artificial, *IEEE Trans. Neural Networks*, 4: 737–739.

10. C. G. Langton (Ed.) (1989), *Artificial Life*, Vol. 6, Addison-Wesley, Reading, MA.

11. W. Pedrycz (1996), *Fuzzy Sets Engineering*, CRC Press, Boca Raton, FL, pp. 73–106.

12. W. Pedrycz and F. Gomide (1998), *An Introduction to Fuzzy Sets: Analysis and Design*, MIT Press, MA.

13. S. Haykin (1999), *Neural Networks: A Comprehensive Foundation*, Prentice-Hall, NJ.

14. Li. M. Fu (1994), *Neural Networks in Computer Intelligence*, McGraw-Hill, NY.

15. J., Hertz, A. Krogn, and G. R. Palmer (1990), *Introduction to the Theory of Neural Computation*, Addison-Wesley, Reading, MA.

16. R. J. Schalkoff (1997), *Artificial Neural Networks*, McGraw-Hill, NY.

17. S. Kumar (2007), *Neural Networks—A Classroom Approach, Tata,* McGraw-Hill, India.

18. C. M. Bishop (1995), *Neural Networks for Pattern Recognition*, Oxford University Press.

19. T. Kohonen (1988), *Self-Organization and Associative Memory,* Springer-Verlag, NY.

20. Zadeh, L. A. (1965), *Fuzzy Sets, Information and Control*, Vol. 8: pp. 338–353.

21. G. J. Klir and B. Yuan (1995), *Sets and Fuzzy Logic: Theory and Applications*, Prentice-Hall, NJ.

22. B. Kosko (1991), *Neural Networks and Fuzzy Systems: A Dynamical Systems Approach to Machine Intelligence*, Prentice-Hall, Englewood Cliffs, NJ.

23. T. J. Ross (1995), *Fuzzy Logic with Engineering Applications*, McGraw-Hill, NY.

24. H. J. Zimmerman (1996), *Fuzzy Set Theory and Its Applications*, Kluwer Academic, Dordrecht, The Netherlands, pp. 131–162.

25. A. Abraham (2001), Neuro-Fuzzy Systems: State-of-the-Art Modeling Techniques, Connectionist Models of Neurons, Learning Processes, and Artificial Intelligence, Lecture Notes in Computer Science. Mira J. and Prieto A. (Eds.), Vol. 2084, Springer-Verlag Germany, pp. 269–276.

26. T. Back, D. B. Fogel, and Z. Michalewicz (Eds.) (1997), *Handbook of Evolutionary Computation*, Oxford University Press.

27. D. B. Fogel (1995), *Evolutionary Computation: Toward a New Philosophy of Machine Intelligence*, IEEE Press, Piscataway, NJ.

28. L. J., Fogel, A. J. Owens, and M. J. Walsh (1966), *Artificial Intelligence through Simulated Evolution*, John Wiley & Sons, NY.

29. J. H. Holland (1975), *Adaptation in Natural and Artificial Systems*, University of Michigan Press, Ann Arbor, MI.

30. I. Rechenberg (1973), Evolutionsstrategie—Optimierung Technischer Systeme nach Prinzipien der Biologischen Evolution (Ph.D. thesis, 1971), Reprinted by Fromman-Holzboog.

31. H.-P. Schwefel (1974), Numerische Optimierung von Computer-Modellen (Ph.D. thesis). Reprinted by Birkhäuser (1977).

32. J. R. Koza (1992), *Genetic Programming: On the programming of Computers by Means of Natural Selection*, MIT Press, Cambridge, MA.

33. E. Bonabeau, M. Dorigo, and G. Theraulaz (1999), *Swarm Intelligence: From Natural to Artificial Systems,* Oxford University Press Inc.

34. T. M. Martinetz and K. J. Schulten (1991), A neural-gas network learns topologies, T. Kohonen, K. Mäkisara, O. Simula, and J. Kangas (Eds.), *Artificial Neural Networks,* North-Holland, Amsterdam, The Netherlands, pp. 397–402.

35. Z. Kobti, R. Reynolds, and T. Kohler (2003), A multi-agent simulation using cultural algorithms: The effect of culture on the resilience of social systems, IEEE Congress on Evolutionary Computation December 5–12, 2003, Canberra, Australia.

36. K. S. Lee and Z. W. Geem (2005), A new meta-heuristic algorithm for continuous engineering optimization: harmony search theory and practice, Computer Methods in Applied Mechanics and Engineering, Vol. 194, No. 36–38, pp. 3902–3933.

37. D. Dasgupta (Ed.) (1999), *Artificial Immune Systems and Their Applications*, Springer-Verlag, Inc. Berlin.

38. J. Wojtusiak and R. S. Michalski (2006), The LEM3 Implementation of learnable evolution model and Its testing on complex function optimization problems, *Proceedings of Genetic and Evolutionary Computation Conference*, GECCO 2006, Seattle, WA.

39. J. Pearl (1997), *Probabilistic Reasoning in Intelligent Systems: Networks of Plausible Inference,* Morgan Kaufmann Publishers.

40. J. Pearl (1987), Distributed revision of composite beliefs, *Artificial Intelligence,* Vol. 33, pp. 173–213.

41. J. Pearl (1986), Fusion, propagation and structuring in belief networks, *Artificial Intelligence*, Vol. 29, pp. 241–288.

42. A. Abraham (2002), Intelligent Systems: Architectures and Perspectives, Recent Advances in Intelligent Paradigms and Applications, A. Abraham, L. Jain, and J. Kacprzyk (Eds.), *Studies in Fuzziness and Soft Computing,* Springer-Verlag Germany, Chapter 1, pp. 1–35.

43. G. Beni and U. Wang (1989), Swarm intelligence in cellular robotic systems, NATO Advanced Workshop on Robots and Biological Systems, Il Ciocco, Italy.

44. I. D. Couzin, J. Krause, R. James, G. D. Ruxton, and N. R. Franks (2002), Collective Memory and Spatial Sorting in Animal Groups, *J. Theor. Biol.*, 218: 1–11.

45. J. Krause and G. D. Ruxton (2002), *Living in Groups,* Oxford University Press, Oxford, UK.

46. B. L. Partridge and T. J. Pitcher (1980), The sensory basis of fish schools: relative role of lateral line and vision. *J. Compar. Physiol.*, 135: 315–325.

47. B. L. Partridge (1982), The structure and function of fish schools. *Sci. Am.*, 245: 90–99.

48. M. M. Milonas (1994), Swarms, phase transitions, and collective intelligence, *Artificial Life III,* Langton CG (Ed.), Addison-Wesley, Reading, MA.

49. J. Kennedy, R. Eberhart, and Y. Shi (2001), *Swarm Intelligence,* Morgan Kaufmann Academic Press.

50. M. Dorigo, V. Maniezzo, and A. Colorni (1996), The ant system: Optimization by a colony of cooperating agents, *IEEE Trans. Systems Man and Cybernetics Part* B, 26.

51. M. Dorigo and L. M. Gambardella (1997), Ant colony system: A cooperative learning approach to the traveling salesman problem, *IEEE Trans. Evolutionary Computing,* 1: 53–66.

52. L. A. Zadeh (1975), The Concept of a Linguistic Variable and Its Application to Approximate Reasoning–1, Information Sci., 8: 199–249.

53. J. M. Mendel and R. I. John (2002), Type-2 Fuzzy Sets Made Simple, *IEEE Trans. Fuzzy Systems,* 10: 117–127.

54. O. Castillo and P. Melin (2008), *Type-2 Fuzzy Logic Theory and Applications,* Springer-Verlag, Berlin.

55. J. M. Mendel, R. L. John, and F. Liu (2006), Interval type-2 fuzzy logic systems made simple, *IEEE Trans. Fuzzy Systems,* 14: 808–821.

56. Z. Pawlak, S. K. M. Wong, and W. Ziarko (1988), Rough sets: Probabilistic versus deterministic approach, *Inter. J. Man-Machine Studies* 29: 81–95.

57. Z. Pawlak (1991), *Rough Sets: Theoretical Aspects of Reasoning About Data,* Dordrecht: Kluwer Academic Publishing.

58. A. Bargiela and W. Pedrycz (2003), *Granular Computing. An introduction,* Kluwer Academic Publishers.

59. W. Pedrycz, A. Skowron, and V. Kreinovich (Eds.) (2008), *Handbook of Granular Computing,* John Wiley & Sons, Inc., NY.

60. R. Bello, R. Falcón, W. Pedrycz, and J. Kacprzyk (Eds.) (2008), *Granular Computing: At the Junction of Rough Sets and Fuzzy Sets,* Springer-Verlag, NY.

61. D. Dasgupta (Ed.) (1999), *Artificial Immune Systems and Their Applications,* Springer-Verlag, Inc., Berlin.

62. J. O. Kephart (1994), A biologically inspired immune system for computers, Proceedings of Artificial Life IV: The Fourth International Workshop on the Synthesis and Simlation of Living Systems, MIT Press, MA, pp. 130–139.

63. N. K. Jerne (1973), The immune systems, *Sci. Am.,* 229(1): 52–60.

64. N. K. Jerne (1983), The generative grammar of the immune system, *EMBO J.,* 4(4): 847–852.

65. N. K. Jerne (1984), Idiotypic networks and other pre-conceived ideas, *Immunolog. Rev.,* 79: 5–24.

66. R. L. Devaney (2003), *An Introduction to Chaotic Dynamical Systems,* 2nd ed,. Westview Press.

67. E. Ott (2002), *Chaos in Dynamical Systems,* Cambridge University Press, NY.

68. J. J. Buckley (1991), Fuzzy dynamical systems, Proceedings of IFSA'91, Brussels, Belgium, pp. 16–20.

69. P. Grim (1993), Self-Reference and Chaos in Fuzzy Logic, *IEEE Trans. Fuzzy Systems,* 1(4): 237–253.

70. R. Storn, K. V. Price, and J. Lampinen (2005), *Differential Evolution—A Practical Approach to Global Optimization,* Springer, Berlin.

71. U. K. Chakraborty (Ed.) (2008), *Advances in Differential Evolution,* Springer-Verlag, Heidelberg.

72. V. Feoktistov (2006), *Differential Evolution—In Search of Solutions,* Springer, Heidelberg.

73. J. Lampinen (1999), A bibliography of differential evolution algorithm, Technical Report. Lappeenranta University of Technology, Department of Information Technology, Laboratory of Information Processing, 1999. Available at http://www.lut.fi/~jlampine/debiblio.htm.

74. J. Vesterstrøm and R. Thomson (2004), A comparative study of differential evolution, particle swarm optimization, and evolutionary algorithms on numerical benchmark

problems, Proceedings of the Sixth Congress on Evolutionary Computation (CEC-2004), IEEE Press.

75. K. M. Passino (2002), Biomimicry of bacterial foraging for distributed optimization and control, *IEEE Control Systems Mag.,* 52–67.

76. Y. Liu and K. M. Passino (2002), Biomimicry of social foraging bacteria for distributed optimization: models, principles, and emergent behaviors, *J. Optimization Theory App.,* 115(3): 603–628.

77. K. V. Frisch (1976), Bees: *Their Vision, Chemical Senses and Language,* (Revised edition) Cornell University Press, Ithaca, NY.

78. S. Camazine, J. Deneubourg, N. R. Franks, J. Sneyd, G. Theraula, and E. Bonabeau (2003), *Self-Organization in Biological Systems,* Princeton University Press, Princeton, NY.

79. Y. Yonezawa and T. Kikuchi (1996), Ecological Algorithm for Optimal Ordering Used by Collective Honey Bee Behavior, 7th International Symposium on Micro Machine and Human Science, 249–256.

80. T. D. Seeley and S. C. Buhrman (1999), Group decision making in swarms of honey bees, *Behav. Ecol. Sociobiol.,* 45: 19–31.

81. T. Schmickl, R. Thenius, and K. Crailsheim (2005), Simulating swarm intelligence in honey bees: foraging in differently fluctuating environments, Genetic and Evolutionary Computation Conference (GECCO 2005), Washington, DC, pp. 273–274.

82. N. P. P. M. Lemmens (2006), To bee or not to bee: a comparative study in swarm intelligence, Master thesis, Maastricht University, Maastricht ICT Competence Centre, Institute for Knowledge and Agent Technology, Maastricht, Netherlands, 2006.

83. T. Sato and M. Hagiwara (1997), Bee system: finding solution by a concentrated search, Proceedings of the IEEE International Conference on Systems, Man, and Cybernetics, Vol. 4(C), pp. 3954–3959.

84. D. Karaboga (2005), An idea based on honey bee swarm for numerical optimization, Technical Report-TR06, Erciyes University, Engineering Faculty, Computer Engineering Department, Turkey.

85. X. S. Yang (2005), Engineering optimizations via nature-inspired virtual bee algorithms, IWINAC 2005, LNCS 3562, J. M. Yang and J. R. Alvarez (Eds.), Springer-Verlag, Berlin Heidelberg, pp. 317–323.

86. D. T. Pham, E. Kog, A. Ghanbarzadeh, S. Otri, S. Rahim, and M. Zaidi (2006), The bees algorithm—a novel tool for complex optimization problems, IPROMS 2006 Proceeding 2nd International Virtual Conference on Intelligent Production Machines and Systems, Elsevier, Oxford, UK.

87. P. Lucic and D. Teodorovic (2001), Bee system: modeling combinatorial optimization transportation engineering problems by swarm intelligence, Preprints of the TRISTAN IV Triennial Symposium on Transportation Analysis, Sao Miguel, Azores Islands, pp. 441–445.

88. P. Luckic and D. Teodorovic (2002), Transportation modeling: an artificial life approach, ICTAI'02 14th IEEE International Conference on Tools with Artificial Intelligence, pp. 216–223.

89. D. Teodorovic and M. Dell'Orco (2005), Bee colony optimization—a cooperative learning approach to complex transportation problems, Advanced OR and AI Methods in Transportation, pp. 51–60.

90. S. Nakrani and C. Tovey (2003), On honey bees and dynamic allocation in an internet server colony, Proceedings of 2nd International Workshop on the Mathematics and Algorithms of Social Insects, Atlanta, GA.

91. H. F. Wedde, M. Farooq, and Y. Zhang (2004), BeeHive: An Efficient Fault-Tolerant Routing Algorithm Inspired by Honey Bee Behavior, Ant Colony, Optimization and Swarm Intelligence, M. Dorigo (Ed.), Lecture Notes in Computer Science 3172, Springer, Berlin, pp. 83–94.

92. H. Drias, S. Sadeg, and S. Yahi (2005), Cooperative bees swarm for solving the maximum weighted satisfiability problem, IWAAN International Work Conference on Artificial and Natural Neural Networks, Barcelona, Spain, pp. 318–325.

93. D. T. Pham, S. Otri, A. Ghanbarzadeh, and E. Kog (2006), Application of the bees algorithm to the training of learning vector quantization networks for control chart pattern recognition, ICTTA'06 Information and Communication Technologies, pp. 1624–1629.

94. N. Quijano, B. W. Andrews, and K. M. Passino (2006), Foraging theory for multizone temperature control, *IEEE Computational Intelligence Mag.*, 1(4): 18–27.

95. N. Quijano and K. M. Passino (2007), The ideal free distribution: theory and engineering application, *IEEE Transactions Systems, Man, Cybernetics Part B*, 37(1): 154–165.

2

FUNDAMENTALS OF PATTERN ANALYSIS: A BRIEF OVERVIEW

2.1 INTRODUCTION

With the rapid proliferation of the use of computers, a vast amount of data are generated in every area of engineering and scientific disciplines (biology, psychology, medicine, marketing, finance, etc.). This vast amount of data with potentially useful information needs to be analyzed automatically for extraction of hidden knowledge. Pattern analysis is the process of automatically detecting patterns characterizing the inherent information in data. A pattern is defined in [1] as opposite of chaos; *It is an entity, vaguely defined, that could be given a name*. The objective of pattern analysis is to identify the patterns into some known categories–classes or to group the patterns in different categories that are then assigned some tags–class names. The former is known as *supervised pattern classification* and the later is known as *unsupervised pattern classification* or *clustering*.

The area of pattern analysis or pattern classification is not a new one, the research began during the 1950s and varieties of techniques [2–4] have been developed over the years. The survey papers of Unger [5], Wee [6], and Nagy [7] represent an account of the earlier works done in this area. Classical data analysis techniques for pattern discovery are based mainly on statistics and mathematics [8–10]. An excellent overview of statistical pattern recognition techniques is available in [11]. Though statistical techniques are well developed, they seem to be no longer adequate for analyzing an increasingly huge collection of complex data in a variety of domains (e.g., the worldwide web, bioinformatics, healthcare, or scientific research). Recently, new intelligent data analysis technologies are emerging based on soft computing tools (e.g.,

Computational Intelligence and Pattern Analysis in Biological Informatics, Edited by Ujjwal Maulik, Sanghamitra Bandyopadhyay, and Jason T. L. Wang
Copyright © 2010 John Wiley & Sons, Inc.

artificial neural network, fuzzy logic, and rough sets), evolutionary techniques, and genetic algorithm to deal with imprecision and uncertainty in complex data [12–18].

This chapter represents an introduction to the fundamental concept behind pattern recognition techniques and a brief overview of the methodologies developed to date. Section 2.2 introduces the basic concepts behind pattern analysis and different approaches for designing a pattern recognition system. The following sections deal with the key processes of pattern analysis and a brief overview of the presently available techniques. Emphasis has been given to statistical techniques, the pioneering contributor in the field of pattern analysis. Section 2.7 concludes with a discussion of future issues.

2.2   PATTERN ANALYSIS: BASIC CONCEPTS AND APPROACHES

The basic steps of an automatic pattern analysis system are shown in Figure 2.1. The numerical representation of the pattern constitutes the measurement space. The lower dimensional representation of the measurement space constitutes the feature space and the categorization of the pattern represents the decision space. The role of the preprocessing step is to separate the pattern of interest from noisy background, and other necessary operations for suitable processing in the next step. Feature selection or feature extraction is to select–extract discriminatory features for representing the input pattern in a compact way for correct classification in the next stage, while discarding redundant information. The final step classifies input patterns to one of the possible classes or groups the patterns into some categories according to similarities among them. The accuracy of an automatic pattern recognition system depends jointly on the performance of the feature selector and the classifier. The degradation at any stage affect the efficiency of the other stage resulting in an overall inefficient system.

The different approaches for pattern analysis developed so far can be categorized into four areas: which are (1) template matching, (2) statistical approach, (3) syntactic approach, and (4) the soft computing approach. Some attempts also have been made to design hybrid systems with combinations of different approaches. A brief description of the different approaches are presented below.

2.2.1   Template Matching

The simplest and earliest approach to pattern recognition is based on template matching. The input pattern to be classified is matched against the reference patterns called the templates of the available classes. The reference patterns are learned from the

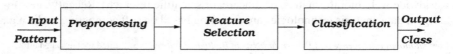

FIGURE 2.1   Basic pattern analysis system.

training samples and matching is done by using a similarity measure, mostly correlation measures. This approach is used mostly in the application of text or string matching. Dynamic programming based techniques [19] are the popular example of template matching [20, 21]. The rigid template matching approach is not suitable for pattern analysis problems where the intraclass variation is large.

2.2.2   Syntactic Approach

For hierarchical patterns, where a pattern is composed of simple subpatterns that are themselves composed of simpler subpatterns, the syntactic approach is efficient for analysis [22]. In syntactic approach, a formal analogy is drawn between the structure of patterns with a syntax of a language. The simplest patterns are called *primitives* and the complex patterns are formed by interconnecting primitives according to some defined rules (e.g., rules of grammar in a language). Thus the patterns are described by primitives and grammatical rules. The grammatical rules for each class are assessed from the training samples. This approach is useful for the non-numeric patterns having definite structure.

2.2.3   Statistical Approach

Among all the approaches, statistical pattern recognition has gained the widest acceptance. In classical statistical pattern analysis [9], a pattern is represented by a set of n features, or attributes, viewed as an n-dimensional feature vector (the points in n-dimensional measurement space R^n) are represented as $x = (x_1, x_2, \ldots x_n)^T$. Feature selection process transforms the pattern vector from n-dimensional measurement space to a d-dimensional feature space, where $d \leq n$. Recognition or classification process classifies or groups the patterns into one of the m possible classes. The statistical techniques for pattern analysis are represented in brief in the following sections.

2.2.4   Soft Computing Approach

Different computing tools (e.g., artificial neural network, fuzzy logic, rough set, genetic algorithm and evolutionary computation, and their integration to deal with impreciseness and uncertainty in real-world pattern analysis problems are collectively known as *soft computing tools*. Recently, these tools are increasingly used for pattern analysis. A brief presentation of soft computing approaches is presented in the later section.

2.3   FEATURE SELECTION

Feature selection or extraction is one of the major steps in an automatic pattern analysis system. The main objective of feature selection is to retain the optimum discriminatory information and to reduce the dimensionality of the measurement space from n to d $(d \leq n)$ to facilitate classification or recognition processes. The pioneering works on feature selection deals mostly with statistical tools and the major techniques developed so far can be broadly classified into two categories:

Feature selection in measurement space in which the feature set is reduced by discarding redundant or unimportant features.

Feature selection in transformed space in which the higher dimensional pattern vector is mapped to a lower dimensional space.

2.3.1   Feature Selection in Measurement Space

Feature selection in measurement space or feature subset selection selects a subset of d features from a set of n features on the basis of their quality in discriminating classes. Feature subset selection techniques are based on the design of a *criterion function* and the selection of a *search strategy*. The criterion function evaluates the goodness of a feature and ranks them. The best two features may not be the best feature subset of two features when used in combination [23]. So, we need a search strategy to decide the best possible feature subset among a number of candidates.

2.3.1.1 Feature Evaluation Measures.   There are several approaches to evaluate the *goodness* of a feature subset. Some of the popular measures are listed here. The details can be found in [8].

2.3.1.1.1 Measures Based On Error Probability.   Pattern classification is a decision-making process in which an input pattern in an n-dimensional feature space, defined by $f = [f_1, f_2, \ldots, f_n]$, is assigned to one of a number of possible classes w_i, where $i = 1, 2, \ldots, m$, depending on the value of the feature vector. Let the *a priori* probability of occurrence of a class w_i be $P(w_i)$, and let the multivariate class-conditional probability density function of class w_i be $p(f \mid w_i)$. The mixture density function $p(f)$ is given by

$$p(f) = \Sigma_{i=1}^{m} p(f \mid w_i) P(w_i) \tag{2.1}$$

According to Bayes' rule [2], the *a posteriori* probability for the ith class is

$$P(w_i \mid f) = p(f \mid w_i) P(w_i) p(f) \tag{2.2}$$

and according to Bayes' decision procedure, an unknown input pattern is assigned to class w_i if

$$P(w_i \mid f) \geq P(w_j \mid f) \text{ for all } i, j = 1, 2, \ldots, m. \quad i \neq j \tag{2.3}$$

The objective of any pattern recognition process is to classify unknown patterns with the lowest possible probability of misrecognition. The objective for designing the feature selection criterion should be such that the error probability p_e is minimized. In an n-dimensional feature space f, the error probability p_e is given by

$$p_e = \int [1 - \max_i P(w_i|f)] p(f) df \qquad (2.4)$$

Although the *error probability* is, from the theoretical viewpoint, the ideal measure for designing the feature selection criterion, it is not easy to evaluate from the practical computational point of view. Therefore a number of alternative criteria for feature evaluation have been suggested so far. Most of the indirect measures have been developed based on the concept of distance, separability, overlap, or dependence between the probability distributions characterizing the pattern classes.

2.3.1.1.2 Measures Based On Class Separability. The discriminatory power of any feature is associated with the concept of class separability. The *interclass distance* between two classes w_1 and w_2 is the simplest concept of class separability and can easily be used to assess the discriminatory potential of a feature in pattern representation. This measure is not defined explicitly by class-conditional probability density functions. Its estimate based on elements of the training set can be computed directly without prior determination of the probabilistic structure of the classes. Thus, separability measures based on this concept cannot serve as true indicators of the mutual overlap of the classes,though it is very simple to evaluate. The measures derived from the concept of class separability that are normally used in practice are divided into the following three groups:

1. *Measures Derived from the Probabilistic Distance* To obtain a realistic picture of mutual class overlap, measures have been developed based on the concept of the measure of distance between the probability density functions characterizing the pattern classes. These measures are termed as *probabilistic distance measures.* They do not bear any exact relationship to p_e. Hence, upper and lower bounds expressed in terms of these measures have been derived to provide an indication of the accuracy of the estimate of p_e. The error probability p_e in the two-class case is easily shown as, for $m = 2$,

$$p_e = 0.5[1 - \int |p(f|w_1)P(w_1) - p(f|w_2)P(w_2|df]] \qquad (2.5)$$

Now, p_e is maximum when the integrand is zero (i.e., the density functions are completely overlapping, and p_e is zero when the functions do not overlap. The integral in Eq. (2.5) can be considered to quantify the "probabilistic distance" between the two density functions. The greater the distance, the smaller the error, and vice versa. Any other measure of "distance" between the two density functions, such as

$$J = \int f[p(f|w_i), P(w_i) \quad i = 1, 2]df \qquad (2.6)$$

satisfying $J \geq 0$ can be used as a feature evaluation criterion. Here $J = 0$ when $p(f|w_i), i = 1, 2$ are overlapping and J is maximum when $p(f|w_i), i = 1, 2$ are nonoverlapping.

The most commonly used probabilistic distance measure are given below:

Bhattacharya Distance. The Bhattacharya distance function is defined as follows:

$$J_B = -\ln \int [p(f|w_1)p(f|w_2)]^{1/2}df \qquad (2.7)$$

For multivariate Gaussian distributions where

$$p(f|wi) = N(\mu_i, \Sigma_i), i = 1, 2, \ldots, \qquad (2.8)$$

J_B becomes,

$$J_B = 1/8(\mu_1 - \mu_2)^T \left(\frac{\Sigma_1 + \Sigma_2}{2}\right)^{-1} (\mu_1 - \mu_2)$$

$$+ 1/2\ln\left\{\frac{\det(\Sigma)}{\sqrt{\det(\Sigma_1)\det(\Sigma 2)}}\right\} \qquad (2.9)$$

μ_i and Σ_i represent a mean vector and covariance matrix for the probability distribution of the feature for the ith class, respectively.

The Jeffreys–Matsusita Distance Measure. The Jeffreys–Matushita distance measure J_M is defined to be

$$J_M = [\int (\sqrt{p(f|w_1)} - \sqrt{p(f|w_2)})^2 df] \qquad (2.10)$$

Note that the Jeffreys–Matushita and Bhattacharya distance are two different variations of the same measure and the relationship between them is given by

$$J_M = \{2[1 - \exp(1 - J_B)]\}^{1/2} \qquad (2.11)$$

Divergence Function. The divergence function was first introduced by Jeffreys and is defined by

$$J_D = \int [p(f|w_1) - p(f|w_2)] \ln \frac{p(f|w_1)}{p(f|w_2)} df \qquad (2.12)$$

Later it was developed by Toussaint and for the multivariate Gaussian distribution, the divergence function becomes

$$J_D = \frac{1}{2}\text{tr}(\Sigma_1^{-1}\Sigma_2 + \Sigma_2^{-1}\Sigma_1 - 2I)$$
$$+ \frac{1}{2}\text{tr}[(\Sigma_1^{-1} + \Sigma_2^{-1}(\mu_1 - \mu_2)^T(\mu_1 - \mu_2)]. \tag{2.13}$$

Mahalanobis Distance. For two multivariate distributions with common dispersion matrix, the Mahalanobis distance is given as

$$D^2 = (\mu_1 - \mu_2)^T \Sigma^{-1}(\mu_1 - \mu_2) \tag{2.14}$$

This distance function is very easy to compute though it is difficult to make theoretical assessment of the accuracy in a distribution-free case.

Kolmogorov Variational Distance. The Kolmogorov variational distance is defined to be

$$J_K = \frac{1}{2}E\{|(P(w_1|f) - P(w_2|f)|\} \tag{2.15}$$

From this measure, the probability of error p_e can be determined directly by the equation

$$p_e = \frac{1}{2} - J_K \tag{2.16}$$

but the computational difficulty associated with this measure is the same as that for p_e.

There are several other measures, developed from time to time, by the researchers. A complete discussion on their relative merits and demerits in evaluating feature quality is available in [24].

2. *Measures Derived from Probabilistic Dependence.* The degree of dependence between the feature vector and the class membership can be used as a measure of the effectiveness of any feature in distinguishing different classes. The degree of dependence between the variables f and w_i can be measured by the distance between the conditional density $p(f|w_i)$ and the mixture density $p(f)$. Any of the probabilistic distance measure can be used for evaluating the probabilistic dependance between f and w_i simply by replacing one of the class-conditional density functions with the mixture density. By computing the weighted average of the class-conditional distance, the overall dependency can be used that will

indicate the effectiveness of any feature in a multiclass environment. Some of the measures are given below:

Bhattacharyya

$$I_B = \Sigma_{i=1}^c P(w_i)[- \ln \int \sqrt{p(f|w_i)p(f)}df \qquad (2.17)$$

Matushita Distance

$$I_M = \Sigma_{i=1}^c P(w_i)\{ \int [\sqrt{p(f|w_i)} - \sqrt{p(f)}]^2 df\}^{0.5} \qquad (2.18)$$

Patric–Fisher Distance

$$I_P = \Sigma_{i=1}^c P(w_i)\{ \int [p(f|w_i) - p(f)]^2 df\}^{0.5} \qquad (2.19)$$

3. *Measure Derived from Information Theoretic Approach.* These measures are generally derived from the generalizations of Shannon's entropy [25], based on probabilistic measures. From information theory, information gain is analogous to reduction in uncertainty, which in turn is quantified by *entropy*. From the *a posteriori* probabilities $P(w_i|f)$, one can gain information about the dependance of f on w_i. Thus the expected value of the generalized entropy function can be used as a measure of feature quality, considering that the smaller the uncertainty, the better the feature vector. The average generalized entropy of degree α is defined as

$$J_E^\alpha = \int (2^{1-\alpha} - 1)^{-1}[\Sigma_{i=1}^m P^\alpha(w_i|f) - 1]p(f)df, \qquad (2.20)$$

where α is a real, positive parameter. For $\alpha = 1$, the measure becomes

$$J_s = - \int \Sigma_{i=1}^m P(w_i|f) \log_2 P(w_i|f)df \qquad (2.21)$$

which is the separability measure based on the well-known Shannon entropy. The optimal feature set can be obtained by minimizing the above criterion.

Entropy can also be used without the knowledge of densities as in decision tree algorithm [26], where the information gain with the inclusion–deletion of features are independently computed.

2.3.1.2 Search Strategies.

The selection of an optimal feature subset of d features from a set of n features on the basis of a feature evaluation measure becomes a difficult search problem when n is large. The two main approaches by which suboptimal solutions to the problem can be achieved are *forward* and *backward selection* [8]. A lot of search algorithms of different variants (sequential search, random search [27], etc.) of the two main approaches and their combinations have been developed for feature subset selection process. One of the popular techniques is *branch and bound* developed by Narendra and Fukunaga [28] and its variants [29]. A good survey of search strategies for feature subset selection can be found in [2, 30, 31].

2.3.1.3 Feature Selection Algorithms. The existing approaches of a feature subset selection can also be viewed as broadly classified into two categories: *filter* and *wrapper* approaches. Filter approaches [32, 33] are based on a criterion function that is classifier independent, while wrapper approaches [34] use the classifier accuracy as the criterion function and depends on the learning algorithm of the specific classifier. The two approaches have basic merits and demerits. While classifier dependant methods produce good results, especially when the classifier is designed to solve the particular problem, it is not computationally attractive when the number of input features are large. The computational burden is more heavy when a nonlinear classifier with complex learning algorithms are used.

2.3.2 Feature Selection in Transformed Space

The feature selection in transformed space is commonly known as a feature extraction method that uses all the information contained in a pattern vector and maps the higher dimensional pattern vector to a lower dimensional one. The objective of transformation, linear or nonlinear, is also to make original features uncorrelated to remove redundancy. The mathematical mapping techniques are computationally simpler than the probabilistic criteria and produce satisfactory results in practical situations, but unlike the probabilistic criteria they do not have any relationship with the error probability.

Linear transformation (e.g., principal component analysis, PCA), factor analysis, linear discriminant analysis, independent component analysis, and projection pursuit [2] are widely used in pattern analysis. The PCA or K-L transform is the most popular one in which d largest eigenvectors of the covariance matrix of the n-dimensional patterns are used for representation of the pattern. A lot of transforms [e.g., Fourier transform (FT) and its variants DFT, FFT, Harr transform, direct cosine transform (DCT)] are popular in spatial pattern analysis. Kernel PCA [35], multidimemsional scaling (MDS) [36], and artificial neural network-based [37, 38] methods are examples of nonlinear transformation. A comparative study of feature selection algorithms can be found in [39].

2.3.3 Soft Computing Approaches for Feature Selection

Recently, many feature selection algorithms based on soft computing approaches [40, 41], mainly artificial neural network, fuzzy set, genetic algorithm, and evolutionary computation and their hybrids [17], have been developed for solving real-world problems, where statistical methods are difficult to apply. Artificial neural network-based approaches are found in [38, 42–44]. In [45], a fractal neural network architecture is proposed and is used as a feature selector. The self-organization map (SOM) [46] or autoassociative networks [47] can be used as a nonlinear feature extractor. A comparative review of neural network feature extractor is found in [48].

In [49], fuzzy set theoretic measure based on the index of fuzziness and fuzzy entropy is developed for feature evaluation and ranking. Some hybrid neuro-fuzzy approaches are reported in [50–52]. Feature selection algorithm based on rough set theory and hybrid approaches are reported in [53–56]. Genetic algorithm (GA, widely used in optimization problems, is also a good candidate for feature subset selection and a number of GA based and hybrid algorithms are developed in this different application area. Some of them are reported in [57–63]. Other evolutionary computational techniques, like particle swarm optimization (PSO) and their hybrids with other soft computing tools, recently have been used for feature selection problems [64–69].

2.4 PATTERN CLASSIFICATION

The final and ultimate goal of pattern analysis is to classify the input patterns to known classes or to group them in different categories depending on their similarity. When the class information is available, the pattern analysis system learns from the training samples. The unknown input pattern, when presented to the learned system, is identified as a member of one of the known classes. This paradigm, known as *supervised classification*, is represented in this section.

2.4.1 Statistical Classifier

In supervised classification, a set of patterns having known class information are used as training samples by which the classifier learns the decision rule with some suitable algorithm. The learned classifier then categorizes the unknown input pattern to one of the classes with the help of the learned decision rule. Lots of learning algorithms using statistical concepts have been developed and are based on them and a variety of classifiers now have been designed. Statistical classification methods can be broadly classified into three groups [11]. The simplest and most intuitive approach is based on similarities measured by some distance function [70]. Here the proximity of a pattern to a class serves as the measure for its classification. Minimum distance classifier, nearest-neighbor algorithm [8], and its variants are the popular techniques in this category. The most advanced techniques for computing prototypes are vector and learning vector quantization [46].

2.4.1.1 k-NN Classifier. The k nearest-neighbor (k-NN) classifier is one of the earliest, simpliest, and most popular classifier. The algorithm known as the k-NN decision rule, can be stated as follows: Given an unknown pattern vector x and a distance measure,

Out of n training patterns, k nearest neighbors, irrespective of the class labels, are chosen, where k is always odd.
Assign the unknown vector x to the class w_i, $i = 1, 2, \ldots, m$ for which $\sum_i k_i$ is maximum, where k_i denotes the neighboring pattern belonging to class w_i.

For $k = 1$ the algorithm is simply known as the *nearest-neighbor* rule. Various distance measures can be used including the simplest Euclidean and Mahalanobis. For large values of n, this simple classifier can show quite a good performance.

2.4.1.2 Bayes Classifier and Discriminant Analysis. The main approachs of statistical methods are the probabilistic approach and the famous Bayes classfier [2,8], based on Bayes decision rule, which has been developed for a known class of conditional probability densities $p(x|w_i)$. A number of well-known decision rules, including Bayes decision rule, the maximum likelihood rule, and the Neyman–Pearson rule are available to generate the decision boundary. First, according to the Bayes decision rule, an input pattern x is assigned to class w_i for minimum error or minimum risk of classification if,

$$P(w_i|x) \geq P(w_j|x) \quad \text{for all} \quad i, j = 1, 2, \ldots, m. \quad i \neq j \qquad (2.22)$$

$P(w_i|x)$ is the *a posteriori* probability for class w_i.

Using Bayes rule of probability, the above rule can be effectively expressed using class conditional probability densities.

In practice, the estimates of densities are used in place of true densities. The density estimates are either *parametric,* where the distribution of the feature vectors are known, *nonparametric*, or *distribution free* methods. Commonly used parametric models are Gaussian distributions given as

$$p(x|w_i) = \frac{1}{(2\pi)^{n/2}|\Sigma_i|^{1/2}} \exp\left[-\frac{1}{2}(x - \mu_i)^T \Sigma_i^{-1}(x - \mu_i)\right] \qquad (2.23)$$

where $i = 1, 2, \ldots, m$, $\mu_i = E[x]$ denotes the mean value of class w_i, Σ_i denotes the $n \times n$ covariance matrix defined as $\Sigma_i = E[(x - \mu_i)(x - \mu_i)^T]$.

A variety of density estimators for the nonparametric approach from simple histogram estimators, followed by window estimators and kernel estimators, are available in the literature [2,8].

The equation for the decision surface of the two regions containing the ith and jth class is given by

$$P(w_i|x) - P(w_j|x) = 0 \qquad (2.24)$$

Now $g_i(x)$, a monotonically increasing function representing $f(P(w_i|x))$, is known as *discriminant function*. Thus the decision rule can be stated as follows in Eqs. (2.25) and (2.26).

Classify the pattern x in class w_i if

$$g_i(x) \geq g_j(x) \,\forall j \neq i \qquad (2.25)$$

and the equation of decision surface separating two regions becomes

$$g_i(x) - g_j(x) = 0, i, j = 1, 2 \ldots, m, \quad i \neq j \qquad (2.26)$$

Linear discriminant analysis is another category of approaches to construct decision boundaries or decision surface by optimizing certain error criterion. When the estimate of densities are difficult, it is preferable to compute decision surfaces directly by alternative costs. Such approaches gives rise to linear discriminant analysis and design of many linear classifiers. Linear discriminant analysis (LDA) approximates boundaries between classes by placing hyperplanes optimally assuming the classes to be linearly separable. The limitations of linear classifiers for nonlinearly separable classes prompted the development of nonlinear classifiers. A comparative study of various statistical classifiers can be found in [71].

2.4.1.3 Decision Tree Classifier. Decision tree classifiers [26] are a special type of nonlinear classifier. They are multistage decision systems that iteratively select an individual feature to partition the feature space generating a tree structure. The leaf nodes represent the final classification. Selection of a feature at each node is done according to some criterion function (e.g., information content). Though these classifiers are suboptimal, they are popular due to the fast classification ability and the rule generation with individual features making the classification process transparent to users.

2.5   UNSUPERVISED CLASSIFICATION OR CLUSTERING

When class information is not available, the input patterns are grouped into some classes or clusters according to their similarity. This paradigm of classification is known as *unsupervised classification* or *cluster analysis* in the context of pattern analysis. Clustering is one of the primitive mental activities of humans to deal with huge amounts of information they receive every day. Remembering every piece of information is difficult and humans tend to categorize entities into clusters. Cluster analysis is applied to different areas and has a long history of research. The early works can be found in [72, 73]. More recent algorithms can be found in [74]. Like the case of supervised classification, a pattern here is also represented in terms of n-dimensional vectors. The basic steps of the clustering task are as follows:

1. *Preprocessing.* As in the supervised classification, noise reduction and normalization is to be done first before any processing.
2. *Feature Selection.* Features must be properly selected to retain discriminatory information and to reduce the dimension of the pattern vectors to ease computational burden in later stages. Most of the methodologies for feature selection described in earlier sections can be used also for feature selection in this case. Some works on feature selection for unsupervised classification have been reported in [75–77].
3. *Proximity or Similarity Measure.* The measure for computing the similarity of two pattern vectors is to be selected from a variety of similarity metrics.

4. *Clustering Criterion.* The clustering criterion is expressed as an objective function or cost function that evaluates the goodness of a cluster based on the intended objective of clustering.

5. *Clustering Algorithms.* A specific algorithm to obtain the cluster using proximity measure and the clustering criterion is needed for formation of clusters.

6. *Validation of the Clusters.* The process of evaluating the correctness of the generated cluster through some measure is known as validation [78–80].

7. *Interpretation.* The process of attaching meaning to the generated clusters or naming the clusters is known as interpretation.

2.5.1 Definition of Clustering and Proximity Measure

Let X be a set of N pattern vectors, that is, $X = (x_1, x_2, \ldots, x_N)$. An m clustering of X partitions the pattern space into m sets $C_1, C_2, \ldots, C_m$, such that

$$C_i \neq \Phi, i = 1, 2, \ldots, m$$

$$\bigcup_{i=1}^{m} C_i = X$$

$$C_i \cap C_j = \Phi, i \neq j, i, j = 1, 2, \ldots, m$$

As there is an overlapping of categories for real-world data, crisp clustering defined above cannot handle them. Fuzzy clustering [81] of X into m clusters in which all the patterns can belong to several clusters with a varying degree of membership functions u_j can be defined below as:

$$u_j : X \to [0, 1] \quad j = 1, 2, \ldots, m$$

and

$$\sum_{j=1}^{m} u_j(x_i) = 1 \quad i = 1, 2, \ldots, N$$

$$0 \leq \sum_{i=1}^{N} u_j(x_i) \leq N \quad j = 1, 2, \ldots, m$$

A *proximity measure* can be defined in terms of either a dissimilarity measure (DM) or a similarity measure (SM). A similarity measure is intuitively opposite to a DM. Now, a DM d on X is a function

$$d : X \times X \to R$$

where R is the set of real numbers, such that

$$\exists d_0 \in R : -\infty \le d_0 \le d(x, y) \le +\infty \quad \forall x, y \in X$$
$$d(x, x) = d_0 \; \forall x \quad \in X$$
$$d(x, y) = d(y, x) \; \forall x \quad y \in X$$
$$d(x, z) \le d(x, y) + d(y, z) \quad \forall x, y, z \in X$$

The simplest dissimilarity metric is the Euclidean distance and is widely used as DM in clustering applications. There are also other DMs (Manhattan distance, point symmetric metric etc.).

The most common SM is an inner product

$$S_i n(x, y) = x^T y = \sum_{i=1}^{n} x_i y_i$$

The Hamming distance, Tanimoto measure, and so on, are other examples of SMs.

2.5.2 Clustering Algorithms

Clustering algorithms available in the literature can be divided into the following major categories:

Sequential Algorithms. These algorithms are simple and fast and produce single clustering. The patterns are presented in order, the clusters produced are compact, and are hyperspherical and hyperellipsoidal an shaped.

Hierarchical Clustering Algorithms. These algorithms are further divided into *agglomerative* and *divisive* algorithms. Agglomerative clustering produces a sequence of clustering with a decreasing number of clusters in each step, merging two clusters from the previous step into one. Divisive algorithms work in just the opposite direction. They produce a sequence of clustering with an increasing number of clusters in each step, splitting one cluster from the previous step to two clusters in the next steps.

Clustering Algorithm Based on Cost Function Optimization. This category contains algorithms in which a cost function is optimized to evaluate the clustering process. Generally, the number of cluster is fixed, the algorithm iteratively produces successive clusters with the objective of improving cost function, and finally stops when the optimal value is reached. This category includes the following subcategories:

1. Hard or crisp clustering algorithms, where a pattern belongs exclusively to a specific cluster. The most famous ISODATA [3] belongs in this category.
2. Fuzzy clustering algorithm, where a pattern can belong to multiple clusters with a certain membership value lying within (0,1). Fuzzy ISODATA [82] is an example of this category.

3. Probabilistic clustering algorithm where the cost function follows Bayesian theory.

4. Possibilistic clustering algorithm based on a measure of possibility of a pattern vector belonging to a certain cluster.

5. Boundary detection algorithms detect the boundary of a cluster region instead of determining the clusters by feature vector.

Soft Computer-Based Clustering Algorithms. An artificial neural network with competitive learning, fuzzy logic, and genetic algorithm-based clustering techniques [83, 84] are the popular successful clustering approaches from a soft computing paradigm.

A comparative performance analysis of several clustering algorithm can be found in [85].

2.6 NEURAL NETWORK CLASSIFIER

Artificial neural networks, the most widely used soft computing paradigm, have recently emerged as an important tool for data analysis and pattern classification. Their effectiveness in both supervised and unsupervised classification has been tested empirically and many applications in a variety of real-world classification tasks have been developed [12, 14, 86]. A survey of neural network classifiers can also be found in [87]. Links between neural and other conventional classifiers are discussed in [47, 88]. Performance comparisons of neural network classifiers and conventional statistical classifiers also have been studied in a number of works. Some of them are reported in [89, 90]. Riplay [91] compared neural networks with various classifiers (e.g., classification tree, projection pursuit, linear vector quantization, and nearest-neighbor methods).

Although many types of neural networks are used in classification problem, the most widely studied neural network for classification purposes is the *feedforward multilayer perceptrons (MLP).* One of the pioneer works on the use of MLP for pattern classification is studied in [92]. In [93], fractal neural network architecture is proposed and its performance as a classifier has been studied in comparison to MLP. It was found that it is well suited for classification of fractal patterns. Other architectures (e.g., *radial basis function, RBF,* networks [94], *support vector machines (SVM)* [96] and are also developed for supervised classification. *Self-organizing map (SOM)* or a *Kohonen Network* [46] is applied to unsupervised classification.

Although significant progress has been made in neural network-based classification for real-world problems, there are still some unresolved issues. Though neural networks do not require explicit knowledge of underlying distribution of patterns like statistical classifiers, their classification process in most of the cases is not transparent. This blackbox characteristics of neural architecture poses problem for generating explicit decision rules. To avoid this, some hybrid approaches combining neural network with a rough set or fuzzy logic have also been studied recently [17].

2.7   CONCLUSION

This chapter presents a brief overview of the fundamental techniques of pattern analysis. Pattern analysis is an important process for knowledge extraction from raw data generated everyday in different areas of human interest. With the progress of computing technologies, large amounts of data in recently discovered areas (e.g., molecular biology or genomic research), is now becoming available daily. This huge amount of data needs to be processed in order to extracting hidden information. Though the techniques of pattern analysis have grown for a long time and well-known tools are available, the demand for development of newer and more powerful techniques is also increasing due to the generation of newer and newer varieties of data.

Thus, the importance of research for improving pattern analysis techniques is ever increasing. For the development of new techniques, one should be fully aware of the basic concepts of fundamental pattern analysis techniques. This chapter attempts to represent the basic concepts and approaches behind pattern analysis techniques. A brief overview of the important and most popular statistical tools are explained. Recent approaches based on the soft computing paradigm are also introduced with a brief representation of the promising neural network classifiers as a new direction toward dealing with imprecise and uncertain patterns generated in newer fields.

REFERENCES

1. S. Watanabe (1985), *Pattern Recognition: Human and Mechanical*, New York, Jonh Wiley & Sons, Inc., NY.

2. R. O. Duda and P. E. Hart (1973), *Pattern Classification and Scene Analysis*, Wiley, NY.

3. R.O. Duda, P. E. Hart, and D. G. Stork (2001), *Pattern Classification*, 2nd ed., John Wiley & Sons, Inc., NY.

4. S. Theodoridis and K. Koutroumbas (1999), *Pattern Recognition*, Academic Press, San Diego.

5. S. H. Unger (1959), Pattern detection and recognition, *Proc. IR*, 47: 1737–1752.

6. W. G. Wee (1968), A survey of pattern recognition, *IEEE Proc. Seventh Symp. Adaptive Proc.*, 2.e.1–2.e.1.

7. G. Nagy (1968), State of the art in pattern recognition, *Proc. IEEE*, 56: 836–862.

8. P. A. Devijver and J. Kittler (1982), *Pattern Recognition: A Statistical Approach*, Prentice-Hall, London.

9. K. Fukunaga (1990), *Introduction to Statistical Pattern Recognition*, Academic Press, NY.

10. L. Devroye, L. Gyorfi and G. Lugosi (1996), *A Probabilistic Theory of Pattern Recognition*, Springer, NY.

11. A. K. Jain, R. P. W. Duin, and J. Mao (2000), Statistical Pattern Recognition : A Review, *IEEE Trans. PAMI*, 22(1): 4–37.

12. C. M. Bishop (1995), *Neural Networks for Pattern Recognition*, Oxford University Press, NY.

13. C. M. Bishop (2006), *Pattern Recognition and Machine Learning*, Springer Science+ Business Media, NY.

14. B. D. Ripley (1996), *Pattern Recognition and Neural Networks*, Cambridge University Press, NY.

15. Y. H. Pao (1989), *Adaptive Pattern Recognition and Neural Networks*, Addison-Wesley, NY.

16. S. K. Pal and D. Dutta Majumder (1986), *Fuzzy Mathematical Approach to Pattern Recognition*, Wiley (Halsted Press), NY.

17. S. K. Pal and S. Mitra (1999), *Neuro-Fuzzy Pattern Recognition: Methods in Soft Computing*, John Wiley & Sons, Inc., NY.

18. S. K. Pal and A. Pal (eds.) (2001), *Pattern Recognition: From Classical to Modern Approaches*, World Scientific, NY.

19. R. E. Bellman (1957), *Dynamic Programming*, Princeton University Press, Princeton, NY.

20. H. Sakoe and S. Chiba (1978), 'Dynamic programming algorithm optimization for spoken word recognition', *IEEE Trans. Acous, Speech Signal Proc.*, 26:(2): 43–49.

21. H. Silverman and D. P. Morgan (1990), The application of the dynamic programming to connected speech recognition, *IEEE Signal Proc. Mag.*, Vol. 7(3): 7–25.

22. K. S. Fu (1982), *Syntactic Pattern Recognition and Applications*, Prentice-Hall, NJ.

23. T. M. Cover (1974), The Best Two Independent Measurements are not the Two Best, *IEEE Trans. SMC*, 4: 116–117.

24. C. B. Chittineni (1980), Efficient feature subset selection with probabilistic distance criteria, *Infor Sci.*, 22: 19–35.

25. M. Ben-Bassat (1982), Use of Distance Measures, Information Measures and Error bounds in Feature Evaluation, *Handbook of Statistics*, 2: 773–791, North-Holland.

26. J. R. Quinlan (1993), *Programs for Machine Learning*, Morgan Kaufman, CA.

27. H. Liu and H. Motoda (1998), *Feature Selection for Knowledge Discovery and Data Mining*, Kluwer Academic Publishers, London.

28. P. Narendra and K. Fukunaga (1977), A Branch and Bound Algorithm for Feature Subset Selection, *IEE Trans. Computer,* C-26(9): 917–922.

29. I. Foroutan and and J. Sklansky (1987), Feature selection for automatic classification of non-gaussian data, *IEEE Trans. SMC*, 17(2): 187–198.

30. W. Siedlecki and J. Sklansky (1988), On Automatic Feature Selection, *Inter. J. Pattern Recogn. Art. Intell.*, 2: 197–220.

31. M. Dash and H. Liu (1997), Feature Selection for Classification, *Intelligent Data Analysis*, 1: 131–156.

32. H. Almuallim and T. G. Dietterich (1994), Learning boolean concepts in the presence of many irrelevant features, *Arti. Intell.*, 69: 279–305.

33. K. Kira and L. A. Rendell (1992), The feature selection problem: Traditional methods and a new algorithm, *Proceedings of Ninth National Conference on Artificial Intelligence*, MIT Press, Cambridge, MH, pp. 129–134.

34. G. H. John, R. Kohavi, and K. Pfleeger (1994), Irrelevant feature and the subset selection problem, *Machine Learning: Proceedings of the Eleventh International Conference*, pp. 121–129.

35. B. Scholkopf, A. Smola, and K. R. Muller (1998), Nonlinear Component analysis as a Kernel Eigenvalue Problem, *Neural Comput.*, 10(5): 1299–1319.

36. I. Borg and P. Groenen (1977), *Mordern Multidimensional Scaling*, Springer-Verlag, Berlin.

37. S. Haykin (1999), *Neural Networks, A Comprehensive Foundation*, Prentice-Hall, NJ.

38. R. Setiono and H. Liu (1997), Neural Network Feature Selector, *IEEE Trans. NN*, 8(3): 654–662.

39. M. Kudo and J. Sklansky (2000), Comparison of Algorithms that Select Features for Pattern Recognition, *Pattern Recog.*, 33(1): 25–41.

40. N. R. Pal (1999), Soft computing for feature analysis. *Fuzzy Sets Systems*, 103: 201–221.

41. B. Chakraborty (2002), Integration of Soft Computing Approaches for Feature Selection in Pattern Recognition Problems, *J. IETE*, 48(5): 403–413.

42. D. W. Ruck, S. K. Rogers, and M. Kabrisky (1990), Feature selection using a multilayer perceptron, *Neural Network Comput.*, 20: 40–48.

43. A. Verikas and M. Bacauskiene (2002), Feature selection with neural networks, *Pattern Recog. Lett.*, 23(11): 1323–1335.

44. N. Kwak and C.-H. Choi (2002), Input feature selection for classification problems, *IEEE Trans. Neural Networks*, 13(1): 143–159.

45. B. Chakraborty and Y. Sawada (1999), Fractal Neural Network Feature Selector for Automatic Pattern Recognition System, *IEICE Trans. Fund. Elect. Commun. Comput. Sci.*, E82-A(9): 1845–1850.

46. T. Kohonen (2001), *Self Organizing Maps*, Springer, NY.

47. E. Oja (1997), The Nonlinear PCA Learning Rule in Independent Component Analysis, *Neurocomputing*, 17(1): 25–45.

48. B. Lerner, H. Guterman, M. Aladjem, and I. Dinstein (1999), A comparative Study of Neural Network based Feature Extraction, *Pattern Recogn. Lett.*, 20(1): 7–14.

49. S. K. Pal and Basabi Chakraborty (1986), Fuzzy set Theoretic Measure for Automatic Feature Selection, *IEEE Trans. Sys, Man Cybernetics*, SMC-16(5): 754–760.

50. S. K. Pal, R. K. De, and J. Basak (2000), Unsupervised feature evaluation: a neuro-fuzzy approach, *IEEE Trans. Neural Networks*, 11(2): 366–376.

51. B. Chakraborty and G. Chakraborty (2001), A Neuro Fuzzy Algorithm for Feature Subset Selection, *IEICE Trans. Fund. Elect. Commun. Comput. Sci.*, E84-A(9): 2182–2188.

52. B. Chakraborty (2000), Feature Selection by Artificial Neural Network for Pattern Classification, *Pattern Recognition in Soft Computing Paradigm*, Vol. 2 of FLSI Soft Computing Series, World Scientific, NY. pp. 95–109.

53. M. Quafafou and M. Boussouf (2000), Generalized rough set based feature selection, *Intelligent Data Anal.*, 4(1) 3–17.

54. M. Zhang and J. T. Yao, (2004), A rough set based approach to feature selection, *Proc. NAFIPS*, 1: 434–439.

55. R. Jensen and Q. Shen (2007), Rough set based feature selection: A review, *Rough Computing: Theories, Technologies and Applications*, IGI Global, pp. 70–107.

56. R. B. Bhatt and M. Gopal (2005), On fuzzy-rough set approach to feature selection, *Pattern Recog. Lett.*, 26(7): 965–975.

57. W. Siedlecki and J. Sklansky (1989), A note on genetic algorithms for large-scale feature selection, *Pattern Recog. Lett.*, 10(5): 335–347.

58. M. L. Raymer, W. F. Punch, E. D. Goodman, L. A. Kuhn, and A. K. Jain (2000), Dimensionality reduction using genetic algorithms, *IEEE Trans. EC*, 4(2): 164–171.

59. J. S. Lee, I. S. Oh, and B. R. Moon (2004), Hybrid Genetic Algorithm for Feature Selection, *IEEE Trans. PAMI*, 26(11): 1424–1437.

60. F. Hussein, N. Kharma, and R. Ward (2001), Genetic algorithms for feature selection and weighting, a review and study, *Proccedings of Sixth International Conference on Document Analysis and Recognition*, pp. 1240–1244.

61. B. Chakraborty (2002), Genetic Algorithm with Fuzzy Operators for Feature Subset Selection, *IEICE Trans. Fund. Electr. Commun. Comput. Sci.*, E85-A(9): 2089–2092.

62. J. Huang, Y. Cai, and X. Xu (2007), A hybrid genetic algorithm for feature selection wrapper based on mutual information, *Pattern Recog. Lett.*, 28(13): 1825–1844.

63. J. Lu, T. Zhang, and Y. Zhang (2008), Feature selection based-on genetic algorithm for image annotation, *Knowledge Based Systems*, 21(8): 887–891.

64. Y. Liu et al. (2005), Feature Selection with Particle Swarms, *LNCS*, 3314: 425–430.

65. B. Chakraborty (2009), Binary Particle Swarm Optimization based Algorithm for Feature Subset Selection, *Proceedings ICAPR09 (International Conference on Advances in Pattern Recognition 2009)*, pp. 145–148.

66. C. J. Tu, L. Y. Chuang, J. Y. Chang, and C. H. Yang (2006), Feature Selection using PSO-SVM, *Proceedings of International Multiconference Engineers and Computer scientist*, Association of Engineers, Hong Kong, pp. 138–143.

67. T. F. Lee, M. Y. Cho, and F. M. Fang (2007), Feature Selection of SVM and ANN using Particle Swarm Optimization for Power Transformers Incipient Fault Symptom Diagnosis, *Intern. J. Comput. Intel. Res.*, 3(1): 50–65.

68. M. Shoorehdeli, M. Teshnehlab, and H. A. Moqhaddam (2006), Feature Subset Selection for face detection using genetic algorithms and particle swarm optimization, *Proceedings of International Conference on Networking Sensing and Control, IEEE Internaltional Conference Networking, Sensing and Control*, Ft. Louderdale, FL, pp. 686–690.

69. X. Wang, J. Yang, X. Teng, W. Xia, and R. Jensen (2007), Feature Selection based on Rough Sets and Particle Swarm Optimization, *Pattern Recog. Lett.*, 28(4): 459–471.

70. J. T. Tou and R. C. Gonzalez (1974), *Pattern Recognition Principles*, Addison-Wesley, London.

71. S. Aeberhand, D. Coomas, and O. Devel (1994), Comparative analysis of statistical pattern recognition methods in high dimensional setting, *Pattern Recog.*, 27(8): 1065–1077.

72. M. R. Anderberg (1973), *Cluster Analysis for Applications*, Academic Press, NY.

73. J. A. Hartigan (1975), *Clustering Algorithms*, Wiley, New York.

74. B. S. Everitt, S. Landau, and M. Leese (2001), *Cluster Analysis*, Arnold, London.

75. J. G. Dy and C. E. Brodly (2004), Feature Selection for Unsupervised Learning, *J. Machine Learning Res.*, 5: 845–889.

76. J. Handl and J. Knowles (2006), Feature Subset Selection in Unsupervised Learning via Multiobjective Optimization, *Inter. J. Comput. Intel. Res.*, 2(3): 217–238.

77. P. Mitra, C. A. Murthy, and S. K. Pal (2002), Unsupervised feature selection using feature similarity, *IEEE Trans. PAMI*, 24(3): 301–312.

78. M. Halkidi, Y. Batistatikis, and M. Vazirgiannis (2002), Cluster validity methods: part I, *SIGMODD Rec.*, 31(2): 264–323.

79. M. Halkidi, Y. Batistatikis, and M. Vazirgiannis (2002), Cluster validity methods: part II, *SIGMODD Rec.*, 31(3): 19–27.

80. X. L. Xie and G. Beni (2001), A validity measure for fuzzy clustering, *IEEE Trans. PAMI*, 23(6): 674–680.

81. J. C. Bezdek (1981), *Pattern Recognition with Fuzzy Objective Function Algorithm*, Plenum Press, New York.

82. J. C. Dunn (1973), A fuzzy relative of the ISODATA process and its use in detecting compact well separated clusters, *J. Cybernetics*, 3: 32–57.

83. U. Maulik and S. Bandyopadhyay (2000), Genetic Algorithm based Clustering Technique, *Pattern Recog.*, 33(9): 1455–1465.

84. S. Saha and S. Bandyopadhyay (2007), A fuzzy genetic clustering technique using a new symmetry based distance for automatic evolution of clusters, *Proceedings of ICCTA, IEEE Computer Society*, pp. 309–314.

85. U. Maulik and S. Bandyopadhyay (2002), Performance evaluation of some clustering algorithms and validity indices, *IEEE Trans. PAMI*, 24(12): 1650–1654.

86. C. G. Loony (1997), *Pattern Recognition using Neural Networks*, Oxford University Press, NY.

87. G. P. Zhang (2000), Neural Networks for Classification: A Survey, *IEEE Trans. SMC Part C*, 30(4): 451–462.

88. B. Cheng and D. Titterington (1994), Neural networks: A review from statistical perspectives, *Stat. Sci.*, 9(1): 2–54.

89. W. Y. Huang and R. P. Lippmann (1987), Comparisons between neural net and conventional classifiers, *Proc. IEEE 1st. Int. Conf. NN*, 485–493.

90. D. Michie et al. (1994), *Machine Learning, Neural and Statistical Classification*, Ellis Horwood, London.

91. A. Riplay (1994), Neural networks and related methods for classification, *J. R. Statis. Soc B*, 56(3): 409–456.

92. R. P. Lippmann (1989), Pattern classification using neural networks, *IEEE Commun. Mag.*, 47–64.

93. B. Chakraborty, Y. Sawada, and G. Chakraborty (1997), Layered Fractal Neural Net: Computational Performance as a Classifier, *Knowledge-Based Systems*, 10(3): 177–182.

94. M. J. D. Powell (1985), Radial basis functions for multivariable interpolation: A review, *IMA Conference on Algorithms for the Approximations of Functions and Data, IEEE Communication Sociaty*, pp. 143–167.

95. W. A. Light (1992), Some aspects of radial basis function approximation, *Approximations Theory, Spline Functions and Applications*, Boston, Kluwer Academic Publishers, Boston, pp. 163–190.

96. V. N. Vapnik (1998), *Statistical Learning Theory*, Jonh Wiley & Sons, Inc., NY.

3

BIOLOGICAL INFORMATICS: DATA, TOOLS, AND APPLICATIONS

KEVIN BYRON, MIGUEL CERVANTES-CERVANTES, AND JASON T. L. WANG

3.1 INTRODUCTION

Biological informatics (BI) has emerged as one of the most important interdisciplinary fields in the last decade. Major research efforts in BI include nucleotide sequence and structure alignment, gene finding and genome assembly, gene expression and regulation, protein and ribonucleic acid (RNA) structure prediction, biological networks and pathway analysis, genome-wide association studies, computational proteomics and biomarker detection, molecular evolution and population genetics, to name a few. These efforts are often concurrent with the development of software tools for data analysis, leading to new discoveries in diverse areas of the biological sciences [1–4].

This chapter presents a case study in BI, focusing on locating noncoding RNAs (ncRNAs) in *Drosophila* genomes using software tools, in particular the Infernal package [5–7]. Noncoding RNAs are functional RNA transcripts that are not messenger RNAs (mRNAs) and therefore are not templates in protein biosynthesis. Recent experiments have shown that ncRNAs perform a wide range of cellular functions [8]. In particular, RNA on the X-1 (*roX1*) plays an essential role in the dosage compensation system, which increases the transcription level on the X chromosome in *Drosophila* males (XY) with respect to that of females (XX) [9]. Experiments have shown *roX1* functionality in some species of *Drosophila* whose genomes have been annotated [10–12]. Our working hypothesis is that RNA transcripts of the *roX1* genes across *Drosophila* species possess conserved secondary structures. Advances in genomic sequencing from 12 *Drosophila* species [13] will contribute to support this hypothesis.

Computational Intelligence and Pattern Analysis in Biological Informatics, Edited by Ujjwal Maulik, Sanghamitra Bandyopadhyay, and Jason T. L. Wang
Copyright © 2010 John Wiley & Sons, Inc.

The software package Infernal has implemented covariance models for the prediction of ncRNA functional conservation and it is considered to be one of the most accurate tools for this purpose [14]. A covariance model is a statistical representation or profile of a family of related RNAs that share a consensus RNA secondary structure [15]. Infernal [6, 7] contains the utility cmbuild for the production of a covariance model from a multiple sequence alignment in Stockholm format. Another utility, cmsearch, is used to search for sequences that are similar to the model. The cmsearch process is computationally expensive when using a single-processor approach. However, by utilizing a parallel-processing approach, search results can be obtained expeditiously.

We have used a covariance model to demonstrate its capabilities in genome-scale searching. The *roX1* sequences were experimentally obtained from eight *Drosophila* species, namely, *D. ananassae*, *D. erecta*, *D. melanogaster*, *D. mojavensis*, *D. pseudoobscura*, *D. simulans*, *D. virilis*, and *D. yakuba*. We focused on obtaining evidence of conserved RNA secondary structures within *roX1* sequences on the entire genomes of these eight organisms. To this effect, we used a covariance model derived from several *roX1* sequences at hand. We found conserved RNA secondary structures within *roX1* genes of six of the eight *Drosophila* species. We then used the same covariance model to search for evidence of conserved RNA secondary structures in the complete genomes of the four remaining sequenced *Drosophila* species for which we have no experimentally obtained *roX1* genes. These four species are *D. grimshawi*, *D. persimilis*, *D. sechellia*, and *D. willistoni*. Our results show strong evidence for the presence of *roX1* functional domains encoded in the genome of *D. sechellia*.

3.2   DATA

There is a wide variety of biological data stored in open access databases. Herbert et al. [16] surveyed the many bioinformatic databases accessible on the worldwide web. In this case study, we use two categories of data: *roX1* genes and *Drosophila* genomes (cf. Tables 3.1 and 3.2). We used a "slide-and-fold" method to construct thermodynamically stable RNA secondary structures in the *roX1* genes. Gene subsequences of 100 nucleotides (nt) long or less were folded according to thermodynamic properties using the Vienna RNA package [17, 18]. Adjacent subsequences were overlapped by 50 nt. With this method, RNA secondary structures can be derived accurately and efficiently for two reasons: (1) predicting the formation of small secondary structures is more accurate and efficient than for large ones; and (2) secondary structures with size <50 nt are folded twice as subsequences of two different larger secondary structures, further increasing the chance of getting accurate RNA secondary structures. We also used the setting in the Vienna package that yielded multiple RNA secondary structures with the same minimum energy for a given sequence to further improve the folding accuracy. The number of predicted RNA secondary structures for each *roX1* gene is shown in the last column of Table 3.1. A total of 773 RNA secondary structures was obtained for all eight species examined.

TABLE 3.1 Description of *roX1* Genes Used in This Case Study

Species	Length	FlyBase Region	Region Coordinates	No. of Structures
D. ananassae	3493	scaffold_13117	695557–693154	77
			693089–692300	
			692143–692065	
			692247–692215	
D. erecta	3462	scaffold_4690	1139892–1137083	98
			1140318–1139928	
			1137036–1136857	
D. melanogaster	3468	chromosome X	3755987–3754338	106
			3754043–3753143	
			3756379–3756024	
			3754304–3754082	
			3753108–3752929	
D. mojavensis	3768	scaffold_6328	3900419–3899115	99
			3901467–3900566	
			3901937–3901499	
			3902390–3902000	
			3898736–3898624	
			3898929–3898874	
			3898845–3898810	
			3947396–3947375	
			246881–246900	
			700541–700522	
D. pseudoobscura	3469	XL_group 1e	6901185–6898994	92
			6898915–6897910	
			6897801–6897717	
			1352025–1352045	
			10880750–10880730	
			476212–476239	
			2910133–2910114	
D. simulans	3439	chromosome X	2761962–2759151	101
			2762379–2761996	
			2759122–2758943	
			9903425–9903446	
D. virilis	3623	scaffold_13042	4639617–4638455	97
			4637622–4636608	
			4638333–4637894	
			4636532–4636064	
			4637736–4637672	
			4637835–4637787	
			4636035–4635995	
			4638396–4638367	
D. yakuba	3433	chromosome X	4658396–4661828	103
			3710814–3710795	

TABLE 3.2   Description of *Drosophila* Genomes Downloaded from FlyBase

Species	Release No.	Release Date	No. of Nucleotides	No. of Sequences	No. of Files
D. ananassae	1.3	7/24/08	230,993,012	13,749	1
D. erecta	1.3	7/24/08	152,712,140	5,124	1
D. grimshawi	1.3	7/24/08	200,467,819	17,440	1
D. melanogaster	5.18	5/16/09	130,430,583	7	7
D. mojavensis	1.3	7/24/08	193,826,310	6,841	1
D. persimilis	1.3	7/24/08	188,374,079	12,838	1
D. pseudoobscura	2.4	5/19/09	152,738,921	4,896	1
D. sechellia	1.3	7/24/08	166,577,145	14,730	1
D. simulans	1.3	7/24/08	137,828,247	10,005	1
D. virilis	1.2	7/24/08	206,026,697	13,530	1
D. willistoni	1.3	7/24/08	235,516,348	14,838	1
D. yakuba	1.3	7/24/08	165,693,946	8,122	1

Table 3.2 presents details of the 12 *Drosophila* genomes used in our case study. Genome data were downloaded from FlyBase, accessible at http://flybase.org/. The number of files these sequences reside in is indicated in the last column. There is a total of 2,161,185,247 nucleotides in the 12 genomes, which collectively contain 122,120 sequences residing in 18 files. Most of the genomes have not been separated into clearly defined chromosomes. As sequencing efforts continue for species of *Drosophila*, we expect that in time all 12 specie genomes will be annotated regarding specific chromosome identification.

3.3   TOOLS

In the case study presented here, we used two software tools to analyze the genomic data at hand. The first tool, called RSmatch and developed in our lab [19–21], is capable of aligning structure-annotated RNA sequences so that both sequence and structure information are taken into consideration during the alignment process. The second tool, Infernal [6, 7], was designed for genome-wide searching for conserved RNA secondary structures. Since the secondary structure of RNA determines its function, the Infernal tool is capable of predicting ncRNA functional conservation in genomes.

RSmatch [21] decomposes an RNA secondary structure into a set of components that are further organized by a tree model to capture the peculiarities of this RNAs framework. RSmatch can find the optimal global or local alignment between two RNA secondary structures using two scoring matrices, one for single-stranded regions and the other for double-stranded regions. The time complexity of RSmatch is $O(mn)$, where m is the size of the query structure and n that of the subject structure.

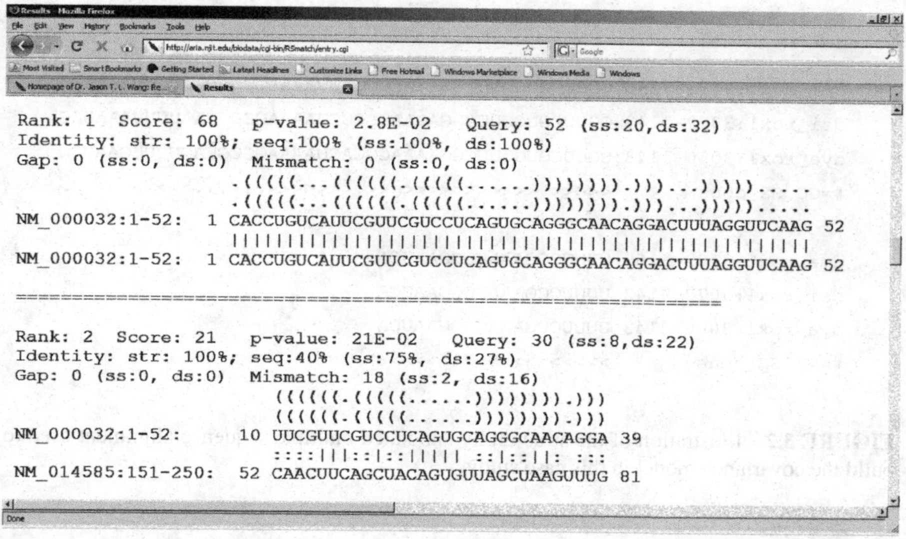

```
Rank: 1   Score: 68    p-value: 2.8E-02    Query: 52 (ss:20,ds:32)
Identity: str: 100%; seq:100% (ss:100%, ds:100%)
Gap: 0 (ss:0, ds:0)   Mismatch: 0 (ss:0, ds:0)
                .(((((...(((((.(((((......)))))))).)))...))))).....
                .(((((...(((((.(((((......)))))))).)))...))))).....
NM_000032:1-52:   1 CACCUGUCAUUCGUUCGUCCUCAGUGCAGGGCAACAGGACUUUAGGUUCAAG 52
                    |||||||||||||||||||||||||||||||||||||||||||||||||||
NM_000032:1-52:   1 CACCUGUCAUUCGUUCGUCCUCAGUGCAGGGCAACAGGACUUUAGGUUCAAG 52


===================================================================

Rank: 2   Score: 21    p-value: 21E-02    Query: 30 (ss:8,ds:22)
Identity: str: 100%; seq:40% (ss:75%, ds:27%)
Gap: 0 (ss:0, ds:0)   Mismatch: 18 (ss:2, ds:16)
                (((((((.(((((......)))))))).)))
                (((((((.(((((......)))))))).)))
NM_000032:1-52:   10 UUCGUUCGUCCUCAGUGCAGGGCAACAGGA 39
                     ::::|||::|::||||| ::|::||: :::
NM_014585:151-250: 52 CAACUUCAGCUACAGUGUUAGCUAAGUUUG 81
```

FIGURE 3.1 Screenshot showing a partial output from the local alignment function of RADAR.

The RSmatch program is implemented into a web server called RADAR (acronym for RNA Data Analysis and Research) [19, 22]. This web server can perform a multitude of functions related to RNA structure comparison, including pairwise structure alignment, constrained structure alignment, multiple structure alignment, database search, clustering, and consensus structure prediction. The goal behind establishing this web server is to develop a versatile tool that provides a computationally efficient platform for performing tasks related to RNA structure analysis. Figure 3.1 shows a partial output obtained from aligning a query RNA structure with a set of subject RNA structures using the local alignment function of RADAR. The figure lists the top two ranked subject structures that receive the largest alignment scores, where the structures are represented in the Vienna style dot bracket format [17, 18].

A program component of Infernal, cmbuild, takes a structurally annotated multiple sequence alignment as input, and outputs a profile, whereas the program cmsearch uses the profile to search a nucleic acid sequence database for homologous RNAs. In addition, Infernal contains a program called cmalign, which uses the profile to align any number of unaligned RNA sequences to the profile, producing a structure-based multiple sequence alignment [6, 7].

Infernal employs profile stochastic context-free grammars, which include both sequence and RNA secondary structure consensus information. This tool is used for constructing and maintaining the Rfam database of structurally annotated RNA multiple alignments [8]. The Rfam database contains hundreds of RNA sequence families, where each family has a hand-curated representative alignment, called a

```
# STOCKHOLM 1.0

dme_rox1:3102-3165  GGUUCGUGUUUCGGAAAACGCAUUAAAAGGCGUAAUUUUAAAUCG
dsi_rox1:3079-3142  GGUUCGUGUUUCGGAAAACGCUCUAAAAGGCGCAAUUUUAAAUCG
dya_rox1:3080-3143  GGUUCGUGUUUCGGAAAACGCACUAAAAGGCGUAGUUUUGAAUCG
#=GC SS_cons        <<<<<.<<<<<<<<<<<<<<.<<<<<<<..<...>>>>>>>>.>>

dme_rox1:3102-3165  UUUUCCGAAAUGGGAAUCA
dsi_rox1:3079-3142  UUUUCCGAAAUGGGAAUCA
dya_rox1:3080-3143  UUUUCCGAAAUGGGAAUCA
#=GC SS_cons        >>>>>>>>>>>.>>>>>.
//
```

FIGURE 3.2   Illustration of the structurally annotated multiple sequence alignment used to build the covariance model in this case study.

seed alignment. This seed alignment is used to make a profile, which can be aligned to new RNA sequences, obtained when nucleic sequence databases grow, to obtain a large, more complete alignment, called a full alignment. The Rfam sequence contains the seed alignments, full alignments, and consensus secondary structures of all the RNA families stored in its database.

3.4 APPLICATIONS

We applied RSmatch and Infernal to mining *roX1* genes in *Drosophila* genomes as follows: We carried out species-against-species pairwise comparisons of all 773 RNA secondary structures obtained from the *roX1* genes shown in Table 3.1 using the local alignment function of RSmatch. This required ~520,000 pairwise comparisons of RNA secondary structures, each comparison yielding an alignment score. Then, we selected local matches across the species that received the largest alignment scores and that were the longest among all the local matches. We obtained one sequence from each of the following three species: *D. melanogaster*, *D. simulans*, and *D. yakuba*. Then, we used the MXSCARNA tool [23] to align the three sequences and obtain a multiple alignment in Stockholm format with predicted structure annotation. Figure 3.2 illustrates the multiple sequence alignment; the numeric range following the species code represents the portion of the *roX1* gene from which the sequence was extracted. In Figure 3.3, the consensus secondary structure for the alignment in Figure 3.2 is portrayed using RNAz [24]. This structurally annotated alignment was input to the cmbuild program of Infernal 1.0 [7] to create a covariance model.

Then, we used the cmsearch program of Infernal 1.0 to locate homologs in the genomes of *Drosophila* species that have been sequenced to date (shown in Table 3.2) using the covariance model (CM) we constructed. Table 3.3 presents a summary of

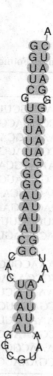

FIGURE 3.3 Illustration of the consensus structure used to build the covariance model in this case study.

TABLE 3.3 Summary of Homologs Found in the *Drosophila* Species Analyzed

ID	Genome Searched	CM Score	FlyBase Region	Region Coordinates	Strand	Within *roX1*
1	*D. ananassae*	32.26	scaffold_13117	692432–692373	−	Y
2	*D. erecta*	72.78	scaffold_4690	1137235–1137172	−	Y
3	*D. melanogaster*	88.84	chromosome X	3753295–3753232	−	Y
4	*D. pseudoobscura*	29.4	Unknown_group_410	14965–14898	−	N
5	*D. pseudoobscura*	29.11	Unknown_group_260	63165–63089	−	N
6	*D. pseudoobscura*	28.28	XL_group 1e	6898105–6898042	−	Y
7	*D. sechellia*	88.1	scaffold_4	2954091–2954154	+	N/A
8	*D. simulans*	88.1	chromosome X	2759303–2759240	−	Y
9	*D. yakuba*	88.69	chromosome X	4661475–4661538	+	Y

TABLE 3.4   Homologous RNA Sequences Found in the *Drosophila* Species Analyzed

ID	RNA Sequence[a]	Length
1	UUC- -GUGUUUCGGGAAAUGCUUUGAAAAGCG-C UUUUGAAACGUUUUCCGAGACGACAGAAA	60
2	GAUUUGUAUUUCGGAAAACGCACCAAAAGGCGUAA UUUAGAAUCGUUUUCCGAAAUGGGAAUCA	64
3	GGUUCGUGUUUCGGAAAACGCAUUAAAAGGCGUAA UUUUAAAUCGUUUUCCGAAAUGGGAAUCA	64
4	GACCACUCCUUCGGGUACCUCAAAAAAAaagGGCA UAGgUAUUUGGGAGGUACCCGAAGGAGUGGUCU	68
5	UCCACACGUUUCCAACUUCGUUUCCACACGC**** **********GUGUGGAAACGAAGUUGGAAACGCg uGUGGAA	77
6	CGUUCGGGUUUCGGAAAACGCGUCGA********* *****UUGAAACGUUUUCCGAAAC-AGAA- -A	64
7	GGUUCGUGUUUCGGAAAACGCUCUAAAAGGCGCAA UUUUAAAUCGUUUUCCGAAAUGGGAAUCA	64
8	GGUUCGUGUUUCGGAAAACGCUCUAAAAGGCGCAA UUUUAAAUCGUUUUCCGAAAUGGGAAUCA	64
9	GGUUCGUGUUUCGGAAAACGCACUAAAAGGCGUAG UUUUGAAUCGUUUUCCGAAAUGGGAAUCA	64

[a] An asterisk (*) indicates a base that is left unaligned with a CM counterpart; a minus (−) sign indicates that no base is present to align with a CM counterpart (not included in the sequence length); and a lowercase letter represents a base on the genome that has been added with respect to the CM.

the homologs with the largest scores found in each species, and Table 3.4 lists the homologous RNA sequences.

It was observed that for the three sequences used to build the covariance model, each of them received the largest score on its respective genome (*D. melanogaster*, *D. simulans*, and *D. yakuba*, respectively). In addition, we found high-score hits in three other species, namely, *D. ananassae*, *D. erecta*, and *D. pseudoobscura*. Note that in *D. pseudoobscura*, the homolog with the largest score is not within the *roX1* gene in that species. Instead, we found a homolog with the third largest score that is within the *roX1* gene in *D. pseudoobscura*. These homologs found in the above six species for which *roX1* genes have been experimentally obtained fall within the known *roX1* genes. The homologous RNAs are similar in their structure. This confirms our hypothesis that there are conserved RNA secondary structures within *roX1* genes across these species. Finally, note that a homolog was found in the genome of *D. sechellia* for which we have not experimentally obtained a *roX1* gene. Figure 3.4 illustrates the secondary structure of the homologous RNA discovered from *D. sechellia*; this secondary structure is similar in structure to the consensus structure in Figure 3.3. This uncovering may help compensation dosage researchers in locating *roX1* functional domains in *D. sechellia*.

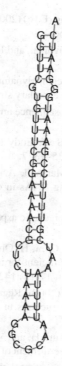

FIGURE 3.4 Secondary structure of the homologous RNA found in *Drosophila sechellia*.

3.5 CONCLUSION

This chapter presents a case study of biological informatics, showing how software tools are applied to the analysis of genomic data arising in the biological sciences. In particular, this chapter showed how the widely used Infernal and RSmatch tools can be combined to mine *roX1* genes in 12 species of *Drosophila* for which entire genomic sequencing data are available. As more genomes are sequenced, new techniques are needed to perform genome-wide discovery of functional elements that play essential roles in metabolic processes. This opens many new research directions in both the biological sciences and computing sciences, while bringing them together.

REFERENCES

1. S. Bandyopadhyay, U. Maulik, and J. T. L. Wang (Eds.) (2007), *Analysis of Biological Data: A Soft Computing Approach*, World Scientific, Singapore.
2. J. T. L. Wang, B. A. Shapiro, and D. Shasha (Eds.) (1999), *Pattern Discovery in Biomolecular Data: Tools, Techniques and Applications*, Oxford University Press, NY.

3. J. T. L. Wang, C. H. Wu, and P. P. Wang (Eds.) (2003), *Computational Biology and Genome Informatics*, World Scientific, Singapore.

4. J. T. L. Wang, M. J. Zaki, H. T. T. Toivonen, and D. Shasha (Eds.) (2005), *Data Mining in Bioinformat.*, Springer, London.

5. S. R. Eddy (2002), A memory-efficient dynamic programming algorithm for optimal alignment of a sequence to an RNA secondary structure, *BMC Bioinformat.*, 3:18.

6. S. Eddy and R. Durbin (1994), RNA sequence analysis using covariance models, *Nucleic Acids Res.*, 22:2079–2088.

7. E. P. Nawrocki, D. L. Kolbe, and S. R. Eddy (2009), Infernal 1.0: inference of RNA alignments, *Bioinformat.*, 25(10):1335–1337.

8. S. Griffiths-Jones, S. Moxon, M. Marshall, A. Khanna, S. R. Eddy, and A. Bateman (2005), Rfam: annotating non-coding RNAs in complete genomes, *Nucleic Acids Res.*, 33:D121–D124.

9. Y. Park and M. I. Kuroda (2001), Epigenetic aspects of X-chromosome dosage compensation, *Science*, 293:1083–1085.

10. S. Park, Y. I. Kang, J. G. Sypula, J. Choi, H. Oh, and Y. Park (2007), An evolutionarily conserved domain of *roX*2 RNA is sufficient for induction of H4-Lys16 acetylation on the Drosophila X chromosome, *Genetics*, 177(3):1429–1437.

11. S. Park, M. I. Kuroda, and Y. Park (2008), Regulation of histone H4 Lys16 acetylation by predicted alternative secondary structures in *roX* noncoding RNAs, *Mol. Cell. Biol.*, 28(16):4952–4962.

12. Y. Park, R. L. Kelley, H. Oh, M. I. Kuroda, and V. H. Meller (2002), Extent of chromatin spreading determined by *roX* RNA recruitment of MSL proteins, *Science*, 298:1620–1623.

13. A. Stark, et al. (2007), Discovery of functional elements in 12 Drosophila genomes using evolutionary signatures, *Nature (London)*, 450:219–232.

14. A. Wang, W. Ruzzo, and M. Tompa (2007), How accurately is ncRNA aligned within whole-genome multiple alignments? *BMC Bioinformat.*, 8:417.

15. R. Durbin, S. Eddy, A. Krogh, and G. Mitchison (1998), *Biological Sequence Analysis: Probabilistic Models of Proteins and Nucleic Acids*, Cambridge University Press, Cambridge UK.

16. K. G. Herbert, J. Spirollari, J. T. L. Wang, W. H. Piel, J. Westbrook, W. C. Barker, Z. Z. Hu, and C. H. Wu (2008), Bioinformatic databases, *Wiley Encyclopedia of Computer Science and Engineering*, B. Wah (Ed.), John Wiley & Sons, Inc., NY, pp. 561:1–561:10.

17. A. R. Gruber, R. Lorenz, S. H. Bernhart, R. Neubock, and I. L. Hofacker (2008), The Vienna RNA websuite, *Nucleic Acids Res.*, 36:W70–W74.

18. I. L. Hofacker (2003), Vienna RNA secondary structure server, *Nucleic Acids Res.*, 31:3429–3431.

19. M. Khaladkar, V. Bellofatto, J. T. L. Wang, B. Tian, and B. A. Shapiro (2007), RADAR: a web server for RNA data analysis and research, *Nucleic Acids Res.*, 35:W300–W304.

20. M. Khaladkar, J. Liu, D. Wen, J. T. L. Wang, and B. Tian (2008), Mining small RNA structure elements in untranslated regions of human and mouse mRNAs using structure-based alignment, *BMC Genomics,* 9:189.

21. J. Liu, J. T. L. Wang, J. Hu, and B. Tian (2005), A method for aligning RNA secondary structures and its application to RNA motif detection, *BMC Bioinformat.*, 6:89.

22. M. Khaladkar, V. Patel, V. Bellofatto, J. Wilusz, and J. T. L. Wang (2008), Detecting conserved secondary structures in RNA molecules using constrained structural alignment, *Comput. Biol. Chem.*, 32:264–272.

23. Y. Tabei, H. Kiryu, T. Kin, and K. Asai (2008), A fast structural multiple alignment method for long RNA sequences, *BMC Bioinformat.*, 9:33.

24. A. R. Gruber, R. Neubock, I. L. Hofacker, and S. Washietl (2007), The RNAz web server: prediction of thermodynamically stable and evolutionarily conserved RNA structures, *Nucleic Acids Res.*, 35:W335–W338.

PART II

SEQUENCE ANALYSIS

4

PROMOTER RECOGNITION USING NEURAL NETWORK APPROACHES

T. Sobha Rani, S. Durga Bhavani, and S. Bapi Raju

4.1 INTRODUCTION

Currently, huge amount of genome data is available due to fast sequencing methods. Similar fast annotation methods of the genome are not available and current technologies consume a lot of time. Hence, machine annotation methods are required to tackle the major problems of promoter recognition and gene recognition.

Promoters occur upstream of a gene and are regions at which ribonucleic acid (RNA) polymerase binds and initiates transcription. Promoters also act as switches specifying the location in the organism, as well as the time at which the transcription can occur at that gene. The location where transcription begins is known as the transcription start site (TSS). A majority of the promoters of genes that transcribe large amounts of messenger RNA (mRNA) have a set of binding sites or regions [1,2]. One of these sites is a TATA sequence, a hexamer, upstream from TSS. Promoter also contains one or more binding regions further upstream and downstream. The eukaryotic and prokaryotic promoter recognition problems have to be dealt with independently. For example, the promoter structure for *Escherichia coli* has two binding regions present at −10 and −35 positions with respect to TSS (position of which is taken as +1). These are indicated as a −35 motif and a −10 motif. The patterns at these binding sites are known to be conserved. In general, patterns (TATA box, CAAT box, Initiator, etc.) are known to be conserved in the promoter sequences within and across species in some cases.

Computational Intelligence and Pattern Analysis in Biological Informatics, Edited by Ujjwal Maulik,
Sanghamitra Bandyopadhyay, and Jason T. L. Wang
Copyright © 2010 John Wiley & Sons, Inc.

The distinct feature in case of eukaryotic transcription is that the RNA polymerase does not bind to the promoter directly. A number of transcription-binding proteins bind to the binding sites and form a complex before RNA polymerase binds. Also, there are three kinds of RNA polymerase in eukaryotes unlike the prokaryotes. For the proteins to bind to deoxyribonucleic acid (DNA), it has to have a physical structure wherein the proteins can come and bind. Special proteins that are used for this purpose are Helix turn Helix, and Zn^{++} fingers.

Promoter recognition is not a trivial problem due to the following reasons: Promoter recognition unlike other recognition problems (e.g., exon prediction and gene recognition) does not yield good results with methods of alignment or sequence similarity searches, since promoters have very low sequence similarity. Though the patterns (e.g., TATA box) are known to be conserved, there exist many exceptions to this rule. Nonconservation and distance between the patterns, the presence or absence of the patterns themselves make the task of promoter prediction an even more complex problem. Also, the occurrence of a promoter is not restricted to the 5' end of a gene alone, but could in fact be found in a coding region or may overlap with another promoter [3] in the case of prokaryotes. Additionally, in the case of eukaryotes, promoters additionally may exist in an intron or in the untranslated region of 3'. Hence, the problem of recognition of promoter against various backgrounds gains importance computationally.

Recently, there has been a deluge of sequencing information due to efficient sequencing methods. Several mammalian, bacterial, and plant species have been sequenced. One can use experimental methods [e.g., DNA footprinting, DNA protein cross-linking, X-ray crystallography, and nuclear magnetic resonance (NMR) spectroscopy] to identify a promoter or a gene. Typically, there are millions of protein sequences, but experimentally determined protein structures are only on the order of 1000. Experimental methods to determine a promoter, a gene, or a protein structure are time-consuming processes. Hence, annotation of important regions (e.g., genes) is not very fast. To overcome this handicap, computational techniques or algorithms that can automatically identify these regions are required.

4.2 RELATED LITERATURE /BACKGROUND

The crux of the problem is to identify a promoter irrespective of its place of occurrence in the genome, by extracting features that are unique to it. Different research groups have been trying to identify these patterns or features specific for promoters by various feature extraction methods and different classifiers.

Machine learning techniques can be used to address the issues mentioned above by modeling the recognition–prediction problem as a pattern recognition problem. To properly classify the promoter sequences *in silico*, one should get features that capture the essence of promoters. Some of the popular feature extraction methods are based on genetic algorithms [4], statistical models (e.g., hidden Markov models [5] and position weight matrices [6–8]), syntactic recognition algorithms [9], expectation, and maximization method [10, 11].

Methods based on features extracted from the binding sites or local consensus regions can be termed as *local signal*-based methods. Position weight matrices, expectation and maximization algorithm, and hidden Markov models have been used in the literature to extract local signals for the promoter recognition problem [5, 6, 10]. Local signal-based methods for eukaryotic promoter recognition use specific motifs like the four binding sites: The TATA box, the initiator (Inr) region, an upstream activating element (UPE), and a downstream promoter element (DPE). The detection of transcription factor binding sites forms the core of the local signal-based methods.

The techniques that use the whole promoter sequence to extract features can be categorized as *global signal*-based methods. Techniques like Fourier transform (FT), sequence alignment method, and so on, fall under this category. Global signal-based methods use properties, such as GpC content, secondary structure elements, and cruciform DNA structure, for eukaryotic promoter recognition [12]. The literature is abundant with local signal-based methods. Global signal-based methods are also catching up. Some of the work on the promoter recognition problem of both these kinds, which were carried out in the last few years, is presented in Section 4.3.

Das and Dai [13] present a comprehensive literature survey on the DNA motif finding algorithms. Motifs generally searched in the promoter sequences of coregulated genes and more recently integrated approaches that include phylogenetic footprinting are being used to find motifs. This survey gives a view of the local signal-based methods that are used to extract conserved patterns in the DNA promoter sequences. Huerta and Collado-Vides created an *E. coli* promoter data set called Regulon database [14]. They extracted and aligned motifs in a given set of unordered sequences producing a frequency matrix. A set of 96 different weight matrices were created for promoter, coding, and noncoding regions. A score is computed using these weight matrices and the best weight matrix is used to predict a promoter. The predictive capacity of the method is 86%, however, accuracy defined as the average of sensitivity and positive predictive rate, is 53%. An important contribution of this work is that they predict a high number of putative promoters (promoter-like signals) in the vicinity of a true promoter, which show a better score than the true promoter. The authors suggest that these putative promoters may be trying to bring Ribonucleic polymerase (RNAP) closer to the functional promoter.

Bajic et al. designed a local signal-based algorithm that combines a nonlinear promoter recognition model with signal processing, artificial neural networks (ANNs), and a set of sensors in Dragon fly (*Drosophila melanogaster*) promoter prediction [6]. These sensors are based on the statistical concept of oligonucleotide positional distributions in specific functional regions of DNA. Each sensor models a particular functional region (e.g., promoter, coding-exon, and intron). These distributions are modeled as a set of position weight matrices of the most significant oligonucleotides. Pentamers (regions of length 5) that most significantly contribute to the separation between the promoter and nonpromoter regions are chosen by determining the significance using their statistical relevance. The signals of a sequence using the positional weight matrices for the three functional regions are fed to a signal processing block.

The output is fed to ANN, which performs multisensor integration. Scores that make the ANN output greater than the selected threshold are to be treated as positive predictions in the promoter region. They have obtained a sensitivity rate of 67%. The authors have shown that their methods predict less false positives compared to the then existing algorithms.

Levitsky and Katokhin [4] have used the genetic algorithm based on iterative discriminant analysis, which is based on a global signal to classify eukaryotic (*Drosophila*) promoters. The negative set is obtained by shuffling the promoters. Two promoter sample TATA and DPE containing sets are formed. The cross-correlation (CC) for TATA containing promoters is reported to be 0.92 and for DPE is shown to be 0.82.

Pedersen et al. characterized the promoters of prokaryotes (*E. coli*) and eukaryotes (*human*) using self-organizing parallel HMMs [5]. They considered a set of three states (the main, the delete, and the insertion states), in addition to start and end states. The set of emissions are the four nucleotides A,T,G,C. Main and insertion states always emit a nucleotide, whereas the deletion state is a no-emission state (i.e., a mute state). Given a set of K training sequences, the parameters of HMM are iteratively modified to optimize the data fit using a measure based on the log-likelihood. A set of HMMs trained on 38 σ^{70}, and 3 σ^{54} sequences are combined in parallel to create a super HMM for *E. coli* promoter recognition. Similarly, human promoter sequences are used to train another HMM model. Clear patterns of well-known consensus signals (TATA box, etc.) could be obtained from the emission probabilities of main states of the HMM model. Their model is able to classify 162 σ_{70} out of 166 sequences as σ^{70} and 3 σ^{54} out of 166 as σ^{54} sequences. Only one σ^{70} sequence out of 166 is misclassified. They have not been tested on nonpromoter sequences.

It is said that DNA encodes two levels of functional information. The first level is for proteins and targets for activators, enhancers, repressors, transcription factor binders, and so on. The second level of information is contained in the physical and structural properties of the DNA itself [15, 16]. In the literature, several groups have exploited these properties to distinguish between features specific to a particular set of a DNA sequences and sequences that do not belong to a particular set. Physico-chemical parameters of a DNA double strand are available in the literature [16]. Kobe et al., reviewed the work of other groups that have considered the structural properties specific to mammals and plants [17]. There are some groups who have encoded the DNA independent of these properties in terms of binary values. Whatever encoding is used, the whole sequence is considered for modeling in global signal-based methods. Conformational and physicochemical properties of B-DNA dinucleotides [16] tabulated by the author and are used as global features for promoter recognition.

This chapter presents our work, which is based on global signal-based methods using a neural network classifier. For this purpose, we considered two global features: n-gram features and features based on signal processing techniques. It is shown that the n-gram features extracted for $n = 2, 3, 4, 5$ efficiently discriminate promoters from nonpromoters.

4.3   GLOBAL SIGNAL-BASED METHODS FOR PROMOTER RECOGNITION

Promoter recognition has been conventionally attempted using binding-site prediction algorithms that are primarily based on motif search techniques. We believe that along with binding sites, the upstream and downstream regions contribute to the function of the promoter, and hence we do an indepth study of the entire promoter region. There is an indication that codons that are triplets constitute useful features [18] in a DNA sequence and also the promoter regions are shown to have conserved hexamers [19]. On the other hand, to compute hexamers that will be 4^6 in number for every DNA sequence is computationally expensive. We present our study of the promoter region using n-gram features that are contiguous blocks of n characters from a sequence for $n = 2, 3, 4$, and 5.

Traditionally, biomedical signals have been analyzed by signal processing techniques [e.g., FT and wavelet transforms]. Biological data sets consist mostly of sequences made up of either nucleotides or amino acids. Hence, an encoding system is required to convert these sequences into numerical series. Once a numerical series is obtained, FT or wavelet transform (WT) can be applied. Wavelets have been used in the literature to analyze biological signals (e.g., genome sequences, protein structures, and gene expression data) [20]. It is assumed that the promoter signal that is responsible for the binding is retained by the promoter whether it occurs in an inter-genic portion or in a coding region [21]. To start with, FT of the sequences is used to analyze the promoter region to gain knowledge in the frequency domain. Fourier transform *per se* cannot be used for promoter recognition. Hence, its power spectrum computed using the Fourier coefficients are used as features. Since in FT, positional information is lost, WT is being used to retain that information. Promoter recognition is posed as a binary classification problem. So far FT has been used by quite a few groups, but there is no work, as far as we know, which uses wavelets for promoter recognition.

4.3.1   Data Set

This section describes the prokaryotic and eukaryotic data sets that are used for promoter recognition problem and the n-gram feature extraction methods used for experimentation.

The prokaryotic data set of *E. coli* is built by taking 669 σ-70 promoter sequences of length 80 with 60 base pairs (bp) upstream of the TSS and the rest downstream as is proposed in the literature from RegulonDB and Promec data bases [22]. Both the positive and the negative data sets are obtained from Gordon et al. [22]. There is no standard negative data set available. Gordon et al., build the negative data set by choosing sequence fragments outside the promoter region. This is a biologically meaningful data set that consists of 709 sequence fragments from the coding region and 709 sequence segments from intergenic portions.

The eukaryotic promoter data set of *Drosophila* is obtained from Ohler et al. [23], which is taken from the eukaryotic promoter database (EPD) [24]. A negative data set is built by them from the *Drosophila* genome [23]. Sequences from both positive and negative data sets are of length 300 bp with 250 bp upstream of the TSS and the rest is downstream. The data set contains 1864 promoter sequences, 2859 from coding and 1799 sequences from intron portions.

4.3.2   Promoter Recognition Using n-Gram Features

A few research papers on protein sequence classification and gene identification that use n-grams are seen, but very few are available in the literature that are applied to promoter recognition. A new class of variable-order Bayesian network models (VOBN) is proposed by Ben-gal et al. [25]. These models generalize the widely used position weight matrix (PWM), Markov, and Bayesian network models. Instead of considering a fixed subset of the positions to model dependencies, in VOBN models, these subsets may vary based on the specific nucleotides observed, which are called the context. The VOBN model is applied to a set of 238 $\sigma 70$ binding sites in *E. coli*. The authors show that the VOBN model can distinguish those 238 sites from a set of 472 intergenic nonpromoter sequences with higher accuracy than fixed-order Markov models or Bayesian trees. They consider the statistical dependencies between adjacent base pairs of nucleotides in *E. coli* to achieve a true positive recognition rate of 47.56% [25].

Leu et al. used n-gram features for $n = 6–20$ to predict promoters for vertebrates [26]. They consider sequences of length 550 bp. Each sequence segment of length 200 bp is given a cumulative score using all these n-grams with the individual n-gram score designed based on its occurrence only in promoter or in nonpromoter or in both promoter and nonpromoter. They achieve an accuracy rate of 88% with this method. Ji et al. implemented support vector machine using n-gram features ($n = 4,5,6,7$) for target gene prediction of Arabidopsis [27].

Wang and Hannenhalli proposed a position specific propensity analysis model (PSPA), which extracts the propensity of DNA elements at a particular position and their cooccurrence with respect to TSS in mammals [28]. They considered a set of top ranking k-mers ($k = 1–5$) at each position ± 100 bp relative to TSS and computed the cooccurrence with other top-ranking k-mers at other downstream positions. The PSPA score for a sequence is computed as the product of scores for the 200 positions of ± 100 bp relative to TSS. They found many position-specific promoter elements that are strongly linked to gene product function.

Li and Lin considered position-specific weight matrices of hexamers at 10 specific positions for the promoter data of *E. coli* [29]. The position correlation scoring matrix (PCSM) is computed for promoter as well as the nonpromoter set of training sequences. If the score is higher for positive than in the negative PCSM, then the test sequence is identified as a promoter and similarly nonpromoters are identified. Li and Lin [28] report performance of sensitivity being 91% and specificity 81% for nonpromoter data consisting of coding regions alone and 90 and 77% for nonpromoter data taken from inter-genic portions only. Applying these scores to the whole genome to predict the promoters, all 683 experimentally verified σ-70 promoters are successfully predicted and 1567 predictions as probable promoters.

More recently, Sonnenburg et al. introduced the positional oligomer importance matrices (POIMs) that are k-mer based scoring schemes and proposed an efficient algorithm to compute the scores for k-mers [30]. The POIMs can be utilized to recognize transcription start, trans-splicing sites (TRSSs) and acceptor splice sites. They showed that POIMs can recover many known motifs whose length, location, and typical sequences of motifs can be obtained accurately by these matrices.

Rani and Bapi carried out a study of different n-grams ($n = 2,3,4$, and 5) and their suitability as features for the promoter recognition problem posed as a binary classification problem [31]. The authors have chosen genomes of *E. coli* from prokaryotes and the method is extended to the eukaryote *D. melanogaster* promoter prediction. In [32], an investigation was made using dinucleotide frequencies as features in promoter recognition. The emphasis here was on analyzing misclassified sequences in both promoter and nonpromoter data sets. Further, in [31], a global view of the whole promoter is attempted using a systematic study of n-grams as features for promoter recognition. The whole promoter sequence is considered for the prediction and no position specific information is used. In Section 4.3.2.1, details of this work are presented.

4.3.2.1 *n-Gram Extraction*

A global signal is extracted from the promoter sequence by looking at the frequency of occurrence of n-grams in the promoter region. The set of n-grams for $n = 2$ is 16 possible combinations of features (AA, AT, AG, AC, TA, etc.) and the set of n-grams for $n = 3$ are 64 triples (AAA, AAT, AAG, AAC, ATA, etc.). The frequency of occurrence of n-grams is calculated on the DNA alphabet A,T,G,C for $n = 2, 3, 4,$ and 5. Let $f_i(n)$ denote the frequency of occurrence of the ith feature of n-grams for a particular n value and let L denote the length of the sequence. The feature values $v_i(n)$ are normalized frequency counts given in the following equation:

$$v_i(n) = \frac{f_i(n)}{L - n + 1} \quad 1 \le i \le 4^n \quad \text{for} \quad n = 2, 3, 4, 5$$

Here, the denominator denotes the number of n-grams that are possible in a sequence of length L. Hence, $v_i(n)$ denotes the proportional frequency of occurrence of ith feature for a particular n value. Thus each promoter and nonpromoter sequence of the data set is represented as a 16-dimensional feature vector $(v_1(2), v_2(2), \ldots, v_{16}(2))$ for $n = 2$, as a 64-dimensional feature vector $(v_1(3), v_2(3), \ldots, v_{64}(3))$ for $n = 3$, and so on, and a 1024-dimensional feature vector $(v_1(5), v_2(5), \ldots, v_{1024}(5))$ for $n = 5$.

The feature vectors for promoter and nonpromoter sequences constitute the entire data set. A portion of the data set is used as the training set and the remaining as a test set in this binary classification problem. The data sets are well separated in the feature spaces $f_i(n)$ for $n = 2, 3, 4,$ and 5. As an illustration, the average separation between promoter and nonpromoter sequences for 3-grams is shown in Figure 4.1. A neural network classifier is trained using n-grams of the training set as input feature vectors and then the test set is evaluated using the same network.

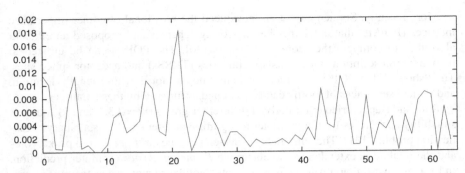

FIGURE 4.1 Average separation between promoter and nonpromoter sequences for 3-grams for *E. coli*. On the x-axis, 0,...,63 denotes 3-grams AAA, AAT, AAG, AAC, . . . , CCG, CCC.

4.3.2.2 Neural Network Classification Performance Promoter classification is obtained using a multilayer perceptron having three layers, namely, an input, a hidden, and an output layer. The output layer has one node to give a binary decision as to whether the given input sequence is a promoter or nonpromoter. The input layer contains 16, 64, 256, and 1024 nodes corresponding to the n-gram features for $n = $ 2,3,4, and 5, respectively. Different experiments are carried out to find the optimal number of hidden nodes that give the best classification performance. In a fivefold cross-validation, 80% of the data set is used for training the network and the remaining 20% is used as the test data set. Average performance of the neural network over fivefolds is reported in order to evaluate the efficacy of the various n-gram features for promoter classification. These simulations are done using the Stuttgart neural network simulator [33].

The classification results are evaluated on the test data set using different performance measures (e.g., precision, specificity and sensitivity, and positive predictive value). Precision is the proportion of the correctly classified sequences of the entire test data set. Specificity is the proportion of the negative test sequences that are correctly classified and sensitivity is the proportion of the positive test sequences that are correctly classified. Positive predictive value (PPV) is defined as the proportion of true positives with respect to the total number of sequences that are predicted as positive (true positives + false positives).

Using this architecture of the neural network, promoter classification is carried out for *E. coli* and *Drosophila* for $n = $ 2,3,4, and 5 grams. It is found in *E. coli* that PPV for 2, 3, 4, and 5-grams is 81.29, 82.97, 80.03, and 81.09, respectively, and the percentage of PPV obtained for *Drosophila* is 85.5, 89.28,89.35, and 91.2, respectively. In the case of *Drosophila*, as the sensitivity value for 5-grams is less than that of 4-grams, hence 4-grams is chosen as the best n-gram features. The classification results for the best n-grams are presented in Table 4.1.

The results show that 3-grams are the best discriminators in *E. coli*, whereas, 4-grams are good in discriminating promoters from nonpromoters in *Drosophila*. It can be seen that the identification of nonpromoters being 85% is much higher than

TABLE 4.1   Classification Performance for *E. coli* and *Drosophila* Promoter Recognition: Best *n*-gram results are shown

Species	Positive Predictive Value	Specificity	Sensitivity
E. coli (**3-gram**)	82.97	86.1	67.75
Drosophila (**4-gram**)	89.35	91.0	75.86

the promoter recognition results at 67%. The ratio of the positive-to-negative data sets is chosen to be 1:2. With the ratio of 1:1, the precision turns out to be 77.1%, specificity 75.69%, and sensitivity 80.47%. It can be seen that even though a much better recognition of promoters is achieved, false positives increase compared to the case when the training data set is in the ratio of 1:2. Hence, only the 1:2 case is used.

We had also experimented with random negative data sets that are obtained by generating nucleotide sequences randomly with 60 and 50% A+T composition used by some research groups [11]. Exceptionally good promoter classification results are obtained with precision, sensitivity, and specificity values being 95.5, 98.18 and 93.0%, respectively, with a single-layer perceptron [32]. Promoter classification with an accuracy of near 96% is achieved by a single-layer perceptron for synthetic negative data sets, potentially indicating the linear separability of the promoter data sets. But then these experiments cannot be used for the whole genome promoter prediction where the predictor has to annotate each nucleotide as belonging to a promoter or a nonpromoter based on the neighboring bases. Hence, it is important to carry on studies of promoter classification with nonpromoters obtained from the genome.

An indepth analysis is carried out in Section 4.4.1 to investigate the limitation on the sensitivity of promoter prediction using 3-gram features. A closer look at the misclassified promoter sequences showed that they belong to the reverse strand of the genome. This fact has to be further investigated.

In Section 4.3.3, we explore a global signal-based method that is based on FT and wavelet transform to extract features for the promoter recognition problem.

4.3.3   Investigation of Promoter Recognition in Frequency Domain

This section explores the application of signal processing techniques (e.g., Fast Fourier Transform (FFT) and wavelet transforms) for promoter recognition as well as the possibility of modeling the RNA polymerase–promoter interaction. Various encoding techniques [electron–ion interaction potential (EIIP), enthalpy, roll angle, etc.] are also included in the encoding of a sequence into a numerical format.

Tiwari et al. showned that the FT gene portion often has a prominent peak at $\frac{1}{3}$ position confirming the periodicity of codons [34]. But, nongenes do not have any such peak. They have decomposed the original sequence into a set of four indicator sequences for the four nucleotides A, T, G, C [35]. Each sequence is a binary sequence indicating the presence or absence of a particular nucleotide. Deyneko et al. applied the physical features (e.g., melting enthalpy, roll angle, and minor groove depth of DNA) to find similar promoters that correlate with their transcription regulatory responsiveness to different antibiotic and osmotic treatments [36]. They transformed the *E. coli* promoters into numerical sequences using physical parameters (enthalpy, roll angle, etc.) Fourier Transform of the transformed sequences is used in computing cross-correlation and auto-correlation between different promoters. In particular, they looked for genes responsible for SOS response.

4.3.3.1 Encoding and Decomposition

A DNA sequence is made up of four nucleotides A, T, G, and C. Different kinds of encodings have been used by different groups [37–39]. Nobuyuki et al. [37] used the values A = 1, T = −1, G = 1, and C = −1, whereas Cosic et al. [39] encoded the nucleotides by using the EIIP values: A: 0.1260, G: 0.0806, T: 0.1335, and C: 0.1340.

There are another set of encodings that are based upon dinucleotides. A large number of physicochemical parameters of DNA double strands/reflecting its specific properties have been collected in a public database [16]. Three parameter sets, melting enthalpy, minor groove depth, and roll, are given in Table 4.2. The DNA enthalpy data describes the melting of DNA double strands. The enthalpy data are dependent on the neighboring nucleotide and direction $5' \rightarrow 3'$ is important here. The reason is that enthalpy is not only attributable to the direction invariant hydrogen bonds, but also to the interactions between electrons of neighboring bp. van der Waals forces also contribute to the interactions between the immediate base neighbors [40]. This information is not reversible for the strand direction and must therefore be taken into account in the enthalpy-based conversion of the primary structure into a signal [41]. Roll angle is another structural feature that may help in promoter recognition. A

TABLE 4.2   Physicochemical Properties of DNA [36]

Dinucleotide	Melting Enthalpy (kcaL/mol.)	Minor Groove Depth (Å)	Roll Angle (degree)
AA	9.05	9.03	0.3
AT	8.60	8.91	−0.8
AG	7.84	8.98	4.5
AC	6.54	8.79	0.5
TA	6.00	9.00	2.8
TT	9.14	9.03	0.3
TG	5.84	9.09	0.5
TC	5.64	9.11	−1.3
GA	5.55	9.11	−1.3
GT	6.45	8.79	0.5
GG	10.95	8.99	6.0
GC	11.10	8.98	−6.2
CA	5.75	9.09	0.5
CT	7.75	8.98	4.5
CG	11.90	9.06	−6.2
CC	11.04	8.99	6.0

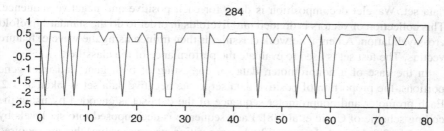

FIGURE 4.2   A sample promoter sequence represented in terms of EIIP values for nucleotides.

dinucleotide step is helically twisted since the distance between sugar–phosphate, backbone is twice the distance between base-stacking distance [42]. If a step is untwisted, the base pairs are pushed apart and the rise distance increases. To regain the stacking, (i.e., to decrease the rise distance) the step then rolls around the major groove [43]. For RNA polymerase to bind to the promoter, an open complex near the −10 site is required. Hence, this particular structural feature may be important in analyzing the dynamics of the DNA segment. The parameters are used to represent the DNA by Kauer and Co-workers [15,36]. Deyneko et al. [36] contend that the mere symbol computations are misleading since AA instead of GA numerically is more significant in terms of melting enthalpy. They claim that by using the physicochemical parameters, they were able to find significant similarity of promoters than with nucleotide comparison.

Here, we followed the EIIP encoding system of Cosic et al. for promoter–RNA polymerase interaction computations, since they also provide EIIP values for amino acids [39]. In the FT case, we used binary indicator sequences [35], enthalpy and roll angle encoding [36], and EIIP encoding [39]. Each sequence is encoded into a numerical sequence by using the encoding scheme. This numerical series is normalized to zero mean and unit standard deviation. Figure 4.2 depicts a sample sequence from the promoter data set that is converted into a numerical sequence using the EIIP values.

4.3.3.2 Feature Extraction   Using one of these encodings, the original sequence is converted into a numerical series. This numerical series is transformed using FTs and WTs.

In FT, discrete fourier transform (DFT) is applied to the promoter, as well as nonpromoter sequences to cull out the dominant components in frequency space. Discrete FT is computed by using FFT in MATLAB. The FFT coefficients are complex, hence the power spectrum is computed using the FFT coefficients.

In wavelet transform, this series is decomposed using a discrete wavelet transform into a number of levels [44]. Bior3.3 biorthogonal wavelets are used to decompose the numerical promoter sequence.

As described earlier, a major portion of the data set is used for training the classifier and the rest that is not exposed to the classifier is used as the test data set. We denote the set of promoters as positive data set and the set of nonpromoters as the negative data set. Wavelet decomposition is done for each positive and negative sequence. This collection of vectors is divided into fivefolds in order to do the standard fivefold cross-validation. A neural network classifier is then trained using the wavelet feature vectors. The test set is used to evaluate the performance of the classifier.

In the case of a nonpromoter, data set consisting of both gene and inter-gene portions, the proportion of positive data set to the negative data set is taken as 1:2. Each promoter and nonpromoter sequence of the data set is encoded by using the coding scheme of Cosic et al [38]. Each sequence is decomposed into six levels by using Bior3.3. In total, there are 120 decomposition structure values that are required to decompose the original numerical sequence. The original wave is decomposed into six detail waves, namely, D1, D2, D3,D4, D5, D6, and one smooth component A6, each of length 80. The classification is based upon various features that are extracted from these decomposition structure values and decomposed wavelet coefficients.

4.3.3.3 Classification
A multilayer feedforward neural network with three layers, namely, an input layer, one hidden and an output layer, is used for promoter classification in the following classification sections with various features based upon signal analysis techniques. The number of nodes in the input layer is dependent on particular features that are used. A hidden layer consists of a certain number of hidden nodes, the number found by trial and error that gives optimal classification performance. The output layer has one node to give a binary decision as to whether the given input sequence is a promoter or a nonpromoter. These simulations are done using Stuttgart neural network simulator [33].

Neural network is trained on the training set and then the classification performance is evaluated on the test set. All the classification experiments are carried out using a fivefold cross validation procedure [45, 46]. The classification results are evaluated using performance measures (e.g., *Precision*, *Specificity*, and *Sensitivity*).

4.3.3.4 Classification Using Power Spectrum Features
Earlier research using FT showed that the coding region of eukaryotes gave a peak at $\frac{1}{3}$ pointing to a codon bias [34], which could be used in gene recognition in case of eukaryotes. In the case of prokaryotes, the periodicity of 3 is observed not only in coding regions, but also in noncoding regions [47]. If different triplets are responsible for periodicities in coding and noncoding regions, they may become helpful in identifying promoters and nonpromoters. Tiwari et al. [34] showed that the gene portion often has a prominent peak at $\frac{1}{3}$ position confirming the periodicity of codons. But, nongenes do not have any such peak. They have decomposed the original sequence U into a set of four indicator sequences, namely, U_A, U_G, U_T, and U_C for the four nucleotides A, T, G, and C [34]. Each sequence is a binary sequence indicating the presence or absence of a particular nucleotide. Table 4.3 displays the classification results of *E. coli* with the power spectrum values as features for a feedforward neural network. The positive recognition results are not very encouraging even though negative recognition results are good, pointing possibly to the inseparability of coding versus noncoding sequences in this feature space.

TABLE 4.3   Classification Results Using Power Spectrum Values For *E. coli* Using Different Encoding Schemes

Features	Precision (%)	Specificity (%)	Sensitivity (%)
EIIP	75.85	88.72	48.58
Binary indicators	73.98	88.36	43.5
Enthalpy	74.44	86.61	46.91
Roll Angle	No training		

Experimenting with various lengths starting from 80 to 350 bp in steps of 40 bp for coding and noncoding sequences, we found that sequence lengths >200 bp might be needed to get a sizeable distinction near the $\frac{1}{3}$rd peak. Hence, it is possible that the promoters versus nonpromoters are not able to throw up any distinct peak structure, which will be useful in classification of *E.coli* promoters.

In order to check the validity of the ideas, same experimentation is done on the *Drosophila* data set [23] used in Section 4.3.1. Here again the sequence is represented as a set of four binary-indicator sequences, each indicating the presence or absence of a particular nucleotide. Classification results using these encodings are shown in Table 4.4. The sensitivity is 50–60%, even though specificity is 85%. When the intron data is removed from the total data set, where is only consists of promoter and coding sequences, the sensitivity improves to 86%. Further, instead of binary values, if EIIP values are used in place of **1** in binary-indicator sequences, the sensitivity is much higher, (94%), which is supported by Trifonov and Sussman [47] data. Hence, it can be concluded that the intron part is similar to the promoter, which is hindering the classification accuracy. In view of the above arguments, in the case of *E. coli*, there are two factors that are affecting the accuracy: one is the length of the sequence and the second is the similarity of noncoding sequences to the promoter sequences. Thus FFT of the DNA sequence encoded using EIIP encoding, gives a slightly better accuracy compared to the other encodings for *E. coli*, and for *Drosophila* binary-indicator sequences gives a marginal improvement over EIIP encoding.

4.3.3.5 Classification Using Wavelet Coefficients A global signal using wavelet transforms is extracted from both promoter, as well as nonpromoter, sequences and is used as input to a classifier. Basically, there are two operations that can be performed on a signal: decomposition and reconstruction. One set of experiments is done using wavelet coefficients at various scales as features for a feedforward neural network

TABLE 4.4   Classification Results Using Power Spectrum Values for *Drosophila* Using Different Encoding Schemes

Features	Precision (%)	Specificity (%)	Sensitivity (%)
EIIP	77.13	87.68	50.69
Binary indicators	77.98	86.51	56.66

TABLE 4.5 Classification Results Using Wavelet Coefficients as Features for a Neural Network Classifier for *E. coli* Using EIIP Encoding

Features	Precision (%)	Specificity (%)	Sensitivity (%)
All 120 values	63.6	86.52	31.7

to classify the promoter sequence. Another set of experiments is done using the decomposed waves as features to the classifier.

Simple FT is not enough to discriminate a promoter against coding and noncoding backgrounds as seen above. The time or positional information is lost in an FT. Wavelet transform retains the positional, as well as frequency information. The decomposition structure has a total number of coefficients of 120. The values are 8, 8, 9, 11, 16, 25, and 43 for A6, D6, D5, D4, D3, D2, and D6, respectively. The classification accuracy of promoter recognition problem is computed using wavelet coefficients as input to the neural network. The results are given in Table 4.5. The results show that nonpromoter recognition is good compared to promoter recognition.

4.3.3.6 Classification Using Decomposed Signals Each decomposed wave is rebuilt using decomposed structure values into a wave of length 80. In total, there are seven waves, namely, A6, D6, D5, D4, D3, D2, and D1 resulting in 560 values (7 × 80). All waves are used to see whether more information is imparted by transforming one initial signal wave into so many decomposed waves. These 560 values are used as input features to a neural network classifier to identify the promoters. Table 4.6 presents the results of the classifier for these feature values. The results again are showing good nonpromoter recognition rather than promoter recognition. It can be concluded that both experiments using wavelet coefficients and decomposed waves are good for nonpromoter recognition. Increase in the number of features has not helped in gaining more information to classify promoters better. Experiments on the *Drosophila* data set also present similar results. The sensitivity is 50% for *Drosophila* using binary indicator sequence encoding scheme. The results are shown in Table 4.7.

4.3.3.7 Cross-Correlation between Promoter and RNA-Polymerase We also looked at modeling the interaction between promoter and RNA polymerase during promoter recognition [48]. Basically, interactions between protein and DNA can be categorized into four classes: DNA backbone–protein backbone (18%), DNA backbone–protein

TABLE 4.6 Classification Results Using Decomposed Waves as Features to a Neural Network Classifier for *E. coli* Using EIIP Encoding

Features	Precision (%)	Specificity (%)	Sensitivity (%)
All decomposed waves (560)	69.23	87.59	30.21

TABLE 4.7   Classification Results Using Decomposed Waves as Features to a Neural Network Classifier for *Drosophila* Binary Indicators Encoding Scheme

Features	Precision (%)	Specificity (%)	Sensitivity (%)
All decomposed waves (2100)	77.61	89.14	50.62

side chain (51%), DNA side chain–protein backbone (1%) DNA side chain–protein side chain (30%) [49]. Protein–DNA interactions are chemically the same as protein–protein interactions. They consist of electrostatic interactions, hydrogen bonds, and hydrophobic interaction. However, hydrogen bonds constitute the major term for recognition and specificity and a large portion of the binding energy [50, 51]. It has been proposed that matching of periodicities within the distribution of energies of free electrons along the interacting proteins or protein and DNA can be regarded as resonant recognition [38]. The whole process can be observed as the interaction between transmitting and receiving antennaes of a radio system.

The sigma subunit of the RNA polymerase is of 612 aa (amino acids) length. The subunit is converted into a numerical sequence using the EIIP values for the aa [44]. This particular subunit is also decomposed into six levels using the Bior3.3 biorthogonal wavelet. The maximum absolute value of the correlation coefficient at each decomposition level can be treated as the similarity score between the signals. Cross-correlation between RNA polymerase and sample sequence is given Figure 4.3. The number of correlation coefficients is 691. In case of binary encoding, wavelet at a particular level is obtained by taking the norm of four vectors for each i, j, where i is the location and j is the level number as

$$W(j, i) = \sqrt{W_A(j, i)^2 + W_T(j, i)^2 + W_G(j, i)^2 + W_C(j, i)^2} \qquad (4.1)$$

The results of classification using both these encodings are given in Table 4.8.

The results using features of cross-correlation between promoter and RNA polymerase sigma subunit, and cross-correlation between decomposed waves of both

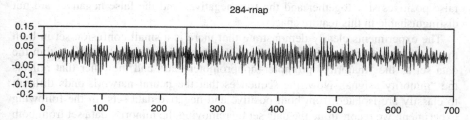

FIGURE 4.3 Cross-correlation between sample promoter and RNA polymerase subunit sigma.

TABLE 4.8   Classification Results Using DNA–RNA Polymerase Sigma Subunit Cross-Correlation Values as Features for a Neural Network Classifier for *E. coli*

Features	Precision (%)	Specificity (%)	Sensitivity (%)
EIIP encoding	66.46	86.18	24.65
Binary encoding	69.67	89.64	27.34

promoter and RNA polymerase sigma subunit have shown a remarkable ability to identify nonpromoters. Finally, the assumption that signal processing methods can capture the interaction between the RNA polymerase sigma subunit and promoter has not fructified well. It is also found that the different encoding schemes, including those that use the structural properties of the genome do not influence the classification performance.

4.4   CHALLENGES IN PROMOTER CLASSIFICATION

4.4.1   Limitations in the Neural Network Performance

Detailed analysis of the classification results of promoters of *E. coli* is carried out with the best features, which are 3-grams as basis. Many experiments are carried out in the training phase of the neural network by varying the network architecture with different number of hidden layers and the number hidden nodes in each hidden layer. Yet, the network could not achieve a training performance beyond 85%. The sets of misclassified and correctly classified sequences are studied closely by keeping the feature extraction and the classifier scheme as described in Sections 4.3.2.1 and 4.3.2.2. For a deeper analysis of promoters classification, a set of sequences is selected randomly from both promoters and nonpromoters (consisting of both gene and intergene portions) in the ratio of 1:2, respectively, for training. That is, a set of 454 sequences are taken from a promoter data set as a positive set, and 454 sequences are taken from each gene and inter-gene sequence sets. The rest of the data set is used as a test data set.

It clearly can be seen from Figure 4.4 and Table 4.9 that the true positives and false positives stay together and the true negatives and the false negatives are not distinguishable in this feature space.

The experiments clearly demonstrate that there is a small confusion set in both the promoter and nonpromoter data sets. We categorize the two classes within the data set as the "majority" promoter–nonpromoter class and the other that reflects the "minority" signal. Now, the sequences that the neural network finds difficult to classify are isolated from both positive and negative data sets. In the following experiment, we reconstitute the data set by removing the minority data set from both the promoter and nonpromoter sets and call it *Major Set* (Maj). It is found that a neural network, which we call NN_{Maj}, without a hidden layer achieves 100% training performance and the results of the test data set are shown in Table 4.10.

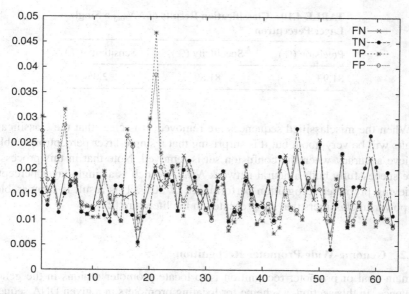

FIGURE 4.4 Plot of 3-gram frequency averages for promoter and negative data sets consisting of segments from gene and inter-gene portions of the DNA.

Similar performance is observed for the neural network NN_{Min} when trained only on Min. That is, the Maj class constituting the majority promoter and the majority nonpromoters is linearly separable. Similarly, the Min set is also linearly separable.

Note that in Table 4.9 the numbers as well as the exact sequences in each of these boxes match. For example, the set of 130 FNs of NN_{Min} is a superset of the 128 TPs of NN_{Maj}. Thus, we see that both promoter and nonpromoter sequences have two distinct patterns, one being recognized by NN_{Maj} and the other by NN_{Min}. But for 5–7 sequences, the NN_{Maj} and NN_{Min} behave in a complementary fashion, which is confusing. A small portion (14%) of the nonpromoter data set is similar to a majority (70%) of the promoter data set. Also, 86% of the nonpromoter data set (TN) is closer to 30% of the promoter data set (FN).

TABLE 4.9 Test Data Results of Neural Networks NN_{Maj} **and** NN_{Min}

Positive Test Data (156)	Negative Test Data (392)
TP of NN_{Maj} = 128	TN of NN_{Maj} = 321
⊆	⊇
FN of NN_{Min} = 130	FP of NN_{Min} = 307
FN of NN_{Maj} = 28	FP of NN_{Maj} = 71
⊇	⊆
TP of NN_{Min} = 26	TN of NN_{Min} = 85

TABLE 4.10   Classification Results of NN_{Maj} a Single Layer Perceptron

Precision (%)	Specificity (%)	Sensitivity (%)
81.93	81.89	82.05

When the misclassified sequences are removed, it is clear that the classification results will be very good, but it is surprising that a single-layer perceptron is able to achieve accuracy when the confusion set is removed. Note that in this process we have successfully built a neural network NN_{Maj}, which is a single-layer perceptron achieving promoter recognition performance of 80%. This result is comparable to the powerful classifiers that are presented in the literature [22].

4.4.2   Genome-Wide Promoter Recognition

A main goal of promoter recognition is to locate promoter regions in the genome sequence. In this section, a scheme for locating promoters in a given DNA sequence segment of *E. coli* genome of length N in a particular direction (say, $5'–3'$) is proposed. The scheme does not address the issue of locating TSS in the promoter region. The NN_{Maj} network is a classifier that is constructed with the negative data set composed of genic and intergenic portions. When the negative data set is a combination of both coding and noncoding segments, it is advantageous in the sense that the promoter and nonpromoter could be classified at the same time. But, the classification accuracy is not 100%, and there is no way one can eliminate the false positives and negatives. To overcome this handicap, instead of using the earlier neural networks, a new set of neural networks based on different combinations of the data sets are designed. One network, NN_{PC}, is trained using promoter and coding data sets as positive and negative data sets, respectively, and another one, NN_{PN}, using promoter and noncoding data sets.

A moving window of length 80 is considered to extract segments from the start of the DNA sequence, that is, 1–80, 2–81, 3–82, and so on. A given sequence segment is classified as promoter by a voting scheme. If NN_{PC} and NN_{PN} both classify the sequence as a promoter sequence, then the sequence is voted as a promoter or otherwise a nonpromoter. Each of the segments thus gets classified as a promoter (P) or nonpromoter (NP). If a segment $m - (m + 79)$ is classified as a promoter, then the nucleotide m is annotated as P and if it is classified as nonpromoter, then m is annotated as NP. This process of annotation is continued for the entire sequence to get a sequence of P's and NPs. A stretch of these outcomes greater than a threshold (e.g., 50 consecutive positive outcomes) is treated as a P or as an NP region.

The whole genome of *E. coli* is divided into 400 sections. The following is a case study on two sections (Sections 1 and 3) of *E. coli* whole genome. The combined outputs of NN_{PC} and NN_{PN}, as described earlier, is used to annotate the promoter regions. The consensus regions can be seen in Figures 4.5 and 4.6. Since NN_{PN} shows many spurious promoters, it is essential to take the consensus result. In the figures,

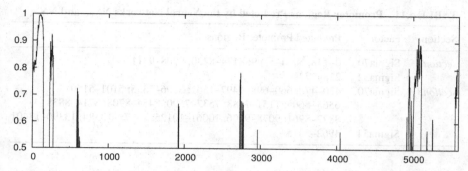

FIGURE 4.5 The combined output of the networks NN_{PC} and NN_{PN} versus the moving window for *section1* of the *E. coli* genome.

the output result of the ensemble of networks of NN_{PC} and NN_{PN} is shown to indicate that a consensus for a stretch of >50 bp will be annotated as a promoter.

Table 4.11 shows the section number, the sigma factor, and the extent of the region identified as promoter from the experiment. In the whole genome annotation, it is considered essential that no true promoter is missed. The *n*-gram based classifier is able to annotate all the existing promoters that are in NCBI in the sections that are considered. On the other hand, a few regions are additionally annotated as promoters. For example in *section3*, 3296–3355, 7537–7590, 8454–8708 which are regions predicted as promoters, are not accounted for in the NCBI data. Only wet lab experiments can verify the validity of this result.

There are not many whole genome promoter prediction programs for prokaryotes. The available tools for prokaryotic promoter prediction are that of Gordon et al. [52] who developed a whole genome promoter prediction based on their sequence alignment kernel (SAK); Bacterial Promoter BPROM is developed by SoftBerry Inc. [53]; Neural network promoter prediction (NNPP) tool developed by Reese [54]. SAK predicts whether the 61st position of a sequence of length 80 is a TSS or not. The legend of SAK says that the more positive the outcome is, the more probable

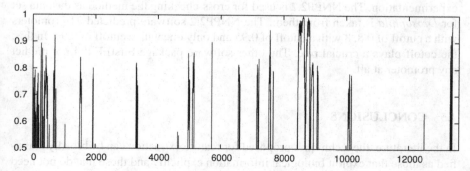

FIGURE 4.6 The combined output of the networks NN_{PC} and NN_{PN} versus the moving window for *section3* of the *E. coli* genome.

TABLE 4.11   Promoter Regions Predicted by the Neural Networks NN_{PC} and NN_{PN}

Section	Factor	Predicted Promoter Regions
section1	Sigma70	0–148; 5004–5109; 8174–8220; 9208–9311
	Sigma32	228–277
section3	Sigma70	420–478; 660–698; 1497–1561; 3296–3355; 5101–5150
		6563–6605; 7151–7188; 7537–7590; 8454–8708; 8714–8838
		8872–8961; 9078–9106; 10061–10125; 13378–13384; 13390–13401
	Sigma54	4962–5015

that segment is a promoter, and a promoter, is denoted by "L". There are no such annotations in the test case. But, it can be seen that most of the peaks coincide. In the case of BPROM, an internal parameter threshold for promoters is set as 0.20 [51]. Bacterial promoter (BPROM) has predicted 31 promoters in this region. Further, BPROM predicts the TSS and determines the binding regions. The NNPP predictions are made with a cut-off rate of 0.80 [55]. A comparative study of promoter recognition by these tools along with 3-grams shows that 3-grams outperform these tools. Classifier based on 3-grams achieves 100% sensitivity, whereas SAK, NNPP, and BPROM achieve 69.23, 76.92, and 38.46, respectively.

The results give a clear indication that cascaded networks based on 3-grams perform significantly well. One more factor is that, unless we know, here a promoter region exists, we cannot say an outcome from these other tools is positive since there are many false positives. In our scheme, wherever we find a stretch of positives, using the cascaded method, we can label them as positive predictions.

The promoter prediction is carried out for the *Drosophila* genome with the ensemble of neural networks of NN_{PC} and NN_{PN} using 4-grams. A stretch of 10 kbp is used that starts with a gene followed by two more genes. For this data, four promoters are identified by the ensemble of which two promoters occur before the genes and one in the intron region and one in the exon region. The stretches of promoter occurring in intron and exon portions are 150 bp in length, whereas the portions identified before the genes are 350 bp in length. The threshold has to be set more rigorously, by more experimentation. The NNPP2.2 is used for cross-checking the method as the data set for *Drosophila* is taken from them. The NNPP2.2 software predicted 21 promoters with a cutoff of 0.8, 8 with a cutoff of 0.95 and only one with a cutoff of 0.99. In this, the cutoff plays a crucial role. The other software package FirstEF did not predict any promoter at all.

4.5   CONCLUSIONS

In the literature, the techniques proposed for feature extraction can be broadly classified as those that exploit biological information explicitly and those that do not need *a priori* biologically based labeling information. In the former category, called the *local methods*, the features are extracted from the binding regions or local motifs, whereas in the latter, *global signal methods*, features are derived utilizing the physic-ochemical and structural properties of the whole promoter region. The recognition methods that exploit the promoter signal like the position weight matrices (PWM), the expectation maximization algorithm, and the techniques like FTs, are proposed in the literature. This chapter presents promoter recognition using n-gram based features and features based on FT and WT. We demonstrate that the n-gram based features perform the best for the whole genome annotation.

Whole genome annotation is a major challenge for promoter prediction tools. The performance of an algorithm on a limited training and test data set may not be really a performance indicator of how well it may identify promoters in a whole genome. Methods that are proposed giving good accuracies on training and test data sets, may or may not perform better on the whole genome.

The binding regions are important in assisting the RNA polymerase to bind the promoter, but that information alone is not sufficient to recognize a promoter. Local features are calculated from binding sites that are available in Harley's data [19]. Global features are extracted from the whole promoter sequence aligned with respect to TSS and nonpromoter data sets. If we compare the results that are obtained using a signal extracted from motifs–binding regions in the promoter with the signal obtained from the whole promoter sequence, it is evident that the local signal has a handicap in extending to a whole genome promoter prediction process. The signal from the entire promoter sequence without segmenting it into important and nonimportant portions will lead to better generalization in the case of *E. coli*. The PWM based features, as well as n-grams from the whole promoter, give better genome promoter annotation results than the other local signal extraction schemes.

Experiments are carried out to find a signature of the promoter present at any particular resolution. If the characteristic signal of a promoter that is supposed to be conserved irrespective of place of occurrence of the genome promoter is not preserved, then promoter recognition based on the signal processing techniques will not be very helpful. The results of *E. coli* and *Drosophila* show that features using FFT and wavelets are not sufficient to recognize a promoter against a coding and noncoding background. This fact is evident from the results where the negative data seems to be recognized better than a promoter. The promoter data set seems to have no pattern in the FT, WT feature space that can be learned by the classifier. In summary, it turns out that signal processing techniques cannot be used as general classification algorithm. The conjecture that structural properties are underlying principles for base selection is not evident from the current experiments.

This chapter shows that in an n-gram feature space, recognition rate of *Drosophila* promoters is better than *E. coli* promoter recognition. Best performance for *Drosophila* is 87% compared to *E. coli's* 80% with a very good positive predictive rate as shown in Section 4.3.2.2. Promoter architecture of eukaryotes is in general much more complex than a prokaryote promoter architecture. It is found that n-gram preferences for *Drosophila* is stronger in a discriminating promoter versus a non-promoter than for *E. coli*. The prediction of the negative data set is higher possibly because the intron portions are similar to nongene segments in eukaryotes. In fact, the results of promoter recognition using FT give only ~50% positive identification.

From these results, we can conclude that different adjacency preferences are shown for promoter and nonpromoter regions. One major advantage of using n-gram based whole genome promoter annotation is that one does not need any prior information about the promoter, the location of binding sites, the spacer lengths, and so on. The additional advantage of using n-gram features is that the input vectors computed for neural network classifier will not change irrespective of the length of the promoter sequence.

4.6   FUTURE DIRECTIONS

The techniques described in this chapter can be developed to build a full-fledged automated whole genome promoter annotation tool. Whole genome promoter prediction using 3-grams has been applied to the forward strand only. The same scheme needs to be applied to the reverse strand with appropriate preprocessing so that the method can achieve whole genome promoter recognition.

Signal processing techniques need to be explored further to enhance the recognition rates. Since RNA polymerase is an enzyme, which is a protein, three-dimensional structure information of RNA polymerase can be used to characterize promoter–RNA polymerase interaction. It is to be explored if instead of using Bior3.3 as the mother wavelet, RNA polymerase itself can be used as a mother wavelet to imitate the biological mechanism closely. This line of application of wavelets would be quite novel.

Proteins are believed to be responsible for most of the genetically important functions in all cells. Hence, the focus has been entirely on gene recognition. Recent studies indicate that ncRNAs (noncoding RNAs), which do not code for proteins, affect transcription and the chromosome structure, in RNA processing and modification, regulation of mRNA stability and translation, and also affect protein stability and transport [56, 57]. An effort to look for them in typically 95% of the total DNA is a huge task. By suitably modeling the promoters of these ncRNAs, they can be predicted much more easily. Some of the techniques that are developed here can be extended to do this work.

REFERENCES

1. R. Grosschedl and M. L. Birnstiel (1980), Identification of regulatory sequences in the prelude sequences of an h2a histone gene by the study of specific deletion mutants *in vivo*, *Proc. Natl. Acad. Sci.*, **77**(12): 7102–7106.

2. S. L. McKnight and K. R. Yamamoto (1992), *Transcriptional regulation*, Cold Spring Harbor Laboratory Press, MA.

3. FANTOM Consortium (2005), RIKEN Genome Exploration Research Group and Genome Science Group (Genome Network Project Core Group), The transcriptional landscape of the mammalian genome *Science*, **309**: 1559–1563.

4. V. G. Levitsky and A. V. Katokhin (2003), Recognition of eukaryotic promoters using a genetic algorithm based on iterative discriminant analysis, *In Silico Biol.* **3**.

5. A. G. Pedersen, P. Baldi, Y. Chauvinb, and S. Brunak (1999), The biology of eukaryotic promoter prediction—a review, *Comput. Chem.,* **23**: 191–207.

6. V. B. Bajic, S. H. Seah, A. Chong, G. Zhang, J. L. Y. Koh, and V. Brusic (2002), Dragon promoter finder: recognition of vertebrate RNA polymerase II promoters, *Bioinformatics,* **18**(1): 198–199.

7. J. M. Claverie and S. Audic (1996), The statistical significance of nucleotide position-weight matrix matches, *CABIOS,* **12**(5): 431–439.

8. N. I. Gershenzon, G. D. Stormo, and I. P. Ioshikhes (2005), Computational technique for improvement of the position-weight matrices for the DNA/protein binding sites, *Nucleic Acids Res.,* **33**(7): 2290–2301.

9. S. W. Leung, C. Mellish, and D. Robertson (2001), Basic gene grammars and DNA-chart parser for language processing of Escherichia coli promoter DNA sequences, *Bioinformatics,* **17**: 226–236.

10. L. R. Cardon and G. D. Stormo (1992), Expectation maximization algorithm of identifying protein-binding sites with variable lengths from unaligned DNA fragments, *J. Mol. Biol.,* **223**: 159–170.

11. Q. Ma, J. T. L. Wang, D. Shasha, and C. H. Wu (2001), Dna sequence classification via an expectation maximization algorithm and neural networks: a case study, *IEEE Transactions on Systems,Man and Cybernetics, Part C: Applications and Reviews, Special Issue on Knowledge Management,* **31**: 468–475.

12. T. Werner (1999), Models for prediction and recognition of eukaryotic promoters, *Mammalian Genome,* **10**: 168–175.

13. M. K. Das and H. K. Dai (2007), A survey of DNA motif finding algorithms, *BMC Bioinformat.,* **8**: (7:S21).

14. A. M. Huerta and J. Collado-Vides (2003), Sigma70 promoters in escherichia coli: Specific transcription in dense regions of overlapping promoter-like signals, *J. Mol. Biol.,* **333**: 261–278.

15. G. Kauer and B. Helmut (2003), Applying signal theory to the analysis of biomolecules, *Bioinformatics,* **19**(16): 2016–2021.

16. J. V. Ponomarenko, M. P. Ponomarenko, A. S. Frolov, D. G. Vorobyev, G. C. Overton, and N. A. Kolchanov (1999), Conformational and physicochemical DNA features specific for transcription factor binding sites, *Bioinformatics,* **15**: 654–668.

17. F. Kobe, S. Yvan, D. Sven, R. Pierre, and Y. P. Peer (2005), Large-scale structural analysis of the core promoter in mammalian and plant genomes, *Nucleic Acids Res.,* **33**(13): 4255–4264.

18. W. Li (1997), The study of correlation structures of DNA sequences: a critical review, *Comp. Chem.,* **21**: 257–271.

19. C. B. Harley and R. P. Reynolds (1987), Analysis of e.coli promoter sequences, *Nucleic Acids Res.,* **15**(5): 2343–2361.

20. L. Pietro (2003), Wavelets in bioinformatics and computational biology: state of art and perspectives, *Bioinformatics,* **19**(1): 2–9.

21. J. D. Alicia, D. J. Bradley, L. Michael, and A. G. Carol (1996), The sigma subunit of escherichia coli RNA polymerase senses promoter spacing, *Proc. Nat. Acad. Sci.,* **93**: 8858–8862.

22. L. Gordon, A. Y. Chervonenkis, A. J. Gammerman, I. A. Shahmurradov, and V. Solovyev (2003), Sequence alignment kernel for recognition of promoter regions, *Bioinformatics,* **19**: 1964–1971.

23. U. Ohler, G. C. Liao, H. Niemann, and G. M. Rubin (2002), Computational analysis of core promoters in the drosophila genome, *Genome Biology* 2002, **3**(12):research0087.1-0087.12.

24. Eukaryotic Promoter Database (EPD). Available at *http://www.epd.isb-sib.ch/index.html*

25. I. Ben-Gal, A. Shani, A. Gohr, J. Grau, S. Arviv, A. Shmilovici, S. Posch, and I. Grosse (2005), Identification of transcription factor binding sites with variable-order Bayesian networks, *Bioinformatics,* **21**; 2657–2666.

26. F. Leu, N. Lo, and L. Yang (2005), Predicting vertebrate promoters with homogeneous cluster computing, In *Proc. 1st International Conference on Signal-Image Technology and Internet-Based Systems (SITIS)*, pp. 143–148.

27. H. Ji, D. Xinbin and Z. Xuechun (2006), A systematic computational approach for transcription factor target gene prediction, in *IEEE Symposium on Computational Intelligence and Bioinformatics and Computational Biology CIBCB '06*, pp. 1–7.

28. J. Wang and S. Hannenhalli (2006), A mammalian promoter model links cis elements to genetic networks, *Biochem. Biophys. Res. Commun.* **347**: 166–177.

29. Q. Z. Li and H. Lin (2006), The recognition and prediction of $\sigma 70$ promoters in Escherichia coli K-12, *J. Theor. Biol.,* **242**: 135–141.

30. S. Sonnenburg, A. Zien, P. Philips, and G. Ratsch (2008), POIMs: positional oligomer importance matrices—understanding support vector machine—based signal detectors, *Bioinformatics,* **24**: i6–i14.

31. T. Sobha Rani and Raju S. Bapi (2008), Analysis of n-gram based promoter recognition methods and application to whole genome promoter prediction, *In Silico Biol.,* **9**: s1–s16.

32. T. S. Rani, S. D. Bhavani, and R. S. Bapi (2007), Analysis of *E. coli* promoter recognition problem in dinucleotide feature space, *Bioinformatics,* **23**: 582–588.

33. Stuttgart Neural Network Simulator. Available at http://www-ra.informatik.uni-tuebingen.de/SNNS/

34. S. Tiwari, S. Ramachandran, A. Bhattacharya, S. Bhattacharya, and R. Ramaswamy (1997), Prediction of probable genes by fourier analysis of genomic sequences, *Comput. Appl. Biosci.,* **13**: 263–270.

35. R. F. Voss (1992), Evolution of long-range fractal correlations and 1/f noise in DNA base sequences, *Phys. Rev. Lett.,* **68**(5): 3805–3808.

36. I. V. Deyneko, E. K. Alexander, B. Helmut, and G. Kauer (2005), Signal-theoretical DNA similarity measure revealing unexpected similarities of *E. coli* promoters, *In Silico Biol.,* **5**.

37. K. Nobuyuki, O. Yashurio, M. Kazuo, M. Kenichi, K. Jun, C. Piero, H. Yoshihide, and K. Shoshi (2002), Wavelet profiles: Their application in Oryza Sativa DNA sequence analysis, In *Proc. IEEE computer society Bioinformatics conference(CSB02)*, pp. 345–348.

38. A. Arneodo, E. Bacry, P. V. Graves, and F. Muzy (1995), Characterizing long-range correlations in DNA sequences from wavelet analysis, *Phys. Rev. Lett.,* **74**(16): 3293–3297.

39. I. Cosic (1994), Macromolecular bioactivity(is it resonant interaction between macromolecules?-theory and applications, *IEEE Trans. Biomed. Eng.,* **41**(12): 1101–1114.

40. M. Suzuki, N. Yagi, and J. T. Finch (1996), Role of base-backbone and base-base interactions in alternating DNA conformations, *FEBS Lett.,* **379**: 148–152.

41. T. V. Chalikian, J. Volkner, G. E. Plum, and K. J. Breslauer (1999), A more unified picture for the thermodynamics of nucleic acid duplex melting: A characterization by calorimetric and volumetric techniques, *Proc. Natl. Acad. of Sci. USA,* **96**: 7853–7858.

42. C. R. Calladine and D. R. Drew 1992, *Molecular Structure and Life,* CRC Press.

43. A. A. Gorin, V. B. Zhurkin, and W. K. Olson (1995), B-DNA twisting approach correlates with base-pair morphology, *J. Mol. Biol.,* **247**: 34–48.

44. H. T. Chafia, F. Qian, and I. Cosic (2002), Protein sequence comparison based on the wavelet transform approach, *Protein Eng.,* **15**(3): 193–203.

45. E. Alpaydin (2004), *Introduction to Machine Learning,* MIT Press.

46. T. M. Mitchell, *Machine Learning,* McGraw Hill, Singapore, 1997.

47. E. N. Trifonov and J. L. Sussman (1980), The pitch of chromatin DNA is reflected in its nucleotide sequence, *Proc. Natl. Acad. Sci. USA* **77**: 3816–3820.

48. T. Sobha Rani and Raju S. Bapi (2008), *E. coli* Promoter Recognition Through Wavelets, *Proc. BIOCOMP 2008,* 256–262.

49. Y. Mandel-Gutfreund, O. Schueler, and H. Margalit (1995), Comprehensive analysis of hydrogen bonds in regulatory protein DNA-complexes: In search of common principles, *J. Mol. Biol.,* **253**: 370–382.

50. N. M. Luscombe, R. A. Laskowski, and J. M. Thornton (2001), Amino-acid base interactions a three-dimensional analysis of protein-DNA interactions at atomic level, *Nucleic Acids Res.,* **29**: 2860–2874.

51. K. Luger, A. W. Mader, R. K. Richmond, D. F. Sargent, and T. J. Richmond (1997), Crystal structure of the nucleosome core particle at 2.8 a resolution, *Nature (London),* **389**: 251–260.

52. Sequence Alignment Kernel. Available at *http://nostradamus.cs.rhul.ac.uk/ leo/sak_demo.*

53. Prediction of Bacterial promoters (BPROM). Available at *http://www.softberry.com/ berry.phtml?topic =bprom*

54. Berkeley Drosophila Genome Project (BDGP). Available at *http://www.fruitfly.org/ seq_tools/promoter.html*

55. Neural Network Promoter Predictor (NNPP). Available at *http://www.fruitfly.org/seq_ tools/promoter. html*

56. J. S. Mattick (2003), Challenging the dogma: the hidden layer of non-protein-coding RNAs in complex organisms, *BioEssays,* **25**: 930–939.

57. S. Gisela (2002), An expanding universe of noncoding rnas, *Science,* **296**: 1260–1263.

5

PREDICTING microRNA PROSTATE CANCER TARGET GENES

Francesco Masulli, Stefano Rovetta, and Giuseppe Russo

5.1 INTRODUCTION

MicroRNAs (or miRNAs) are a class of noncoding RNA (ncRNA) of 18–25 nucleotides (nt) in length regulating gene expression that were first described in 1993 by Lee et al. [1], while the term *microRNA* was first introduced in 2001 [2]. The miRNAs are capable of base pairing with imperfect complementarity to the transcripts of animal protein-coding genes (also termed targets), usually within the 3′ untranslated region (3′–UTR). The miRNAs are involved in several biological and metabolic pathways and play a very important role in many diseases (e.g., cancer [3], alzheimer's disease [4], Parkinson's disease [5], and viral infections [6]).

Because animal miRNAs form base pairing with imperfect complementarity, computational prediction of miRNA targets is not an easy task, and nowadays many miRNA target prediction programs have been developed and applied.

The Mirecords website available at (http://mirecords.umn.edu/miRecords/) shows a continuously updated list of biologically validated gene targets of known miRNAs in humans and other animals (as reported by the scientific literature) together with the miRNA target predictions obtained by various target prediction programs. This list tells us that much more work must be done in order to obtain reliable miRNA target prediction methods. The reason is because (1) at present there are target genes biologically validated that are not predicted by any method; (2) the considered methods seldom agree; (3) even where there is a concordance concerning the target gene between the biological procedure and the prediction of a computational method,

Computational Intelligence and Pattern Analysis in Biological Informatics, Edited by Ujjwal Maulik,
Sanghamitra Bandyopadhyay, and Jason T. L. Wang
Copyright © 2010 John Wiley & Sons, Inc.

this cannot be considered a final validation of the prediction method as the available biological procedures are not able to detect the specific miRNA target site.

This chapter presents an approach to improve the state of the art of computational prediction of target sites, by identifying several refinements of the available algorithms, and providing an optimization of the parameters involved so as to maximize the adherence of results to biological evidence. The increased selectivity of the method may also be used to guide the experimental validation in a more focused direction. The proposed approach applies a genetic algorithm [7] to fine-tune the parameters of the analysis chain exploiting the biological knowledge on miRNA and genes involved in prostate cancer.

The following sections discuss the role of miRNAs in prostate cancer. Sections 5.3 and 5.4, present the most diffused software tools for miRNA gene target prediction. Sections 5.5–5.7 show our approach and the experimental analysis. The discussion and conclusions are in Section 5.8.

5.2   miRNA AND PROSTATE CANCER

MicroRNAs or miRNAs are small noncoding RNAs of 18–25 nucleotides in length. The miRNA genes are generally transcribed by RNA polymerase II [8] even though it was recently documented that RNA polymerase III might be involved as well [9]. MicroRNA is derived from a complex process of maturation of its primary transcript named pri-miRNA, a molecule capped at the 5′ end, polyadenylated at the 3′ end similarly to mRNAs and containing a local stem–loop structure, a terminal loop, and two flanking single-stranded arms. Then, the pri-miRNA is processed into a 70 nt hairpin-like precursor miRNA named pre-miRNA by a multienzymatic complex composed of the RNase III enzyme Drosha and the double-stranded RNA binding protein DGCR8/Pasha [10]. Next, the pre-miRNA is transported from the nucleus to the cytoplasm and diced into miRNA duplexes together with a double-stranded RNA binding-domain protein named TRBP by RNaseIII nuclease Dicer. After Dicer processing, the miRNA duplex is unwound, the released mature miRNA binds to a protein named Argonaute, the RNA strand of the miRNA duplex complementary to the mature miRNA is degraded and the mature miRNA is then free to interact with its mRNA targets. More details about miRNA biogenesis can be found in [11, 12].

The miRNAs are involved in lung, prostate, breast, and colorectal cancer [13–18]. Following a simple view, if a certain miRNA target binds tumor suppressor genes, it is supposed to be an oncogene, but, if a miRNA targets an oncogene, it might be viewed as a tumor suppressor gene. However, things may be far more complicated, as each miRNA can mediate the expression of hundreds of mRNAs. The first evidence that miRNAs may function as tumor suppressors has been reported in [19]. More details about the role of miRNAs in cancer are presented in [20].

This chapter will focus on miRNAs' influence in prostate cancer. Prostate cancer (PC) is the second leading cause of cancer deaths in men [21, 22]. It is not invariably lethal, however, and is a heterogeneous disease ranging from asymptomatic to a rapidly fatal systemic malignancy. The prevalence of PC is so high that it could be considered a normal age-related phenomenon. In spite of the availability of biomarkers for PC, the basic molecular mechanisms regulating its development and progression are still very poorly understood. These observations have led researchers to speculate that other key factors might play a role in PC pathogenesis and/or progression. Different studies demonstrated aberrant expression of several miRNAs in PC cells (e.g., let-7c , miR-19b, miR-20a, miR-29b, miR-100, miR-125b, miR-126*, miR-128b, miR-146a, miR-146b, miR-184, miR-221, miR-222, miR-361, miR-424 miR-663) [23–28]. Although a number of PC related miRNAs were discovered, to date, only five are characterized for their functionalities: three as oncogenes and two as tumor suppressors (miR-20a, miR-125b, miR-126*, miR-146a, and miR-221/222). Oncogenic miRNAs downregulate the expression of apoptosis-related genes, and tumor suppressor miRNAs target the proliferation related genes. Due to the oncogenic or tumor-suppressive properties of PC related miRNAs, they might be considered as new potential biomarkers, but more importantly as therapeutic targets for PC treatment in the near future.

Research efforts are therefore currently focusing on the discovery of more precise markers, which are needed so that appropriate treatment decisions can be made for individual patients, and on the characterization of genetic pathways involved in the development and progression of the disease. However, simply identifying the list of genes involved in a disease is only a first step in the process. There is the need for identifying more refined information (e.g., the interaction between the various steps in the pathway).

5.3 PREDICTION SOFTWARE FOR miRNAs

The discovery of miRNAs acting in PC pathways and the identification of the specific sites where they act is a major advance in the identification of regulatory networks that lead to the development and progress of the disease. The overall activity aims to develop and use novel computational (*in silico*) methods for predicting both novel miRNAs and target genes and sites, with the long-term goal to substantially improve the knowledge about PC, and consequently the development of ad hoc therapies.

The miRNA genes are identified on a large scale using direct biochemical cloning and computational approaches [29, 30]. It has been estimated that there are as many as 1000 miRNAs in the human genome. As miRNA sequences are identified they are collected in several databases including miRBase and MicroRNAdb [31].

The other goal is to identify and experimentally validate mRNA gene targets. Nowadays high-throughput approaches to validate miRNA targets experimentally are lacking. Only few nonhigh-throughput experimental approaches, which are not able to detect the specific miRNA target site, are available, (e.g., using a luciferase reporter construct by cloning the predicted binding site sequence of the miRNA into the 3′–UTR region) [32, 33], and then transfecting the miRNA into a cell line containing the luciferase reporter to access the effect of the miRNA on luciferase expression [34].

Researchers can publish discovered miRNA target data and experimental details into the public domain by submitting they results to some databases recently realized, including miRBase [31] and miRNAMAP [35], Mirecords, Argonaute [36], and TarBase [37, 38].

A large number of target prediction algorithms have been developed to guide the experimental validation in a more focused direction. Presently, the cited databases contain only a limited number of confirmed miRNA targets (i.e., true positives). An even more limited number of known miRNAs do not interact with a target gene (i.e., true negatives), so it is very difficult to develop miRNA target prediction algorithms with high sensibility and selectivity, by using, for example, neural networks or support vector machines [39].

A particular microRNAs can base-pair with perfect or imperfect complementarity to the transcripts of several hundred animal protein-coding genes (also termed targets), generally within the 3′–UTR. A large number of target prediction algorithms have been developed since direct experimental methods for discovering miRNA targets are lacking.

In plants, miRNA targets are computationally identified through the extensive complementarity between miRNAs and their corresponding targets. However, computational identification of miRNA targets in mammalian miRNAs is considerably more difficult because most animal miRNAs only partially hybridize to their mRNA targets.

The miRNA target prediction programs typically rely on a combination of specific base-pairing rules and conservational analysis to score possible 3′–UTR recognition sites and enumerate putative gene targets. Predictions based solely on base-pairing rules yield a large number of false-positive hits. The number of false-positive hits, as estimated by random shuffling of miRNA sequences, can be greatly reduced, however, by limiting hits to only those conserved in other organisms [40, 41]. By systematically varying selected miRNA sequences and testing for their ability to repress a given target, several rules have been established for miRNA:target binding [42–44]. Usually, only the 3′–UTR of the mRNA is considered and sometimes it is possible to find more than one target site prediction for the same miRNA.

The miRNA target prediction tools have been applied in a variety of organisms with two primary aims. The first is to allow researchers to narrow down the list of potential gene targets for experimental confirmation and validation when searching for a particular miRNA target. The second is to predict the number of genes regulated by miRNAs and various global trends in miRNA regulation.

As these algorithms predict between 10 and 30% of all genes that are regulated by miRNAs [45–47] and neither available tool can comprehensively elucidate all possible targets, suggest was for handling a variety of tools [38, 48] together were made.

Anyway, the most important goal is to ensure the selectivity and sensibility of a specific miRNA target prediction software. To this aim, we describe the optimization process we applied to a miRanda [49] tool that nowadays is the most popular miRNA target prediction method. Both the miRanda and our method will be described in the following sections. Here, we report the principal characteristics of other diffused miRNA target programs:

- miTarget [50], based on a support vector machine (SVM) classifier [39], which uses features (e.g., the thermodynamic free energy of binding between the miRNA and possible target site), base complementarity at specific positions, and structural features (e.g., mismatches and bulges as input). This approach is limited, however, by the lack of availability of experimentally validated targets for classifier training.
- PicTar [51] first looks for perfect seed binding of seven nucleotides in the 5′ end starting at either the first or second position. The free energy of miRNA:target binding is then computed for seeds with imperfect matches. To delineate a list of predicted target sites, energy thresholds are imposed and then a maximum likelihood score is computed based on conservation across multiple organisms.
- PITA [52] incorporates the role of target-site accessibility, as determined by base-pairing interactions within the mRNA, in miRNA target recognition.
- RNA22 [53] finds putative miRNA binding sites in the sequence of interest, and then identifies the targeting miRNA.
- RNAhybrid [54] finds the minimum free energy hybridization of a long and a short RNA.
- TargetScan [41] computes seed-binding sites based on perfect complementarity of a seven nucleotide region conserved across five organisms (chicken, mouse, chimp, human, and dog) between bases 2–8 on the 5′ end of the miRNA.
- MicroTar evaluates miRNA–target complementarity and thermodynamic data [55].
- DIANA-microT [44], variant of miRanda, uses a modified initial base-pairing rule that focuses on the sizes of allowable bulges in initial seeds.

5.4   miRanda

In 2003, (available at http://www.microRNA.org/microRNA/home.do) Enright et al. [49] proposed *miRanda* that nowadays is the most popular miRNA target prediction method. The *miRanda* [40,49] splits the target gene prediction task into three distinct steps carried out in sequence: (1) homology evaluation; (2) free energy computation; (3) evolutionary conservation computation. In the following description of *miRanda*, we will present the values of parameters used in the last release of the package (Sept. 2008) (available at http://cbio.mskcc.org/miRanda-sept2008.tar.gz).

5.4.1   Homology Evaluation

The first step in *miRanda* is based on sequence matching: miRNA and 3′–UTR miRNA sequences are aligned in order to find sites with a certain level of

TABLE 5.1   Values of Parameters Used by _miRanda_[a]

Parameters	Notation	_miRanda_	Proposed
A:U and G:C	AU	5	1.5
G:U	GU	1	1.5
Mismatch	M	−3	−1.75
Gap opening	GO	−9	−6.5
Gap extension	GE	−4	−2.25
Scale factor	SF	4	3
Temperature (°C)	T	30	37
Homology score threshold	HT	140	32.92
Free energy threshold (kcal mol^{-1})	ΔF	−7	−5.25

[a] Release of September 2008, and those obtained for the proposed method after GA training.

complementarity, to assess if there are any potential binding sites. Sequence alignment is carried out using a slightly modified version of the Smith–Waterman algorithm [56], a dynamic-programming based technique.

The Smith–Waterman algorithm is usually used to compute subsequence alignment based on matching nucleotides. However, _miRanda_ uses it to compute alignment based on complementarity rather than match: the score matrix assigns positive scores to complementary nucleotides (AU) and G=U "wobble" pairs (GU), which are important for the accurate detection of RNA:RNA duplexes [57], and negative scores (M) to all other base pairs, as reported in Table 5.1; penalties are also applied for gap opening (GO) and extension (GE).

In addition, following observation of known target sites, the algorithm applies a scaling factor (SF) to the first 11 positions of the miRNA, to reflect 5′–3′ asymmetry, and some empirical rules: (a) no mismatches are accepted at position 3–12; (b) at least one mismatch should be present between positions 9 and L-5 (where L is total alignment length); and (c) fewer than two mismatches can be present in the last five positions of alignment. A homology threshold (HT) parameter is defined as the score for a perfect 7 nt match in the 3′–UTR side of the miRNA:

$$HT = 7 \times SF \times AU \tag{5.1}$$

The algorithm computes various nonoverlapping alignments and only those alignments whose score exceeds HT are considered potential binding sites and passed to the subsequent processing step, that is, the free energy computation, as free energy computation is a very demanding task in term of computational complexity.

5.4.2   Free Energy Computation

The second step of the _miRanda_ method is computation of the free energy (ΔG), carried out using the RNA folding routine _RNAfold_ included in the Vienna RNA secondary structure library (RNAlib) (available at http://www.tbi.univie.ac.at/RNA/)

[57]. This routine computes the secondary structure and the free energy of a single RNA sequence folding. To obtain the co-folding of miRNA and the 3'–UTR of miRNA sequences, the two sequences are joined in a single sequence with an artificial, linker sequence containing 5 'X' that cannot base pair. Again only hybridization sites whose free energy is under a given threshold (ΔF) are considered valid.

5.4.3   Evolutionary Conservation Computation

The third step of *miRanda* method is the computation of the evolutionary conservation. This is a third filter applied to binding sites that passed the previous two filtering stages. In order to reduce false positives, only predicted target sites that are conserved among different species are considered valid. The evolutionary conservation computation is carried out using *PhastCons* (available at http://compgen.bscb.cornell.edu/phast) [58, 59] that is a software tool based on a phylogenetic hidden Markov model (phylo-HMM) able to estimate the degree of sequence conservation starting from a multialignment of different sequences. *PhastCons* is not integrated in the *miRanda* code, so this computation is carried out after the execution of the *miRanda* program itself.

5.5   PROPOSED METHOD

Table 5.1 shows the parameters used in the latest release of *miRanda* (Sept. 2008): the rewards and the penalties for match and mismatch, the temperature for free energy estimation, and the thresholds on homology and free energy. All these parameters have been manually optimized in order to reduce the false positives and negatives detection of target genes according to biological knowledge available in 2003–2004, when the method was presented [40, 49], and then updated in the same way in the following years. Moreover, as already reported, the usage of the *RNAfold* function to estimate the free energy of the hybridization is tricky because this routine is optimized to compute the secondary structure folding for a single RNA sequence, and cofolding of the miRNA and miRNA sequence is obtained using an artificial linking sequence.

This chapter presents a complete rewriting and rebuilding of *miRanda*, providing some improvements and updates to the original program. Our work is aimed at obtaining a computational prediction of target sites with higher selectivity to be used for guiding the experimental validation in a more focused direction. To this aim, we exploit the updated knowledge on biologically validated miRNA gene targets available in the *Mirecords* website, using the information related to genes and miRNA involved in human PC only, as reported in the recent literature.

For free energy calculation, instead of *RNAfold*, we use the *RNAcofold* routine recently introduced in the Vienna RNA library [60]. The *RNAcofold* is specifically intended to compute the cofolding of two The RNA sequences. The RNAcofold works much like the RNAfold, but allows us to specify two RNA sequences that are then allowed to form a dimer structure. The *RNAcofold* can compute minimum free energy structures, as well as partition function and base-pairing probability matrix.

Since dimer formation is concentration dependent, *RNAcofold* can be used to compute equilibrium concentrations for all five monomer and (homo/hetero)-dimer species, given input concentrations for the monomers. Using this routine, we can obtain a reliable estimation of free energy, without using the trick related to the usage of the *RNAfold* routine.

Moreover, in our approach we do not include the third step of miRanda evaluating the evolutionary conservation, because while conservation has been a primary aspect used to filter hits in most target prediction algorithms, not all target sites are necessarily conserved [20]. See the case of target human genes for specific miRNAs. Note that other newly developed programs use machine learning approaches instead of reliance on conservation [50,55,61], even if the lack of availability of experimentally validated targets for classifier training limits the validity of their results.

In miRanda, the tuning of parameters involved in computational prediction of target sites is done manually on the basis of recent scientific literature. In our case, we studied a machine learning approach exploiting the Mirecords website. As Mirecords website and other miRNA target genes repositories report only (few) positive examples (i.e., biologically validated *miRNA* gene targets) and an even more limited number of miRNAs known to not interact with a target gene (i.e., true negatives), we decided not to apply machine learning-based methods, like neural networks or support vector machines [39]. We approached this one-class prediction problem by implementing a quick automatic parameter tuning technique based on a genetic algorithm, shown in Section 5.6.

5.6 AUTOMATIC PARAMETER TUNING

The one-class prediction approach we have implemented is based on the following assumption: Given the set U of all genes taken into account, an optimal tuning of parameters should allow us to improve the match between the set S of genes selected as predicted targets and the set V of biologically validated target genes, as reported in Mirecords (see Fig. 5.1).

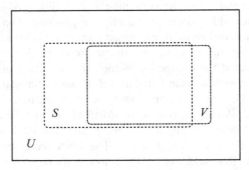

FIGURE 5.1 Here U is the set of all genes taken into account, S is the set of genes selected as predicted targets, and V is the set of biologically validated target genes.

Let us introduce the following notations: $\hat{n} \equiv |S|$, $n_v \equiv |V|$, and $\hat{n}_v \equiv |S \cap V|$, where $|X|$ is the cardinality (size) of set X. In our approach, more emphasis has been put on increasing the size $\hat{n}_v$ of the intersection of S and V (lowering the false negative rate) than on decreasing the size $\hat{n} - \hat{n}_v$ of their difference $S \setminus V$, since the goal is not to miss any of the biologically validated genes. Indeed, predicting some genes that are not validated is a desirable behavior, because these can be submitted for further lab testing, and hopefully could lead to discovery of new, experimentally validated target sites. We can express this goal as the maximization of

$$D \equiv \frac{\hat{n}_v}{n_v} \tag{5.2}$$

subject to a penalty if $\hat{n} > \hat{n}_v$, that can be expressed by a Fermi's sigmoid function:

$$D_1 \equiv \frac{\hat{n}_v}{n_v} \frac{1}{1 + e^{-(\frac{\hat{n}}{\hat{n}_v} - \mu)/s}} \qquad \mu, s \in \Re \tag{5.3}$$

To this aim, we used a genetic algorithm (GA) [7, 62], even if other global search techniques (e.g., simulated annealing [63], particle swarm optimization [64], or harmony [25]) could be employed. Genetic algorithms are global search heuristics to find exact or approximate solutions to minimization or maximization problems, and are based on techniques inspired by evolutionary biology (e.g., selection, crossover, and mutation). Genetic algorithms are implemented as a computer simulation in which a population of abstract representations (chromosomes or genotypes) of candidate solutions (individuals or phenotypes) to an optimization problem evolves toward better solutions. Traditionally, solutions are represented as binary strings (sequences of 0s and 1s), but other encodings are also possible. The evolution usually starts from a population of randomly generated individuals and happens in generations. In each generation, the fitness of every individual in the population is evaluated, multiple individuals are randomly selected from the current population (on the basis of their fitness), and recombined and mutated to form a new population. The new population is then used in the next iteration of the algorithm. The GA terminates when either a maximum number of generations has been produced, or a satisfactory fitness level has been reached for the population.

5.7 EXPERIMENTAL ANALYSIS

5.7.1 Data Set Considered

Candidate target genes have been selected from among those that are involved in pathways related to PC. These targets were obtained from different sources. The first source is [65], where three subtypes of PC are identified at the molecular level and a notable clinical relevance of the subtypes is observed. This study includes a selection of the genes found to be the most discriminative between one subtype and the other two. Another source is [14], where the specific role of two, closely related miRNAs

TABLE 5.2   GA—Genotype/Phenotype

Parameters	Notation	Bits	Interval
A:U and G:C	AU	5	[1,70.75]
G:U	GU	5	[−3, 4.75]
Mismatch	M	5	[−8,−0.75]
Gap opening	GO	5	[−12,−4.75]
Gap extension	GE	5	[−8,−0.25]
Homology score threshold variation	HV	8	[−0.32, 0.32]
Free energy threshold (kcal mol^{-1})	ΔF	8	[−64,0]
Scale factor	SF	3	[2,9]

(miR-15a and miR-16-1) have been experimentally observed in PC. These studies suggest the use of a set of genes from which we have selected an overall data set of 50. We focused on miR-1, a miRNA proven to be involved in mechanisms related to PC [13, 15]. Eight of the genes in the data set are reported as a biologically validated target for miR-1 on the Mirecords website. The available data set of candidate target genes was randomly split into two data sets of 25 each, labeled as A and B, containing four validated targets each. Training was performed with miR-1 on data set B, and the resulting parameters have been used for testing on data set A by cross-validation.

5.7.2   Search Methodology

The tuning of the parameters has been performed by using the GALOPPS 3.2.4 (available at http://garage.cse.msu.edu/software/galopps/) package [66] by Goodman that extends and optimizes the implementation of the simple genetic algorithm (SGA) [7]. We used D_1, Eq. (5.3), as the fitness function. In the third column, Table 5.2 shows the size in bits of the fields of the chromosome assigned to the different parameters of our method (referred to the "genotype"), and in the fourth column the range of the intervals assigned to them (in terms of the "phenotype", i.e., the actual values). All integer values in the genotype, except for the scale factor, are treated as fixed-point numbers with 2 bits for the fractional part. The homology threshold variation (HV) parameter is defined as a percentage variation from the theoretical threshold resulting from Eq. (5.1) and the parameters from the phenotype. The GA parameters have been selected after many attempts and are presented in Table 5.3.

The training task on training set B was repeated several times with different random seeds. In Section 5.2.3, we report the result with the best performances on the test set A.

5.7.3   Results

On a single core Intel laptop with 1600 MHz clock and Linux operating system, the GA finds an optimal solution in 10 min, after 14 generations (iterations) with $\hat{n} = 4$ and $\hat{n}_v = 3$. The values of tuned parameters are shown in column three of Table 5.1.

On the left of Table 5.4, we report the results obtained by the training on data set B and on the test set A. Column three shows the candidate target genes found, column

TABLE 5.3   Selected Parameters for GA Training

Parameter	Value
s Eq. (5.3)	−1
μ Eq. (5.3)	0.69
Probability of mutation	0.01
Crossover probability	0.7
Crossover type	Simple
Selection method	Tournament on five randomly selected individuals
Number of individuals in a generation	50
Maximum number of generations	100

TABLE 5.4   Results on hsa-miR-1[a]

Proposed method on training set ($R = 0.60$)				
Rank	Data Set	Gene	Free Energy	Validated
1	B	CSPG2	−15.1	
2	B	FBLN2	−12.6	v
3	B	EML4	−11.2	v
4	B	MMD	−10.3	v

miRanda on training set ($R = 0.28$)				
Rank	Data Set	Gene	Free Energy	Validated
1	B	CSPG2	−16.59	
2	B	BCL2	−16.53	
3	B	PLS3	−13.73	
4	B	EML4	−12.57	v
5	B	MMD	−12.54	v
6	B	FBLN2	−11.17	v

Proposed method on test set ($R = 0.83$)				
Rank	Data Set	Gene	Free Energy	Validated
1	A	NETO2	−18.2	v
2	A	ARF3	−12.3	v
3	A	COL1A1	−12.2	

miRanda on test set ($R = 0.5$)				
Rank	Data Set	Gene	Free Energy	Validated
1	A	NETO2	−19.49	v
2	A	CCND1	−15.71	
3	A	HDAC9	−12.32	
4	A	ARF3	−11.59	v

[a] Free energies are in kcal/mol^{-1}.

four shows their free energy, and the last column indicates if the gene is reported as biologically validated on the Mirecords website.

On the right side of the same table, we report the results obtained with miRanda using its original parameters [49] presented in column two of Table 5.1.

Note that the 3'–UTR region of a miRNA can contain multiple target sites for an assigned miRNA. In the shown results site, multiplicity is not taken into account.

As in miRanda and the proposed method, the free energies are computed according to two different library routines (*RNAfold* vs *RNAcofold*), and we cannot compare their absolute values. Therefore, we rank the target genes according to their free energy values, so that we can compare ranks instead of actual values. Note that the validated targets with the proposed method are consistently at the highest positions of the list (where the most negative value is the best); this does not hold for miRanda.

To objectively assess this fact, we compare the results obtained by the two methods by using the following performance index ranging in the interval [0, 1]:

$$R \equiv \frac{2}{\hat{n}(\hat{n}+1)} \sum_{i \in S} v(i) \cdot (\hat{n} + 1 - r(i))$$
$$= \frac{2}{\hat{n}} \left(\hat{n}_v - \frac{1}{\hat{n}+1} \sum_{i \in S} v(i) \cdot (r(i)) \right) \tag{5.4}$$

where: $r(i)$ is the rank of the target gene in the list of results, ordered by the value of free energy; $v(i)$ is 1 if the target is validated in miRecords, 0 otherwise. In both data sets, the performance index R of the proposed method is higher than that obtained using miRanda, showing that our method is more selective.

Note that, given the lack of validated miRNA targets (true positives) and validated nontargets (true negatives) in Mirecords and in the other the available databases, it is not possible to perform a depth comparison of the two target prediction algorithms on the basis of more standard metrics for sensitivity and selectivity.

5.8   DISCUSSION AND CONCLUSIONS

As available methods for miRNA discovering miRNA targets are not high throughput, and in general are not completely satisfactory, a large number of target prediction algorithms have been developed, but they show low sensibility and selectivity. Consequently, there are several target genes reported as experimentally validated in databases like miRBase [31] and miRNAMAP [35], Mirecords, Argonaute [36], TarBase [37, 38], that are not predicted by any method or for which the methods seldom agree. Moreover, as the experimental approaches to miRNA targets validation are unable to detect the specific miRNA target site, even when the same target gene is experimentally validated by the biological procedure and predicted by a computational method, this concordance cannot be considered a final validation.

This chapter presented a complete rewriting and rebuilding of the *miRanda* tool [40, 49] aimed at obtaining a more reliable computational prediction of target sites. Our approach makes use of the updated knowledge about biologically validated miRNA gene targets, especially those related to PC, which is available in the *Mirecords* website for tuning the parameters using a GA. We apply the *RNA-cofold* routine for free energy calculation recently introduced in the Vienna RNA library [60], and we do not include the third step of miRanda evaluating the evolutionary conservation, since in the case of target human genes for specific miRNAs not all target sites are necessarily conserved [20].

The proposed approach shows a higher selectivity than *miRanda* and can be considered a good candidate for guiding the experimental validation in a well-focused direction. Moreover, we achieve fast parameter tuning instead of the long manual process needed for other tools, (e.g., *miRanda*), thanks to the application of the GA. Moreover, as the base of known miRNAs grows with new experimentally validated target sites, the procedure presented in this chapter can be used to refine the method to reflect the increased knowledge, in an incremental way.

Note that other criteria than those considered may be important in identifying target sites [67]. Future studies involving other mechanisms may lead to even better reliability of the computational methods with respect to biological evidence.

In the presented work, we used the biological knowledge available on PC. Using the different biological knowledge available, one can extend this approach to the discovering of miRNA target genes for different pathologies.

As larger numbers of validated miRNA targets (true positives) and validated nontargets (true negatives) will become available, methods like the one presented, but developed on a larger scale (more candidate genes, more miRNAs), may lead to even better results. Moreover, it will be possible to develop accurate miRNA target prediction algorithms, using, for example, neural networks or support vector machines [39]. Moreover, it will be possible to perform depth comparisons of target prediction algorithms based on metrics for sensitivity and selectivity.

ACKNOWLEDGMENTS

This work was partially supported by Human Health Foundation, S.H.R.O., and University of Genova. We thank Alessandro Parini for programming support.

REFERENCES

1. R. C. Lee, R. L. Feinbaum, and V. Ambros (1993), The C-Elegans Heterochronic Gene Lin-4 Encodes Small Rnas with Antisense Complementarity to Lin-14, *Cell*, 75:843–54.

2. G. Ruvkun (2001), Molecular biology. Glimpses of a tiny RNA world, *Science*, 294:797–139.

3. R. Ciarapica, G. Russo, F. Verginelli, L. Raimondi, A. Donfrancesco, R. Rota, and A. Giordano (2009), Deregulated expression of miR-26a and Ezh2 in Rhabdomyosarcoma, *Cell Cycle*, 8:172–175.

4. W. J. Lukiw (2007), Micro-RNA speciation in fetal, adult and Alzheimer's disease hippocampus, *Neuroreport*, 18:297–300.

5. J. Kim, K. Inoue, J. Ishii, W. B. Vanti, S. V. Voronov, E. Murchison, G. Hannon, and A. Abeliovich (2007), A microRNA Feedback Circuit in Midbrain Dopamine Neurons, *Science*, 317:1220–1224.

6. D. Eletto, G. Russo, G. Passiatore, L. Del Valle, A. Giordano, K. Khalili, E. Gualco, and F. Peruzzi (2008), Inhibition of SNAP25 expression by HIV-1 Tat involves the activity of mir-128a, *J. Cellular Physiol.*, 216:764–770.

7. D. E. Goldberg (1989), *Genetic Algorithms in Search, Optimization and Machine Learning*, Addison-Wesley, Longman Publishing Co., Inc., Boston.

8. YS. Lee, HK. Kim, S. Chung, KS. Kim, and A. Dutta (2005), Depletion of human microRNA miR-125b reveals that it is critical for the proliferation of differentiated cells but not for the down-regulation of putative targets during differentiation, *J. Biol. Chem.*, 280:16635–16641.

9. X. Z. Cai, C. H. Hagedorn, and B. R. Cullen (2004), Human microRNAs are processed from capped, polyadenylated transcripts that can also function as mRNAs, *RNA*, 10:1957–1966.

10. A. M. Denli, B. B. Tops, R. H. Plasterk, R. F. Ketting, and G. J. Hannon (2004), Processing of primary microRNAs by the Microprocessor complex, *Nature (London)*, 432:231–35.

11. A. Esquela-Kerscher and F. J. Slack (2006), Oncomirs - microRNAs with a role in cancer, *Nat. Rev. Cancer.*, 6:259–69.

12. N. Yanaihara, et al. (2006), Unique microRNA molecular profiles in lung cancer diagnosis and prognosis, *Cancer Cell*, 9:189–198.

13. S. Ambs, R. L. Prueitt, M. Yi, R. S. Hudson, T. M. Howe, F. Petrocca, T. A. Wallace, C.-G. Liu, S. Volinia, G. A. Calin, H. G. Yfantis, R. M. Stephens, and C. M. Croce (2008), Genomic Profiling of microRNA and Messenger RNA Reveals Deregulated microRNA Expression in Prostate Cancer, *Cancer Res*, 68:6162–6170.

14. D. Bonci, V. Coppola, M. Musumeci, A. Addario, L. D'Urso, D. Collura, C. Peschle, R. De Maria, and G. Muto (2008), The miR-15a/miR-16-1 cluster controls prostate cancer progression by targeting multiple oncogenic activities, *Eur. Urol. Suppl.*, 7:271.

15. T. Bagnyukova, I. Pogribny, and V. Chekhun (2006), MicroRNAs in normal and cancer cells: a new class of gene expression regulators, *Exp. Oncol.*, 28:263–269.

16. M. V. Iorio et al. (2005), MicroRNA gene expression deregulation in human breast cancer, *Cancer Res.*, 65:7065–7070.

17. Y. Karube (2005), Reduced expression of Dicer associated with poor prognosis in lung cancer patients, *Cancer Sci.*, 96:111–115.

18. M. Z. Michael, S. M. O'Connor, N. G. van Holst Pellekaan, G. P. Young, and R. J. James (2002), Reduced accumulation of specific microRNAs in colorectal neoplasia, *Mol. Cancer Res.*, 1:882–891.

19. G. A. Calin et al. (2002), Frequent deletions and down-regulation of micro-RNA genes miR15 and miR16 at 13q14 in chronic lymphocytic leukemia, *Proc. Natl. Acad. Sci. USA*, 99:15524–15529.

20. Y. Xi, J. R. Edwards, and J. Jul (2007), Investigation of miRNA Biology by Bioinformatic Tools and Impact of miRNAs in Colorectal Cancer: Regulatory Relationship of c-Myc and p53 with miRNAs, *Cancer Inform.*, 3:245–253.

21. M.L. Gonzalgo and W.B. Isaacs (2003), Molecular pathways to prostate cancer, *MJ Urol.*, 170:2444–2452.

22. A. Jemal, et al. (2003), Cancer statistics, *CA Cancer J. Clin.*, 53:5–26.

23. J. Jiang, E. J. Lee, Y. Gusev, and T. D. Schmittgen (2005), Real-time expression profiling of microRNA precursors in human cancer cell lines, *Nucleic Acids Res.*, 33:5394–5403.

24. AR. Kore, M. Hodeib, and Z. Hu (2008), Chemical Synthesis of LNA-mCTP and its application for MicroRNA detection, *Nucleosides Nucleotides Nucleic Acids*, 27:1–7.

25. K. S. Lee and Z. W. Geem (2005), A new meta-heuristic algorithm for continuous engineering optimization: harmony search theory and practice, *Computer Methods Appl. Mech. Eng.*, 194:3902–3933.

26. S. L. Lin, A. Chiang, D. Chang, and S. Y. Ying (2008), Loss of mir-146a function in hormone-refractory prostate cancer, *RNA*, 14:417–424.

27. A. Musiyenko, V. Bitko, and S. Barik (2008), Ectopic expression of miR-126*, an intronic product of the vascular endothelial EGF-like 7 gene, regulates prostein translation and invasiveness of prostate cancer LNCaP cells. *J. Mol. Med.*, 86:313–322.

28. Y. Sylvestre et al. (2007), An E2F/miR-20avautoregulatory feedback loop, *J. Biol. Chem.*, 282:2135–2143.

29. E. Berezikov, V. Guryev, J. van de Belt, E. Wienholds, RHA. Plasterk, and E. Cuppen (2005), Phylogenetic shadowing and computational identification of human microRNA genes, *Cell*, 120:21–24.

30. I. Bentwich, A. Avniel, Y. Karov, R. Aharonov, S. Gilad, O. Barad, A. Barzilai, P. Einat, U. Einav, E. Meiri, E. Sharon, Y. Spector, Z. Bentwich (2005), Identification of hundreds of conserved and nonconserved human microRNAs, *Natl. Genet.*, 37:766–70.

31. S. Griffiths-Jones (2006), miRBase: the microRNA sequence database, *Methods Mol. Biol.* 342:129–138.

32. B. J. Reinhart et al. (2000), The 21-nucleotide let-7 RNA regulates developmental timing in Caenorhabditis elegans, *Nature (London)*, 403:901–906.

33. X. J. Wang, J. L. Reyes, N. H. Chua, and T. Gaasterland (2004), Prediction and identification of Arabidopsis thaliana microRNAs and their mRNA targets, *Genome Biol.*, 5:R65.

34. S. Davis, B. Lollo, S. Freier, and C. Esau (2006), Improved targeting of miRNA with antisense oligonucleotides, *Nucleic Acids Res.*, 34:2294–304.

35. P. W. Hsu et al. (2006), miRNAMap: genomic maps of microRNA genes and their target genes in mammalian genomes, *Nucleic Acids Res.*, 34:D135–9.

36. P. Shahi et al. (2006), Argonaute: A database for gene regulation by mammalian microRNAs, *Nucleic Acids Res.*, 34:D115–118.

37. M. Megraw, P. Sethupathy, B. Corda, and A. G. Hatzigeorgiou (2007), miRGen: a database for the study of animal microRNA genomic organization and function, *Nucleic Acids Res.*, 35:D149–155.

38. P. Sethupathy, B. Corda, and A. G. Hatzigeorgiou (2006), TarBase: A comprehensive database of experimentally supported animal microRNA targets, *RNA*, 12:192–197.

39. S. Haykin (2008), Neural networks and learning machines, 3rd ed., Prentice-Hall, NY.

40. B. John, A. J. Enright, A. Aravin, T. Tuschl, C. Sander, and D. S. Marks (2004), Human MicroRNA targets, *Plos Biol.*, 2:1862–1879.

41. B. P. Lewis, I.-H. Shih, M. W. Jones-Rhoades, D. P. Bartel, and C. B. Burge (2003), Prediction of Mammalian microRNA Targets, *Cell*, 115:787–798.

42. J. Brennecke, A. Stark, R. B. Russell, and S. M. Cohen (2005), Principles of MicroRNA-target recognition, *Plos. Biol.*, 3:404–418.

43. J. G. Doench and P. A. Sharp (2004), Specificity of microRNA target selection in translational repression, *Genes Dev.*, 18:504–11.

44. M. Kiriakidou, P. T. Nelson, A. Kouranov, P. Fitziev, C. Bouyioukos, Z. Mourelatos, and A. Hatzigeorgiou (2004), A combined computational-experimental approach predicts human microRNA targets, *Genes Dev.*, 18:1165–1178.

45. D. Grun, YL. Wang, D. Langenberger, KC. Gunsalus, and N. Rajewsky (2005), microRNA target predictions across seven Drosophila species and comparison to mammalian targets, *Plos. Comput. Biol.*, 1:e13.

46. B. John, C. Sander, and D. S. Marks (2006), Prediction of human microRNA targets, *Methods Mol. Biol.*, 342:101–113.

47. B. P. Lewis, C. B. Burge, and D. P. Bartel (2005), Conserved seed pairing, often flanked by adenosines, indicates that thousands of human genes are microRNA targets, *Cell*, 120:15–20.

48. P. Sethupathy, M. Megraw, and A. G. Hatzigeorgiou (2006), A guide through present computational approaches for the identification of mammalian microRNA targets, *Nat. Methods*, 3:881–886.

49. A. J. Enright, B. John, U. Gaul, T. Tuschl, C. Sander, and D. S. Marks (2003), microRNA targets in Drosophila, *Genome Biol.*, 5.

50. S.-K. Kim, J.-W. Nam, J.-K. Rhee, W.-J. Lee, and B.-T. Zhang (2006), miTarget: microRNA target-gene prediction using a Support Vector Machine, *BMC Bioinformatics*, 7:411.

51. A. Krek, D. Grün, M. N. Poy, R. Wolf, L. Rosenberg, E. J. Epstein, P. Macmenamin, I. d. da Piedade, K. C. Gunsalus, M. Stoffel, and N. Rajewsky (2005), Combinatorial microRNA target predictions, *Nature Genet.*, 37:495–500.

52. M. Kertesz, N. Iovino, U. Unnerstall, U. Gaul, and E. Segal (2007), The role of site accessibility in microRNA target recognition, *Nat. Genet.*, 39:1278–1284.

53. K. C. Miranda, T. Huynh, Y. Tay, Y.-S. Ang, W.-L. Tam, A. M. Thomson, B. Lim, and I. Rigoutsos (2006), A Pattern-Based Method for the Identification of microRNA Binding Sites and Their Corresponding Heteroduplexes, *Cell*, 126:1203–1217.

54. M. Rehmsmeier, P. Steffen, M. Hochsmann, and R. Giegerich (2004), Fast and effective prediction of microRNA/target duplexes, *RNA*, 10:1507–1517.

55. R. Thadani and MT. Tammi (2006), MicroTar: predicting microRNA targets from RNA duplexes, *BMC Bioinformatics*, 7:S20.

56. T. F. Smith and M. S. Waterman (1981), Identification of common molecular subsequences, *J. Mol. Biol.*, 147:195–197.

57. S. Wuchty, W. Fontana, I. L. Hofacker, and P. Schuster (1999), Complete suboptimal folding of RNA and the stability of secondary structures, *Biopolymers*, 49:145–165.

58. J. Felsenstein and G. A. Churchill (1996), A hidden Markov model approach to variation among sites in rate of evolution, *Mol. Biol. Evol.*, 13:93–104.

59. A. Siepel, G. Bejerano, J. S. Pedersen, A. S. Hinrichs, M. Hou, K. Rosenbloom, H. Clawson, J. Spieth, L. W. Hillier, S. Richards, G. M. Weinstock, R. K. Wilson,

R. A. Gibbs, W. J. Kent, W. Miller, and D. Haussler (2005), Evolutionarily conserved elements in vertebrate, insect, worm, and yeast genomes, *Genome Res.*, 15:1034–1050.

60. S. H. Bernhart, H. Tafer, U. Mückstein, C. Flamm, P. F. Stadler, and I. L. Hofacker (2006), Partition function and base pairing probabilities of RNA heterodimers, *Algorithms for Mol. Biol.*, 1:3.

61. X. Yan, et al. (2007), Improving the prediction of human microRNA target genes by using ensemble algorithm, *FEBS Lett.*, 17:581:1587–93.

62. Z. Michalewicz (1996), Genetic Algorithms + Data Structures—Evolution Programs, Springer-Verlag, NY.

63. C. D. Kirkpatrick, S. Gelatt, and M. P. Vecchi (1983), Optimization by simulated annealing, *Science*, 220:671–680.

64. J. Kennedy, R. C. Eberhart, and Y. Shi (2001), *Swarm Intelligence*, Morgan Kaufmann Publishers, San Francisco.

65. J. Lapointe, C. Li, J. P. Higgins, M. van de Rijn, E. Bair, K. Montgomery, M. Ferrari, L. Egevad, W. Rayford, U. Bergerheim, P. Ekman, A. M. Demarzo, R. Tibshirani, D. Botstein, P. O. Brown, J. D. Brooks, and J. R. Pollack (2004), Gene expression profiling identifies clinically relevant subtypes of prostate cancer, *Proc. Nat. Acad. Sci.*, 101:811–816.

66. E. Goodman (1996), Galopps, the genetic algorithm optimized for portability and parallelism system, users guide, Genetic Algorithms Research and Applications Group (GARAGe), Michigan State University, Tech. Rep.

67. M. Hammell, D. Long, L. Zhang, A. Lee, C. S. S. Carmack, M. Han, Y. Ding, and V. Ambros (2008), mirwip: microRNA target prediction based on microRNA-containing ribonucleoprotein-enriched transcripts, *Nature Methods*.

PART III

STRUCTURE ANALYSIS

6

STRUCTURAL SEARCH IN RNA MOTIF DATABASES

DONGRONG WEN AND JASON T. L. WANG

6.1 INTRODUCTION

Ribonucleic acid (RNA) is transcribed from deoxyribonucleic acid (DNA) and plays a key role in the synthesis of proteins [1]. An RNA structural motif is a substructure of an RNA molecule that has a significant biological function. Well-known RNA structural motifs include the iron response element (IRE) and histone 3'-UTR stem-loop (HSL3) [2, 3]. As increasingly more RNA structural motifs are discovered, it becomes crucial to have databases holding the motifs that can be accessed and used by researchers. For example, Rfam [4] and RNA STRAND [5] are two such databases.

Rfam is a well-annotated, open access database containing information on noncoding RNA (ncRNA) families as well as other RNA structural motifs. The latest version of Rfam 9.0, comprising 603 families in total, is available at http://rfam.sanger.ac.uk/. In Rfam, each ncRNA family is represented by two structure-annotated multiple sequence alignments (MSAs). One MSA is called the seed alignment and the other is called the full alignment. Each multiple sequence alignment is associated with a consensus secondary structure, represented in Stockholm format [6, 7]. The seed alignment consists of functionally related RNA sequences obtained from the literature or wet lab experiments. The seed alignment is used to build a covariance model used by the Infernal program [6] to collect additional functionally related RNA sequences. These additional RNA sequences obtained from the Infernal program are added to the full alignment.

Rfam is equipped with several different search methods. By entering a query sequence, the user can search the covariance models representing the 603 noncoding

Computational Intelligence and Pattern Analysis in Biological Informatics, Edited by Ujjwal Maulik, Sanghamitra Bandyopadhyay, and Jason T. L. Wang

RNA families in Rfam. Since the computational cost involved with covariance models is high, Rfam employs BLAST as a filter to speed up searches. When a search is completed, the search result shows the RNA families that have a high degree of similarity to the input query sequence. The user can view and browse the RNA families displayed in the search result. In addition to the search-by-sequence method, Rfam allows the user to search the ncRNA families stored in its database via keyword and EMBL ID or accession number. The entire Rfam database can also be downloaded in plain text format from the Rfam website and searched offline locally using the Infernal program [6] on the user's own computer.

While Rfam provides keyword- and sequence-based search methods, it lacks structure-based search methods. Many functionally related ncRNAs differ at the sequence level but are similar in their secondary structures. Thus, it is desirable to have structure-based search engines on RNA motif databases. This chapter presents two structural search engines developed in our lab. The first search engine is installed on a database, called RmotifDB [8], which contains secondary structures of the ncRNA sequences in Rfam. The second search engine is installed on a block database, which contains the 603 seed alignments, also called blocks, in Rfam. This search engine employs a novel tool, called BlockMatch, for comparing multiple sequence alignments. We report some experimental results to demonstrate the effectiveness of the BlockMatch tool.

6.2 THE SEARCH ENGINE ON RMOTIFDB

This section presents the structure-based search engine on RmotifDB. This search engine employs our previously developed program, called RSmatch [9], for comparing two RNA sequences taking into account their secondary structures. In what follows, we first review the RSmatch tool and then describe RmotifDB and its structural search engine.

6.2.1 RSmatch

Functional RNA motifs may be detected by aligning the secondary structures of RNA sequences on which the motifs exist. Many software tools have been developed to find the RNA motifs by aligning the RNA secondary structures. However, existing software tools suffer from some drawbacks. They either require a large number of prealigned RNA sequences or have high time complexities. Therefore, these tools have difficulty in processing RNAs without prealigned sequences or in handling large RNA structure databases.

RSmatch is a software tool designed for comparing RNA secondary structures and for motif detection. The RSmatch algorithm is fast; its time complexity is $O(mn)$, where m is the length of a query RNA structure and n is the length of a subject RNA structure. The algorithm decomposes an RNA secondary structure into a collection of structure components. To capture the structural particularities of RNA, RSmatch uses a tree model to organize these structure components. The tool compares a pair of RNA secondary structures using two separate scoring matrices in performing local and global alignments. One scoring matrix is used for single-stranded regions and the other is used for double-stranded regions. When searching an RNA structure database, RSmatch can detect similar RNA substructures, and perform an iterative database search and multiple structure alignment. These operations enable the identification and discovery of functional RNA structural motifs.

By conducting experiments with instances of known RNA structural motifs, including simple stem-loops and complex structures with junctions, we have demonstrated that in detecting the RNA structural motifs, the accuracy of RSmatch is high compared with other software tools [9]. RSmatch is especially useful to scientists and researchers interested in aligning RNA structural motifs obtained from RNA folding programs or wet lab experiments where the size of the RNA structure data set is large. The software is available from http://datalab.njit.edu/biodata/rna/RSmatch/software.htm. Figure 6.1 presents a screenshot illustrating the execution of RSmatch's database search function in the Unix command line environment.

6.2.2   The RmotifDB System

RSmatch offers an efficient algorithm for aligning two RNA structures, along with a basic RNA database search capability, but it must be run offline on a user's local

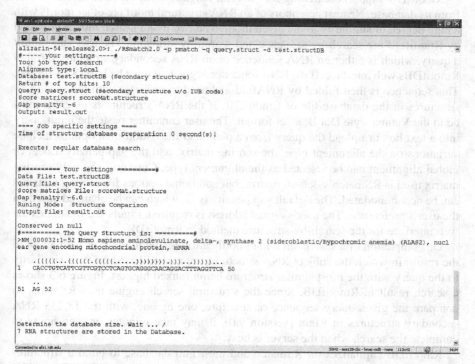

FIGURE 6.1   A screenshot showing the execution of RSmatch in Unix.

machine, which is a major drawback. Even RADAR (http://datalab.njit.edu/biodata/rna/RSmatch/server.htm) [10, 11], a descendant of RSmatch with an excellent web interface for aligning two RNA structures, does not contain a search method for a large database. In Section 6.2.1, we observed that there are provisions for sequence and keyword searching in the Rfam database, but not structure searching. To intensively study RNA structural functions or motifs, a structure-based search engine for RNA motif databases is needed. With this motivation, we have built RmotifDB, which is equipped with a structural search engine and is available at http://datalab.njit.edu/bioinfo/singleseq_index.html.

To build the database for RmotifDB, the plain text seed alignment file with 603 ncRNA families is downloaded from the Rfam 9.0 website. A total of 18,233 ncRNA sequences are extracted from this seed alignment file. Each of these sequences is then folded using the Vienna RNA package's RNAfold [12] to obtain its secondary structure. Finally, the entire 18,233 ncRNA sequences along with their secondary structures are stored in a single plain text file, which constitutes the major database file for RmotifDB. The RSmatch version 2.0 is used by the structural search engine of RmotifDB. The RSmatch 2.0 software is downloaded from the RADAR website. The implementation uses a perl-cgi approach to integrate the system's web interface with RSmatch. This allows the use of the structural search engine over the web via a browser.

RmotifDB supports searching for "nearest neighbors" of RNA structural motifs from its database. Nearest neighbors of an RNA structural motif are other motifs with a high degree of similarity to the given motif. The two major search modes provided by RmotifDB are search-by-sequence and search-by-structure. The user can submit a query, which is either an RNA sequence or an RNA secondary structure, through RmotifDBs web interface. If the RNA sequence is given, it must be in FASTA format. This sequence is then folded by RNAfold and used to compare with the secondary structures in the database file of RmotifDB. If the RNA structure is given, it must be in the Vienna style Dot Bracket format. The user can either paste the input query into a text box or upload the query from a plain text file. Additional options include variations on the alignment type, the scoring matrix, and the gap penalty. Local or global alignment can be selected as the alignment type. Currently, the only scoring matrix used is RSmatch's default matrix, but additional options for scoring matrices can be accommodated. The default gap penalty is -2, which can be changed based on the user's preference. The user's e-mail address is required. Figure 6.2 illustrates the web interface for the search-by-structure method in RmotifDB.

On completion of a search, an e-mail notification is sent to the user with a link to the result, in which the subject RNA structures are ranked based on their similarity to the query with the most similar structure being ranked highest. Figure 6.3 shows a search result in RmotifDB. Since the structural search engine uses RSmatch to compare the given query sequence or structure, one by one, with the 18,233 RNA secondary structures in Rfam (version 9.0), it may take minutes or even hours to complete the search when the server is busy.

RmotifDB capitalizes on RSmatch and the Rfam database to build a structure-based search engine. By providing a convenient browser-style interface, RmotifDB

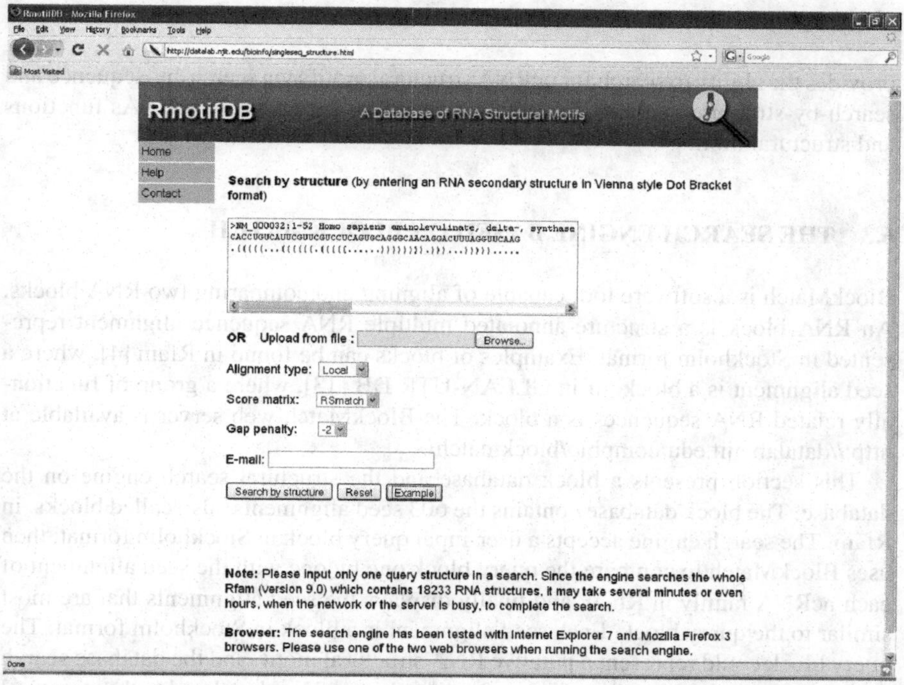

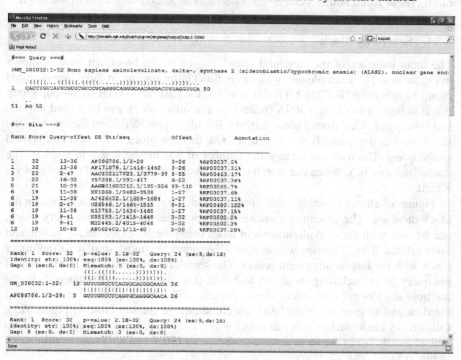

FIGURE 6.2 The web interface of RmotifDBs search-by-structure method.

FIGURE 6.3 An example search result in RmotifDB.

provides the ability to search for ncRNA structural motifs via search-by-sequence and search-by-structure methods, benefiting researchers interested in ncRNAs functions and structural motifs.

6.3   THE SEARCH ENGINE BASED ON BLOCKMATCH

BlockMatch is a software tool capable of aligning and comparing two RNA blocks. An RNA block is a structure-annotated multiple RNA sequence alignment represented in Stockholm format. Examples of blocks can be found in Rfam [4], where a seed alignment is a block, or in GLEAN-UTR DB [13], where a group of functionally related RNA sequences is a block. The BlockMatch web server is available at http://datalab.njit.edu/compbio/blockmatch/.

This section presents a block database and the structural search engine on the database. The block database contains the 603 seed alignments, also called blocks, in Rfam. The search engine accepts a user-input query block in Stockholm format, then uses BlockMatch to compare the query block one by one with the seed alignment of each ncRNA family in Rfam, and finally displays the seed alignments that are most similar to the query block. Each seed alignment is a block in Stockholm format. The query block could represent a putative RNA structural motif, and the database search function allows the detection of Rfam families that are closely related to the structural motif. These Rfam families can be considered as structural neighbors of the motif.

6.3.1   Search by Block

The input interface of the structural search engine on the block database is shown in Figure 6.4. The example query block, in Stockholm format, in the figure is called group 3 taken from GLEAN-UTR DB, which is the Histone $3'$-UTR stem–loop group found in human messenger RNA (mRNAs). The query block can be pasted into the text box or uploaded from a plain text file. If a file is provided, then the block in the file is used as the query. If no file is uploaded, then the block in the text box is used as the query. The user can change the number of hits he/she wants to display. The default number is 5. When the search result is available, the user will be notified via e-mail.

Figure 6.5 shows a sample result obtained from the structural search engine on the block database. The structural search engine compares the user-input query block, one by one, with the seed alignments in Rfam using the BlockMatch algorithm, and finds related Rfam families whose seed alignments are most similar to the query block with the largest alignment scores. The search result consists of a summary of the query block including its length and size, (i.e., the number of sequences in the multiple alignment of the query block, the date and time of query submission, and the date and time of the completed search, shown in the top table in Figure 6.5), followed by the Rfam families that are closely related to the query block, with the top ranked family being the most similar to the query block (shown in the bottom table in Fig. 6.5).

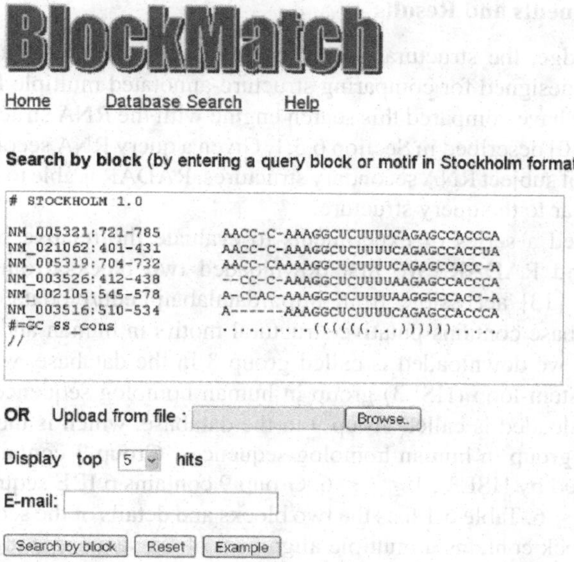

BlockMatch

Home   Database Search   Help

Search by block (by entering a query block or motif in Stockholm format)

```
# STOCKHOLM 1.0

NM_005321:721-785      AACC-C-AAAGGCUCUUUUCAGAGCCACCCA
NM_021062:401-431      AACC-C-AAAGGCUCUUUUCAGAGCCACCUA
NM_005319:704-732      AACC-CAAAAGGCUCUUUUCAGAGCCACC-A
NM_003526:412-438      --CC-C-AAAGGCUCUUUUAAGAGCCACCCA
NM_002105:545-578      A-CCAC-AAAGGCCCUUUUAAGGGCUCACC-A
NM_003516:510-534      A------AAAGGCUCUUUUCAGAGCCACCCA
#=GC ss_cons           .........((((((....))))))......
//
```

OR   Upload from file : [   ] Browse..

Display top [5 ▼] hits

E-mail: [   ]

[Search by block] [Reset] [Example]

FIGURE 6.4   The web interface of the structural search engine based on BlockMatch.

BlockMatch

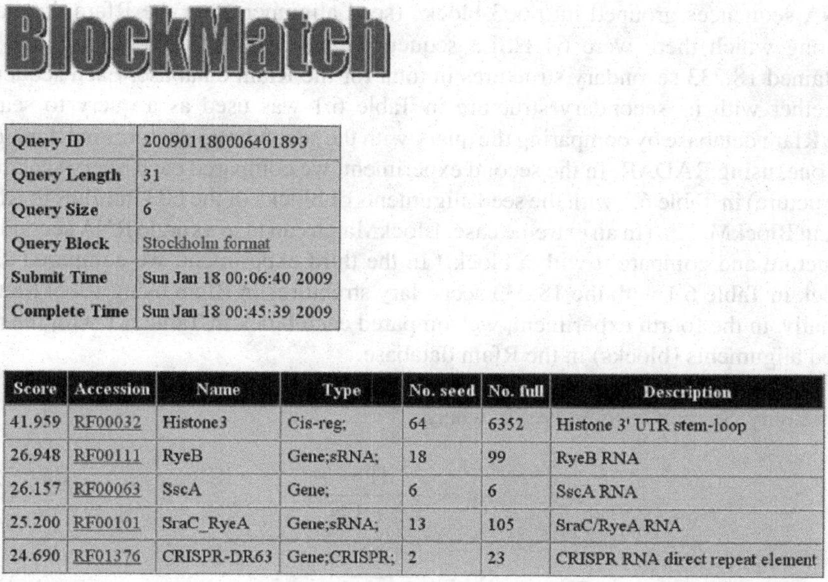

Query ID	200901180006401893
Query Length	31
Query Size	6
Query Block	Stockholm format
Submit Time	Sun Jan 18 00:06:40 2009
Complete Time	Sun Jan 18 00:45:39 2009

Score	Accession	Name	Type	No. seed	No. full	Description
41.959	RF00032	Histone3	Cis-reg;	64	6352	Histone 3' UTR stem-loop
26.948	RF00111	RyeB	Gene;sRNA;	18	99	RyeB RNA
26.157	RF00063	SscA	Gene;	6	6	SscA RNA
25.200	RF00101	SraC_RyeA	Gene;sRNA;	13	105	SraC/RyeA RNA
24.690	RF01376	CRISPR-DR63	Gene;CRISPR;	2	23	CRISPR RNA direct repeat element

FIGURE 6.5   A sample result returned by the structural search engine based on BlockMatch.

6.3.2 Experiments and Results

To our knowledge, the structural search engine based on BlockMatch is the first one of its kind designed for comparing structure-annotated multiple RNA sequence alignments. We have compared this search engine with the RNA structure alignment tool RADAR [10] described in Section 6.3.1. Given a query RNA secondary structure and a database of subject RNA secondary structures, RADAR is able to find the subject structures similar to the query structure.

We conducted a series of experiments to evaluate the relative performance of BlockMatch and RADAR. We first downloaded two blocks from the GLEAN-UTR database [13] accessible from http://datalab.njit.edu/biodata/GLEAN-UTR-DB/. This database contains putative structural motifs in human and mouse UTRs. The first block we downloaded is called group 3 in the database, which is the Histone 3'-UTR stem-loop (HSL3) group in human homolog sequences. The second block we downloaded is called group 9 in the database, which is the Iron response element (IRE) group in human homolog sequences. Group 3 contains 6 HSL3 sequences, denoted by $HSL3_i$, $1 \le i \le 6$. Group 9 contains 6 IRE sequences, denoted by IRE_i, $1 \le i \le 6$. Table 6.1 lists the two blocks and details of the sequences in each block. Each block contains a multiple alignment of six sequences together with the consensus secondary structure of the sequences.

In the first experiment, we used the Vienna RNA package's RNAfold [12,14] to fold each sequence in the two blocks in Table 6.1 to obtain 12 secondary structures, and to fold the sequences in Rfam release 9.0 into secondary structures. There were 18,233 RNA sequences grouped into 603 blocks (seed alignments) in the Rfam database, among which there were 64 HSL3 sequences and 39 IRE sequences; hence we obtained 18,233 secondary structures in total for the Rfam database. Each sequence together with its secondary structure in Table 6.1 was used as a query to search the Rfam database by comparing the query with the secondary structures in Rfam, one by one, using RADAR. In the second experiment, we compared each query sequence (structure) in Table 6.1 with the seed alignments or blocks of the 603 families in Rfam using BlockMatch. (In an extreme case, BlockMatch can take a single RNA secondary structure and compare it with a block.) In the third experiment, we compared each block in Table 6.1 with the 18,233 secondary structures in Rfam using BlockMatch. Finally, in the fourth experiment, we compared each block in Table 6.1 with the 603 seed alignments (blocks) in the Rfam database.

The performance measures used to evaluate the performance of the tools are sensitivity, Sn, and specificity, Sp, where

$$\text{Sn} = \frac{\text{TP}}{\text{TP} + \text{FN}} \tag{6.1}$$

$$\text{Sp} = \frac{\text{TN}}{\text{TN} + \text{FP}} \tag{6.2}$$

where TP is the number of true positives, FN is the number of false negatives, TN is the number of true negatives, and FP is the number of false positives. There were 64

TABLE 6.1   The HSL3 and IRE Blocks Used in Our Experimental Study

Query ID	Block
$HSL3_1$	NM_005321:721-785 AACC-C-AAAGGCTCTTTTCAGAGCCACCCA
	Homo sapiens histone cluster 1, H1e (HIST1H1E), mRNA
$HSL3_2$	NM_021062:401-431 AACC-C-AAAGGCTCTTTTCAGAGCCACCTA
	Homo sapiens histone cluster 1, H2bb (HIST1H2BB), mRNA
$HSL3_3$	NM_005319:704-732 AACC-CAAAAGGCTCTTTTCAGAGCCACC-A
	Homo sapiens histone cluster 1, H1c (HIST1H1C), mRNA
$HSL3_4$	NM_003526:412-438 --CC-C-AAAGGCTCTTTTAAGAGCCACCCA
	Homo sapiens histone cluster 1, H2bc (HIST1H2BC), mRNA
$HSL3_5$	NM_002105:545-578 A-CCAC-AAAGGCCCTTTTAAGGGCCACC-A
	Homo sapiens H2A histone family, member X
$HSL3_6$	NM_003516:510-534 A------AAAGGCTCTTTTCAGAGCCACCCA
	Homo sapiens histone cluster 2, H2aa3 (HIST2H2AA3), mRNA
	#=GC SS_cons .........(((((((....))))))).....
IRE_1	NM_014585:197-237 AACTTCAGCTACAGTGTTAGCTAAGTT
	Homo sapiens solute carrier family 40 (iron-regulated transporter), member 1 (SLC40A1), mRNA
IRE_2	NM_003234:3884-3912 ATTATCGGGAGCAGTGTCTTCCATAAT
	Homo sapiens transferrin receptor (p90, CD71) (TFRC)
IRE_3	NM_003234:3481-3509 ATTATCGGAAGCAGTGCCTTCCATAAT
	Homo sapiens transferrin receptor (p90, CD71) (TFRC)
IRE_4	NM_000032:13-36 GT--TCGTCCTCAGTGCAGGGCA--AC
	Homo sapiens aminolevulinate, delta-, synthase 2 (sideroblastic/hypochromic anemia) (ALAS2), nuclear gene encoding mitochondrial protein, mRNA
IRE_5	NM_000146:20-40 TG---CTTCAACAGTGTTTGGA---CG
	Homo sapiens ferritin, light polypeptide (FTL), mRNA
IRE_6	NM_003234:3430-3460 TTTATCAGTGACAGAGTTCACTATAAA
	Homo sapiens transferrin receptor (p90, CD71) (TFRC)
	#=GC SS_cons (((((.(((((......)))))))))))

HSL3 structures and 39 IRE structures in Rfam. In experiments 1 and 3, a true positive is an HSL3 (IRE, respectively) structure that is returned as one of the top 64 (39, respectively) hits by the tools. A false positive is a non-HSL3 (non-IRE, respectively) structure that is returned as one of the top 64 (39, respectively) hits. A true negative is a non-HSL3 (non-IRE, respectively) structure that is not returned as one of the top 64 (39, respectively) hits. A false negative is an HSL3 (IRE, respectively) structure that is not returned as one of the top 64 (39, respectively) hits.

There was a single HSL3 block (accession RF00032) and a single IRE block (accession RF00037) among the 603 blocks in Rfam. In experiments 2 and 4, TP equals 1 if the HSL3 (IRE, respectively) block is ranked as the top hit by BlockMatch,

TABLE 6.2   Sensitivity and Specificity Values Obtained from Our Experiments

	Experiment 1 (%)		Experiment 2 (%)		Experiment 3 (%)		Experiment 4 (%)	
	Sn	Sp	Sn	Sp	Sn	Sp	Sn	Sp
$HSL3_1$	98.44	99.99	100	100				
$HSL3_2$	98.44	99.99	100	100				
$HSL3_3$	100	100	100	100				
					100	100	100	100
$HSL3_4$	98.44	99.99	100	100				
$HSL3_5$	98.44	99.99	100	100				
$HSL3_6$	100	100	100	100				
IRE_1	56.41	99.91	0	99.83				
IRE_2	64.10	99.92	0	99.83				
IRE_3	48.72	99.89	0	99.83				
					74.36	99.95	100	100
IRE_4	43.59	99.88	0	99.83				
IRE_5	79.49	99.96	100	100				
IRE_6	35.90	99.86	0	99.83				

or 0 otherwise. The FP equals 1 if the HSL3 (IRE, respectively) block is not ranked as the top hit, or 0 otherwise. The TN equals 602 if the HSL3 (IRE, respectively) block is ranked as the top hit, or 601 otherwise. The FN equals 1 if the HSL3 (IRE, respectively) block is not ranked as the top hit, or 0 otherwise.

Table 6.2 summarizes the experimental results. Combining all sequences into a query block and using BlockMatch to align the query block with all the blocks in Rfam yielded the best performance, where BlockMatch achieved a sensitivity value of 100% and a specificity value of 100%. In this case, the tool was able to take into account the characteristics of all sequences in the blocks while aligning them. In experiments 2 and 3, where a sequence (structure) was aligned with a block, partial sequence information was lost, and hence the performance of BlockMatch degraded. In experiment 1, where a query sequence (structure) was aligned with each individual sequence (structure) in the Rfam database, the notion of blocks was completely missing and the RADAR tool yielded the worst performance. These experimental results show that when blocks are available, one should use BlockMatch to do block alignments in performing database searches, hence considering all sequences in an entire block during the alignments, as opposed to using single sequence or structure matching tools to align individual sequences or structures in the blocks.

Note that BlockMatch computes the alignment score of two blocks by considering both the sequence alignment and the consensus structure in each block. We conducted experiments to evaluate the impact of changing the sequence alignment or consensus structure on alignment results. When the sequence alignment or the consensus structure in a block changes, so does the alignment score. The alignment score depends on how many base pairs and single bases occur and what nucleotides are present in each column of the alignment. Suppose there are four sets of blocks $\{A_1, B_1\}$, $\{A_2, B_2\}$, $\{A_3, B_3\}$, and $\{A_4, B_4\}$. Here A_1 and B_1 have similar sequences and similar consensus structures; A_2 and B_2 have similar sequences but different consensus structures; A_3 and B_3 have different sequences but similar consensus structures; and A_4 and B_4 have different sequences and different consensus structures. The alignment score between A_1 and B_1 is generally higher than that of A_2 and B_2 (A_3 and B_3, respectively), which is generally higher than the alignment score between A_4 and B_4.

6.4 CONCLUSION

This chapter presented two structure-based search engines for RNA motif databases. These search engines are useful to scientists and researchers who are interested in RNA secondary structure motifs. The search engine on RmotifDB employs the efficient RSmatch program to perform pairwise alignment of RNA secondary structures. The search engine on the block database uses BlockMatch to perform pairwise alignment of blocks or seed alignments. Both the RNA secondary structures and seed alignments are taken from the widely accessed Rfam database. In future work, we plan to extend the techniques presented here to search for three-dimensional motifs in RNA structure databases [15, 16].

ACKNOWLEDGMENTS

We thank Mugdha Khaladkar, James McHugh, Vandanaben Patel, and Bruce Shapiro for helpful conversations while preparing this manuscript.

REFERENCES

1. J. T. L. Wang and X. Wu (2006), Kernel design for RNA classification using support vector machines, *Inter. J. Data Mining Bioinformat.*, 1:57–76.

2. W. F. Marzluff and R. J. Duronio (2002), Histone mRNA expression: multiple levels of cell cycle regulation and important developmental consequences, *Curr. Opin. Cell Biol.*, 14:692–699.

3. G. Pesole, S. Liuni, G. Grillo, F. Licciulli, F. Mignone, C. Gissi, and C. Saccone (2002), UTRdb and UTRsite: specialized databases of sequences and functional elements of 5′ and 3′ untranslated regions of eukaryotic mRNAs, *Nucleic Acids Res.*, 30:335–340.

4. S. G. Jones, S. Moxon, M. Marshall, A. Khanna, S. R. Eddy, and A. Bateman (2005), Rfam: annotating non-coding RNAs in complete genomes, *Nucleic Acids Res.*, 33:D121–D124.

5. M. Andronescu, V. Bereg, H. H. Hoos, and A. Condon (2008), RNA STRAND: The RNA secondary structure and statistical analysis database, *BMC Bioinformat.*, 9:340.

6. S. R. Eddy (2002), A memory-efficient dynamic programming algorithm for optimal alignment of a sequence to an RNA secondary structure, *BMC Bioinformat.*, 3:18.

7. J. Spirollari, J. T. L. Wang, K. Zhang, V. Bellofatto, Y. Park, and B. A. Shapiro (2009), Predicting consensus structures for RNA alignments via pseudo-energy minimization, *Bioinformat. Biol. Insights*, 3:51–69.

8. D. Wen and J. T. L. Wang (2009), Design of an RNA structural motif database, *Inter. J. Comput. Intell. Bioinformat. Systems Biol.*, 1:32–41.

9. J. Liu, J. T. L. Wang, J. Hu, and B. Tian (2005), A method for aligning RNA secondary structures and its application to RNA motif detection, *BMC Bioinformat.*, 6:89.

10. M. Khaladkar, V. Bellofatto, J. T. L. Wang, B. Tian, and B. A. Shapiro (2007), RADAR: a web server for RNA data analysis and research, *Nucleic Acids Res.*, 35:W300–W304.

11. M. Khaladkar, V. Patel, V. Bellofatto, J. Wilusz, and J. T. L. Wang (2008), Detecting conserved secondary structures in RNA molecules using constrained structural alignment, *Comput. Biol. Chem.*, 32:264–272.

12. I. L. Hofacker (2003), Vienna RNA secondary structure server, *Nucleic Acids Res.*, 31:3429–3431.

13. M. Khaladkar, J. Liu, D. Wen, J. T. L. Wang, and B. Tian (2008), Mining small RNA structure elements in untranslated regions of human and mouse mRNAs using structure-based alignment, *BMC Genomics*, 9:189.

14. A. R. Gruber, R. Lorenz, S. H. Bernhart, R. Neubock, and I. L. Hofacker (2008), The Vienna RNA websuite, *Nucleic Acids Res.*, 36:W70–W74.

15. H. M. Berman, W. K. Olson, D. L. Beveridge, J. Westbrook, A. Gelbin, T. Demeny, S.-H. Hsieh, A. R. Srinivasan, and B. Schneider (1992), The Nucleic Acid Database: a comprehensive relational database of three-dimensional structures of nucleic acids, *Biophys. J.*, 63:751–759.

16. E. Bindewald, R. Hayes, Y. G. Yingling, W. Kasprzak, and B. A. Shapiro (2008), RNA-Junction: a database of RNA junctions and kissing loops for three-dimensional structural analysis and nanodesign, *Nucleic Acids Res.*, 36:D392–D397.

7

KERNELS ON PROTEIN STRUCTURES

SOURANGSHU BHATTACHARYA, CHIRANJIB BHATTACHARYYA,
AND NAGASUMA R. CHANDRA

7.1 INTRODUCTION

Kernel methods have emerged as one of the most powerful techniques for supervised, as well as semisupervised learning [1], and with structured data. Kernels have been designed on various types of structured data including sets [2–4], strings [5], probability models [6], and so on. Protein structures are another important type of structured data [7, 8], which can be modelled as geometric structures or pointsets [9, 10]. This chapter concentrates on designing kernels on protein structures [7, 11].

Classification of protein structures into different structural classes is a problem of fundamental interest in computational biology. Many hierarchical structural classification databases, describing various levels of structural similarities, have been developed. Two of the most popular databases are structural classification of proteins (SCOP) [12] a manually curated database, and class, architecture, topology and homologous superfamilies (CATH) [13], which is a semiautomatically curated database. Since the defining characteristics of each of these classes is not known precisely, machine learning is the tool of choice for attempting to classify proteins automatically. We propose to use the kernels designed here along with support vector machines to design automatic classifiers on protein structures.

Many kernels have been designed to capture similarities between protein sequences. Some of the notable ones include Fisher kernels [6], kernels based on comparison of k-mers [5], and alignment kernels [14]. However, the problem of designing kernels on protein structures remains relatively unexplored. Some of the initial attempts include application of graph kernels [15] and empirical kernel maps

Computational Intelligence and Pattern Analysis in Biological Informatics, Edited by Ujjwal Maulik,
Sanghamitra Bandyopadhyay, and Jason T. L. Wang
Copyright © 2010 John Wiley & Sons, Inc.

131

with existing protein structure comparison algorithms [16]. Reference [17] defines various kernels on substructures using amino acid similarity. However, they fail to capture structural similarity in a principled way. These kernels are used mainly for finding structural motifs and annotating functions.

In a recent paper [18], we proposed several novel kernels on protein structures by defining kernels on neighborhoods using ideas from convolution kernels [19]. These kernels captured the shape similarity between neighborhoods by matching pairwise distances between the constituent atoms. This idea of using only geometric properties to find similarity between proteins is also adopted by many protein structure comparison algorithms [8,11]. We also generalized some of these kernels to *attributed pointsets* [10], and demonstrated their application to various tasks in computer vision.

This chapter reports a detailed exploration of the idea of defining kernels on protein structures using kernels on neighborhoods, which are specific types of substructures. The idea of neighborhoods has been used previously to design protein structure comparison algorithms [11], which performed competitively with the state of the art. Kernels on neighborhoods are subdivided into two types: those using sequence or structure information. Sequence-based kernels on neighborhoods draw ideas from the general set kernels designed in [4] and convolution kernels [19]. Structure-based kernels are motivated from protein structure comparison algorithms using spectral graph matching [11,20]. We show that in a limiting case, the kernel values are related to the similarity score given by protein structure comparison algorithms.

We also explore two different ways of combining sequence- and structure-based kernels, weighting and convex combination, to get kernels on neighborhoods. Finally, we explore two methods of combining the neighborhood kernels, one without using structural alignment, and the other using structural alignment. Interestingly, even though spectrum kernels [5] were defined using feature spaces involving k-mers, we show that they are a special case of our kernels when using only sequence information on sequence neighborhoods.

Extensive experimentation was done to validate the kernels developed here on real protein structures and also to study the properties of various types of kernels. The task chosen was that of classifying 40% sequence nonredundant SCOP [12] superfamilies, which was also demonstrated to be very difficult and relevant. Our kernels outperformed the state of the art protein structure comparison algorithm combinatorial extension (CE) [21]. We also compared our kernels with spectrum kernels [5] and experimentally validated a theoretical property of the structure-based neighborhood kernels.

This chapter is organized as follows: Section 7.2 gives a background of kernel methods and various kernels on structured data. Section 7.3 gives a background on protein structures, describes the protein-structure alignment problem and develops a neighborhood-based algorithm for protein-structure alignment, which is a simplified version of the formulation used in [11]. Section 7.4 proposes kernels for sequence and structure neighborhoods. Section 7.5 defines various kernels on protein structures using the neighborhood kernels defined in Section 7.4. Section 7.6 describes the experimental results obtained with various kernels proposed here and also compares them to existing techniques. We conclude with remarks in Section 7.7.

7.2   KERNELS METHODS

Kernel methods [1, 22, 23] is the collective name for the class of *learning algorithms* that can operate using *only* a real valued similarity function (called *kernel function*) defined for each pair of datapoints. Kernel methods have become popular over the last decade, mainly due to their general applicability and theoretical underpinnings.

A critical step in the effectiveness of a kernel method is the design of an appropriate kernel function. A function $K : \mathcal{X} \times \mathcal{X} \to \mathbb{R}$, is called a positive semidefinite or Mercer kernel if it satisfies the following properties:

Symmetry. $K(x, y) = K(y, x)$, $\forall x, y \in \mathcal{X}$.

Positive Norm. $\mathcal{K}(x, x) \geq 0$, and 0 only if $x = 0$ (a fixed element of $\mathcal{X}$).

Positive Semidefiniteness. $\sum_{i,j} c_i c_j K(x_i, x_j) \geq 0 \forall c_i, c_j \in \mathbb{R}$ and $x_i, x_j \in \mathcal{X}$.

A positive semidefinite kernel K maps points $x, y \in \mathcal{X}$ to a reproducing kernel Hilbert space (RKHS) $\mathcal{H}$. Let $\psi_x, \psi_y \in \mathcal{H}$ be the corresponding points, the inner product is given by:

$$\langle \psi_x, \psi_y \rangle = K(x, y)$$

Also, for a finite dataset $\mathcal{D} = (x_1, \ldots, x_n)$, the $n \times n$ kernel matrix $\mathcal{K}_{ij} = K(x_i, x_j)$, constructed from a positive semidefinite kernel K, can decomposed using eigenvalue decomposition as:

$$\mathcal{K} = \sum_{k=1}^{n} \lambda_k \eta_k \eta_k^T$$

Thus, the feature map ψ_x can be explicitly constructed as

$$\psi_x = (\sqrt{\lambda_1} \eta_1(x), \ldots, \sqrt{\lambda_n} \eta_n(x))^T$$

This effectively embeds the points into a vector space, thus allowing all the vector space-based learning techniques to be applied to points from the arbitrary set $\mathcal{X}$. Some of the common methods to be kernelized are support vector machines, principal component analysis, Gaussian process, and so on (see [1] for details).

7.2.1   Kernels on Structured Data

It is clear from the above discussion that definition of the kernel function is the key challenge in designing a kernel method. This section enumerates some of the well-known kernels that are related to the work described here. We begin by describing operations under which the class of positive semidefinite kernels is closed.

If K is a positive semidefinite (PSD) kernel, so is αK for $\alpha > 0$.

If K_1 and K_2 are PSD kernels, so are $K_1 + K_2$ and $K_1 K_2$.

If $K_n, n = 1, 2, \ldots$ are PSD kernels and $K = \lim_{n \to \infty} K_n$ exists, K is a PSD kernel.

If K_1 is a PSD kernel on $\mathcal{X} \times \mathcal{X}$ and K_2 is a PSD kernel on $\mathcal{Z} \times \mathcal{Z}$, then the tensor product $K_1 \otimes K_2$ and the direct sum $K_1 \oplus K_2$ are PSD kernels on $(\mathcal{X} \times \mathcal{Z}) \times (\mathcal{X} \times \mathcal{Z})$.

For proofs of these closure properties, please see [1,22,23]. From the above properties, it can also be shown that $K'(x, y) = \sum_{i=1}^{\infty} a_i (K(x, y))^i$ is a PSD kernel if K is a PSD kernel.

Intuitively, kernels between arbitrary objects can be thought of as similarity measures. To see this, recall that the inner product $\langle \psi(x), \psi(y) \rangle = K(x, y)$ defined by kernel function K induces a norm $\|\psi(x)\|^2 = \langle \psi(x), \psi(x) \rangle$ in the RKHS $\mathcal{H}$. This norm induces a natural distance metric, defined as $d(x, y) = \|\psi(x) - \psi(y)\|$. It is easy to see that

$$(d(x, y))^2 = K(x, x) + K(y, y) - 2K(x, y)$$

Thus, $d(x, y)$ is a decreasing function of $K(x, y)$. So, $K(x, y)$ can be thought of as a similarity function.

Various kernels between vectors have been used in the literature. Most simple of them is the dot product or linear kernel, given by

$$K_{\text{dot}}(\mathbf{x}, \mathbf{y}) = \mathbf{x}^T \mathbf{y}$$

This kernel uses an identity feature map. Another popularly used kernel between vectors is the Gaussian kernel:

$$K_{\text{Gaussian}}(\mathbf{x}, \mathbf{y}) = e^{\frac{\|\mathbf{x} - \mathbf{y}\|^2}{\sigma^2}}$$

It is useful when one simply wants the kernel to be a decreasing function of the Euclidean distance between the vectors.

One of the most general types of kernels on structured data are the *convolution kernels* [19]. Convolution kernels provide a method of defining PSD kernel on composite objects using kernels on parts. Let $\mathcal{X}$ be a set of composite objects consisting of parts from $\mathcal{X}_1, \ldots, \mathcal{X}_m$. Let R be a relation over $\mathcal{X}_1 \times \cdots \times \mathcal{X}_m \times \mathcal{X}$, such that $R(x_1, \ldots, x_m, x)$ is true if x is composed of $x_1, \ldots, x_m$. Also, let $R^{-1}(x) = \{(x_1, \ldots, x_m) \in \mathcal{X}_1 \times \cdots \times \mathcal{X}_m \mid R(x_1, \ldots, x_m, x) = \text{true}\}$ and K_i be kernels on $\mathcal{X}_i \times \mathcal{X}_i$. The convolution kernel K on $\mathcal{X} \times \mathcal{X}$ is defined as

$$K(x, y) = \sum_{(x_1, \ldots, x_m) \in R^{-1}(x), (y_1, \ldots, y_m) \in R^{-1}(y)} \prod_{i=1}^{m} K_i(x_i, y_i) \qquad (7.1)$$

It can be shown that if $K_1, \ldots, K_m$ are PSD, then so is K. Convolution kernels have been used to iteratively define kernels on strings [14, 19], and applied to processing of biological sequences. They have also been used in natural language processing for defining kernels on parse trees [24]. We use convolution kernels to define kernels on neighborhoods.

Kernels on sets of vectors are the next most general types of kernels and have also been useful in designing kernels for protein structures. It was shown in [25] that given two $d \times c$ matrices X and Y:

$$K_{\text{tr}}(X, Y) = \text{tr}(X^T Y) \text{ and } K_{\text{det}}(X, Y) = \det(X^T Y)$$

are PSD kernels. Both [2] and [25] define kernels on the subspaces spanned by set of vectors. They show that if U_X and U_Y are orthogonal matrices spanning column spaces of X and Y, then the product of cosines of principal angles between the column spaces is given by

$$K(X, Y) = \prod_{i=1}^{k} \cos(\psi_i) = \det(U_X^T U_Y)$$

where ψ_i are the principal angles. This kernel was applied to problems in computer vision [2] (e.g., detection of abnormal motion trajectories and face recognition). These kernels are further generalized in [25]. Shashua et al. also define a general class of kernels on matrices [4]. They show that given two matrices $A_{n \times k}$ and $B_{n \times q}$:

$$K(A, B) = tr(\sum_r (A^T \hat{G}_r B) \hat{F}_r)$$

is a PSD kernel where, zero extensions of $\hat{G}_r$ and $\hat{F}_r$ to $m \times m$, $m = \max\{n, k, q\}$, F_r and G_r, are such that $\sum_r F_r \otimes G_r$ is PSD.

Strings are a type of structured data that find wide applicability in various fields, including biological sequence analysis, text mining, and so on. While the kernels described above can and have been used for string processing, rational kernels, defined in [26] are a general class of kernels defined specifically for strings. Cortes et al. [26] give a general definition of rational kernels and show various theoretical results on conditions for rational kernels to be PSD. A popular special case of these kernels are the k-mer based kernels defined in [5]. Let Σ be the alphabet from which the string is generated, the feature map, ψ, for the kernels are defined by $|\Sigma|^k$ dimensional vector indexed by all k-mers. The value of $\psi_i(x)$ could, for example, be the number of occurrences of the ith k-mer in string x. The spectrum kernel is defined as

$$K(x, x') = \sum_{i=1}^{|\Sigma|^k} \psi_i(x)\psi_i(x')$$

By using $\psi_i(x)$ to be the number of k-mers in x with at most m mismatches from the ith k-mer, we get the mismatch kernel [5]. Section 7.5.1 shows a connection between kernels proposed here and the spectrum kernel. Another kernel defined on strings is the alignment kernels [14], which try to capture the notion of sequence alignment between biological sequences.

Kernels on graphs have been defined in two different settings. The first setting is where the elements of the data set form a (weighted) graph. An example of this type of kernels are the diffusion kernels [27]. Given a graph G with adjacency matrix A, the diffusion kernel matrix K is given as

$$K = e^{\beta A}$$

It can be shown that K is PSD for any A.

Another setting is where each datapoint is a graph. One of the earliest kernels in such a setting used a probability distribution over the paths in the graphs [28]. The kernel is taken as the limiting case of sum over all lengths of paths. Kashima and co-workers [28] provide an efficient way of computing this kernel as a solution of some fixed point equations. Other kernels on graphs include shortest path kernels [29] and cyclic pattern kernels based on subgraphs [30].

7.3 PROTEIN STRUCTURES

7.3.1 Background

Proteins are polymers of small molecules called amino acids. There are 20 different amino acids found in naturally occurring proteins. The polymerized amino acids are also known as *residues*. This chapter uses amino acids and residues interchangeably to mean a unit of the polymer. Polymerization connects each amino acid (residue) with two neighboring ones, thereby forming a sequence order of residues, sometimes also called *chain or topology*. This sequence (a string in computer science parlance) of residues is called the primary structure of a protein.

While the primary structure of a protein has been used by computational biologists to decipher many interesting properties of proteins, higher level descriptions are found to be more informative about protein functions. Protein structure is described on four levels: primary, secondary, tertiary, and quaternary. Secondary structure describes the local hydrogen-bonding patterns between residues, and is classified mainly into α-helixes, β-sheets, and loops. Tertiary structure describes the coordinates of each atom of a polymer chain in three-dimensional (3D) space, and has been found to be directly related to the proteins' properties. Quaternary structure describes the 3D spatial arrangement of many protein chains. This chapter describes a protein by its primary and tertiary structure.

The residues of a protein contain variable number of atoms. However, all the residues have a central carbon atom called the C^α atom. Following common convention, we represent the tertiary structure of a protein as 3D coordinates of C^α atoms. So, a protein P is represented as $P = \{p_1, \ldots, p_n\}$ where $p_i = (\mathbf{x}_i, y_i)$, $\mathbf{x}_i \in \mathbb{R}^3$, $y_i \in \mathcal{Y}$, $1 \leq i \leq n$. Here, $\mathcal{Y}$ is the set of all 20 amino acid residues found in natural proteins.

Definition 7.3.1 *A structural alignment between two proteins P^A and P^B is a 1-1 mapping* $\phi : \{i \,|\, p_i^A \in \bar{P}^A\} \to \{j \,|\, p_j^B \in \bar{P}^B\}$, *where* $\bar{P}^A \subseteq P^A$ *and* $\bar{P}^B \subseteq P^B$.

The mapping ϕ defines a set of correspondences between the residues of the two proteins. The structures $|\bar{P}^A| = |\bar{P}^B|$ is called the *length* of the alignment. Given a structural alignment ϕ between two structures P^A and P^B, and a transformation $\mathcal{T}$ of structure B onto A, a popular measure of the goodness of superposition is the *root-mean-square deviation* (RMSD), defined as

$$\mathrm{RMSD}(\phi) = \sqrt{\frac{1}{|\bar{P}^A|} \sum_{p_i^A \in \bar{P}^A} \|\mathbf{x}_i^A - \mathcal{T}(\mathbf{x}_{\phi(i)}^B)\|^2} \qquad (7.2)$$

Given an alignment ϕ, the optimal transformation $\mathcal{T}$, minimizing RMSD, can be computed in closed form using the method described in [31].

7.3.2 Algorithms for Structural Alignment and a Spectral Method

A typical attempt at designing a structural alignment algorithm involves defining an objective function that is a measure of goodness of a particular alignment, and optimizing the function over a permitted set of alignments. The RMSD is one such possible function. However, calculating RMSD requires calculating the optimal transformation $\mathcal{T}$, which is computation intensive.

Objective functions based on pairwise distances (e.g., distance RMSD) [8], are popular because they don't need computation of optimal transformations. Distance RMSD for an alignment ϕ is defined as

$$\mathrm{RMSD}_D(\phi) = \sqrt{\frac{1}{|\bar{P}^A|^2} \sum_{p_i^A, p_j^A \in \bar{P}^A} (d_{ij}^A - d_{\phi(i)\phi(j)}^B)^2} \qquad (7.3)$$

where, $d_{ij}^A = \|\mathbf{x}_i^A - \mathbf{x}_j^A\|_2$, is the distance between residues p_i^A and p_j^A. The matrix d is also called the *distance matrix* of a protein structure. The RMSD is a distance function since the lower the RMSD, the better the alignment, and hence the closer the proteins in the (hypothetical) protein structure space. Section 7.4.2 proposes a kernel that captures a notion of similarity related to RMSD_D.

One problem in using distance RMSD as an objective function with protein structures, which are inherently noisy, is that it prefers alignments having lower lengths. This problem was addressed in the scoring function used by the popular protein structure comparison algorithm DALI [32]. Given an alignment ϕ between two proteins P^A and P^B, the DALI score function is defined as

$$S_{\mathrm{DALI}}(\phi) = \sum_{p_i^A, p_j^A \in \bar{P}^A} \left(0.2 - \frac{|d_{ij}^A - d_{\phi(i)\phi(j)}^B|}{\bar{d}_{ij}} \right) \exp\left(-\left(\frac{\bar{d}_{lk}}{20}\right)^2 \right) \qquad (7.4)$$

where $\bar{d}_{ij} = (d_{ij}^A + d_{\phi(i)\phi(j)}^B)/2$. This function is relatively robust to differences in distances since any pair of residues for which the difference in distances is $< 20\%$ of the average distance contributes positively to the total score. Another feature of the scoring function is that it penalizes the average distance exponentially. Thus, contribution from relatively distant residues toward the overall score is negligible. This captures the idea that nearby atoms interact with much higher force than distant ones.

The problem of matching pairwise distances can be posed as an inexact weighted graph matching problem [33]. In [20], we used this observation along with observation that interaction between nearby residues are more significant, to propose a new objective function for comparing two protein structures. This objective function is based on *spectral projection vectors*, and can be computed in $O(n)$ time as compared to $O(n^2)$ time needed by the above objective function. Here, we recapitulate the definition briefly, and use it to motivate another kernel on protein structures in Section 7.4.

We start by defining the *adjacency matrix* $\mathcal{A}$ of a protein P as

$$\mathcal{A}_{ij} = e^{\frac{-d_{ij}}{\alpha}}, \quad \alpha > 0 \tag{7.5}$$

Definition 7.3.2   *Let $\mathcal{A}$ be the adjacency matrix of a protein P and $\mathcal{A} = \sum_{i=1}^{n} \lambda_i \zeta_i \zeta_i^T$ be it eigenvalue distribution, such that the eigenvectors are arranged in decreasing order of the eigenvalues. The spectral projection vector $\mathbf{f}$ for P is defined as $f_i = |\zeta_1(i)|$.*

The spectral projection vector has the property of preserving neighborhoods optimally, while also preventing all projection values from being the same and thereby giving a trivial solution. Given spectral projection vectors $\mathbf{f}^A$ and $\mathbf{f}^B$ of two proteins P^A and P^B, respectively, and an alignment ϕ between them, the *spectral similarity score* between the two proteins is defined as

$$S_{\text{spec}}(P^A, P^B) = \max_{\phi} \sum_{i:p_i^A \in \bar{P}^A} T - (f_i^A - f_{\phi(i)}^B)^2 \tag{7.6}$$

where T is a parameter which makes the score function robust to small perturbations in $\mathbf{f}$. The problem of optimizing S_{spec} with respect to all alignments, ϕ, is solvable in polynomial time by posing it as an assignment problem [34]. Reference [20] proposes an efficient heuristic solution to this problem.

Section 7.4 proposes kernels on neighborhoods that capture the notion of similarity defined by the spectral similarity score. The structural alignment algorithm outlined above is very efficient, but does not work satisfactorily when the proteins being compared are of very different sizes. Section 7.3.3, outlines a method of tackling this problem using neighborhoods.

7.3.3   Problem of Indels and Solution Using Neighborhoods

In Section 7.3.2, we posed the problem of protein structure alignment as an inexact weighted graph matching problem, and derived a new similarity score based on spectral projection vectors. At the core of the method is the assumption that all residues in one protein have a matching residue in the second one. However, often proteins showing similar structure or function have many unmatched residues. These unmatched residues are called *indels* (insertions and deletions). Up to 60% indels are encountered in practical situations.

The way in which the algorithm in Section 7.3.2 was derived does not require the number of residues in the two structures to be the same. In fact, it works very well in practice when the number of indels is low. However, for a large number of indels (typically $>40\%$) the method fails to perform as expected. This is due to the fact that the values of the spectral projection vector are changed by addition of extra residues.

Reference [11] proposes to address this problem by applying spectral algorithm to *neighborhoods* for calculating neighborhood alignments and growing the neighborhood alignments to get an alignment of entire structures. In [18] and this chapter, a similar paradigm is followed for designing kernels on protein structures. Here, following [11], we define two types of neighborhoods and give some biological justification behind each of them.

Definition 7.3.3   *The ith structure neighborhood, $N_{str}(i)$, of size l, $1 \le i \le |P|$, of a protein P is a set of l residues closest to residue i in 3D space. So,*

$$N_i = \{p_j \in P \mid p_k \notin N_i \Rightarrow \|p_j - p_i\| \le \|p_k - p_i\| \quad \text{and} \quad |N_i| = l\}$$

The idea behind this definition is that there are highly conserved compact regions in 3D space, which are responsible for structure and functions of a given class of proteins. For example, *structural motifs* are the locally conserved portions of structure, while *core folds* are conserved regions responsible for the fold of the structure [35]. Similarly, *active sites* are conserved regions that are responsible for specfic functions. So, the neighborhoods falling in these conserved regions will have all the residues matched.

The algorithm (see Appendix A) considers all pairs of neighborhoods from both structures, and computes alignment between them. Based on these neighborhood alignments, transformations optimally superposing the aligned residues are computed. Alignment between the two protein structures is then calculated using a similarity measure derived from these transformations. The "best" alignment is reported as the optimal one.

Definition 7.3.4   *The ith sequence neighborhood, $N_{seq}(i)$, of size l, $1 \le i \le |P| - l + 1$, of a protein P is the set of residues contained a sequence fragment of length l starting from residue i. So,*

$$N_{seq}(i) = \{p_i, \ldots, p_{i+l-1}\}$$

Sequence neighborhoods were traditionally used by sequence alignment algorithms, e.g. Blast [36], and have been used in sequence-based kernels described in [5]. They have also been used in some structural alignment algorithms (e.g., CE) [21]. Sequence neighborhoods are sets of residues that are contiguous in the polymer chain, and hence are bonded together by covalent bonds. However, this may not be necessarily compact in 3D space. Also, note that unlike sequence processing algorithms, we include the 3D coordinates of residues along with residue type in the sequence neighborhood. In Section 7.4, we start by defining kernels on the two types of neighborhoods, which are them combined in various ways in Section 7.5 to define kernels on entire protein structures.

7.4 KERNELS ON NEIGHBORHOODS

Neighborhoods are subsets of residues of a protein structure that are compact in 3D space or in the protein sequence space. It is clear from the discussion in Section 7.3.3 that comparing neighborhoods for comparison of protein structures has some theoretical as well as experimental justification. We are interested in extending the same paradigm in design of kernels on protein structures. This section proposes various positive semidefinite kernels on neighborhoods. Section 7.4.1 defines kernels on protein structures using the kernels on neighborhoods defined here.

Each neighborhood N_i (either structure or sequence) is a set of l residues $p_j = (\mathbf{x}_j, y_j)$, where $\mathbf{x}_j \in \mathbb{R}^3$ is the position of the residue in 3D space, and $y_j \in \mathcal{Y}$ is the amino acid type. It may be noted that while defining kernels we do not distinguish between the type of neighborhoods. However, some kernels make more sense with a specific type of neighborhood. We discuss this in more detail in Section 7.4.3.

We begin by defining various kernels capturing similarity between the types of amino acids in the two neighborhoods, then define kernels capturing similarity between 3D structures of the two neighborhoods, and finally describe two methods to combine these two kernels to get kernels on neighborhoods.

7.4.1 Sequence-Based Kernels on Neighborhoods

Amino acid types are one of the most commonly used features in comparison of proteins. There are 20 different types of amino acids are found in proteins. First, we define kernels capturing the similarity between different types of amino acids. The simplest similarity measure is to assign unit similarity between identical amino acids and zero similarity to the rest. This gives us the *identity kernel K_I* on $\mathcal{Y} \times \mathcal{Y}$:

$$K_I(y_1, y_2) = \begin{cases} 1 & \text{if } y_1 = y_2 \\ 0 & \text{otherwise} \end{cases} \quad y_1, y_2 \in \mathcal{Y} \qquad (7.7)$$

Another popular measure of similarity between amino acid types is given by the substitution matrices (e.g., the BLOSUM62 matrix) [37]. BLOSUM matrices give the log of likelihood ratio of actual and expected likelihoods. Unfortunately, the

BLOSUM62 matrix is not positive semidefinite. We use the diffusion kernel [27] technique to construct a positive semidefinite kernel K_{blosum} on $\mathcal{Y} \times \mathcal{Y}$, from the blosum matrix:

$$K_{\text{blosum}} = e^{S_{\text{blosum}}/10} \tag{7.8}$$

where S_{blosum} is the blosum substitution matrix.

Representative Residue Kernel. The amino acid kernels can be combined in various ways to give kernels on neighborhoods. One simple way is to summarize the entire neighborhood by a single representative residue. The choice of representative residue is very natural in the case of a structure neighborhood, since it has a central residue. In case of sequence neighborhoods, the representative residue is taken as the starting residue of the sequence fragment.

Let $K_{AA} : \mathcal{Y} \times \mathcal{Y} \to \mathbb{R}$ be some positive semidefinite kernel on amino acids. The representative residue kernel K_{rep} on neighborhoods is defined as

$$K_{\text{rep}}(N_1, N_2) = K_{AA}(y_{\text{rep}}(N_1), y_{\text{rep}}(N_2)) \tag{7.9}$$

where, $y_{\text{rep}}(N_i)$ is the amino acid type of representative residue of neighborhood N_i chosen as described above.

All Pair Sum and Direct Alignment Kernels. The above kernel is derived by summarizing neighborhoods with their representative residues. Neighborhoods can also be viewed as sets of residues, thus allowing us to use existing set kernels. Many kernels have been proposed on sets (e.g., [2, 3, 5]). Here, we propose two kernels motivated from set kernels.

Let A and B be two $d \times c$ matrices. It was shown in [25], that if k is a PSD kernel on $\mathbb{R}^c \times \mathbb{R}^c$, then $K(A, B) = \text{tr}([k(A^i, B^j)]_{ij}) = \sum_i k(A^i, B^i)$ is a PSD kernel, A^i being the ith column of A. This can be generalized to arbitrary objects (amino acids in this case) rather than vectors in $\mathbb{R}^c$:

Definition 7.4.1   *Let* $N_i = \{p_1^i, \dots, p_l^i\}$, $p_j^i = (\mathbf{x}_j^i, y_j^i)$, $\mathbf{x}_j^i \in \mathbb{R}^3$, $y_j^i \in \mathcal{Y}$ *be a neighborhood, and* $K_{AA} : \mathcal{Y} \times \mathcal{Y} \to \mathbb{R}$ *be any amino acid kernel. The direct alignment kernel* K_{diral} *between neighborhoods* N_i *and* N_j *is defined as*

$$K_{\text{diral}}(N_i, N_j) = \frac{1}{l} \sum_{k=1}^{l} K_{AA}(y_k^i, y_k^j)$$

The fact that K_{diral} is positive semidefinite follows trivially from the above discussion and the fact that l is a positive constant. This kernel assumes a fixed serial ordering of the residues. This is applicable in the case of sequence neighborhoods.

Another case is where such an ordering is not known. For such a case, [4] defines general kernels on matrices that have the same number of rows, but a different number of columns. Let A and B be $n \times k$ and $n \times q$ matrices respectively. Let G and F be $n \times n$ and $q \times k$ matrices, such that G and extension of F to $m \times m$ matrices, $m = \max(n, q, k)$, is a positive semidefinite matrix. Then, $\langle A, B \rangle = tr((A^T G B)F)$ is a PSD kernel. Simplifying this, it can be shown that $K(A, B) = \sum_{i=1}^{q} \sum_{j=1}^{k} k(A^i, B^j)$ is a PSD kernel. Generalizing this result, we can define sequence-based kernels on neighborhoods.

Definition 7.4.2   *Let $N_i = \{p_1^i, \ldots, p_l^i\}$, $p_j^i = (\mathbf{x}_j^i, y_j^i)$, $\mathbf{x}_j^i \in \mathbb{R}^3$, $y_j^i \in \mathcal{Y}$ be a neighborhood, and $K_{AA} : \mathcal{Y} \times \mathcal{Y} \to \mathbb{R}$ be any amino acid kernel. The all pair sum kernel, $K_{allpair}$, between neighborhoods N_i and N_j is defined as*

$$K_{\text{allpair}}(N_i, N_j) = \frac{1}{l^2} \sum_{s=1}^{l} \sum_{t=1}^{l} K_{AA}(y_s^i, y_t^j)$$

The fact that K_{allpair} is PSD follows trivially from the above discussion. This kernel is useful in case of structure neighborhoods where there is no ordering between residues. In Section 7.5, we use a similar technique to define kernels on protein structures.

Permutation Sum Kernel. The set kernel derived above adds up similarity between all pairs of residues in the two neighborhoods. Another interesting kernel is where all possible assignments of one residue to other is considered. In case of neighborhoods of fixed size, this implies considering all permutations of the residues in one of the neighborhoods. We use the idea of convolution kernels [19] to arrive at this notion.

Let $x \in X$ be a composite object formed using parts from $X_1, \ldots, X_m$. Let R be a relation over $X_1 \times \cdots \times X_m \times X$ such that $R(x_1, \ldots, x_m, x)$ is true if x is composed of $x_1, \ldots, x_m$. Let $R^{-1}(x) = \{(x_1, \ldots, x_m) \in X_1 \times \cdots \times X_m | R(x_1, \ldots, x_m, x) = \text{true}\}$ and $K^1, \ldots, K^m$ be kernels on $X_1, \ldots, X_m$, respectively. The convolution kernel K over X is defined as

$$K(x, y) = \sum_{(x_1,\ldots,x_m)\in R^{-1}(x),(y_1,\ldots,y_m)\in R^{-1}(y)} \prod_{i=1}^{m} K^i(x_i, y_i) \qquad (7.10)$$

It was shown in [19], if $K^1, \ldots, K^m$ are symmetric and positive semidefinite, so is K.

In our case, the composite objects are the neighborhoods N_i's and the "parts" are the residues p_j^i, $j = 1, \ldots, l$ in those neighborhoods. The relation R is defined as $R(p_1, \ldots, p_l, N_i)$ is true iff $N_i = \{p_1, \ldots, p_l\}$. Thus, the set $R^{-1}(N_i)$ becomes all permutations of $(p_1^i, \ldots, p_l^i)$. In other words, $R^{-1}(N_i) = \{p_{\pi(j)}^i; j = 1, \ldots, l; \pi \in \Pi(l)$, $\Pi(l)$ being the set of all permutations of l numbers.

Definition 7.4.3   *Let* $N_i = \{p_1^i, \ldots, p_l^i\}$, $p_j^i = (\mathbf{x}_j^i, y_j^i)$, $\mathbf{x}_j^i \in \mathbb{R}^3$, $y_j^i \in \mathcal{Y}$ *be a neighborhood, and* $K_{AA} : \mathcal{Y} \times \mathcal{Y} \to \mathbb{R}$ *be any amino acid kernel. The permutation sum kernel* K_{perm} *between neighborhoods* N_i *and* N_j *is defined as*

$$K_{\text{perm}}(N_i, N_j) = \frac{1}{l!} \sum_{\pi \in \Pi(l)} \prod_{k=1}^{l} K_{AA}(y_{\pi(k)}^i, y_k^j)$$

To see that K_{perm} is a PSD kernel, notice that permuting residues in both neighborhoods will result in all possible assignments being generated $l!$ times. The convolution kernel following the above discussion is

$$K(N_i, N_j) = \sum_{\pi, \pi' \in \Pi(l)} \prod_{k=1}^{l} K_{AA}(y_{\pi(k)}^i, y_{\pi'(k)}^j)$$

$$= l! \sum_{\pi \in \Pi(l)} \prod_{k=1}^{l} K_{AA}(y_{\pi(k)}^i, y_k^j)$$

Since the above kernel is PSD (using theorem 1 in [19]), dividing it by $(l!)^2$, we get K_{perm}, which is also PSD. In Section 7.4.2, we use the same idea to define various structure based kernels on neighborhoods.

7.4.2   Structure-Based Kernels on Neighborhoods

Each residue p_i of a protein structure P can be represented as two parts: the position $\mathbf{x}_i$ and the residue type (attribute) y_i. In Section 7.4.1, we defined many kernels on neighborhoods using kernels on residue type y_i for each residue. Kernels on the residue type are easier to define since the residue types are directly comparable. On the other hand, positions of residues from different protein structures are not directly comparable as they may be related by an unknown rigid transformation.

This section defines kernels on neighborhoods using the structure of the neighborhood described by the position of residues. We begin, by using the *spectral projection vector* derived in Section 7.3.2 (Definition 7.3.2). Note that the spectral projection vector can be thought of as assignment of one real number to each residue in the neighborhood, when used for matching neighborhoods (Section 7.3.3). Also, it can be inferred from Eq. (7.6), that the components of the spectral projection vector can be compared directly.

Spectral Neighborhood Kernel. Let $N_1 = \{p_1^1, \ldots, p_l^1\}$ and $N_2 = \{p_1^2, \ldots, p_l^2\}$ be two neighborhoods, each having l residues. Let $\mathbf{f}^1$ and $\mathbf{f}^2$ be the spectral projection vectors (Definition 7.3.2 for these neighborhoods. The residue kernel, K_{res}, between ith residue of N_1, p_i^1, and jth residue of N_2, p_j^2, is defined as the decreasing function of the difference in spectral projection:

$$\mathcal{K}_{\text{res}}(p_i^1, p_j^2) = e^{\frac{-(f_i^1 - f_j^2)^2}{\beta}} \tag{7.11}$$

β being a parameter. This kernel is PSD since it is essentially a Gaussian kernel. Note that the spectral projection vector trick was used to find a quantity that is comparable between residues of two structures.

Now, we can use the techniques used in Section 7.4.1 to define kernels on neighborhoods. We use the convolution kernel method since it also gives a relation to the spectral similarity score [Eq. (7.6)]. In our case, X is the set of all neighborhoods and $X_1, \ldots, X_m$ are all sets of all the residues p_i's from all the neighborhoods. Here, note that even if the same residue appears in different neighborhoods, the appearances will be considered to be different, since their spectral projection values are different.

Following the discussion in Section 7.4.1, the relation R is defined as $R(p_1, \ldots, p_l, N)$ is true iff $N = \{p_1, \ldots, p_l\}$. Since, all the X_i's have all the residues from N, the cases for which R can hold true are the permutations of residues of N. Since this can happen for both N_1 and N_2, each combination of correspondences occurs $l!$ times. Thus, using $K^i = K_{\text{res}}, i = 1, \ldots, l$ in Eq. 7.10, the kernel becomes

$$K(N_1, N_2) = l! \sum_{\pi \in \Pi(l)} \prod_{k=1}^{l} K_{res}(p_k^1, p_{\pi(k)}^2)$$

$$= l! \sum_{\pi \in \Pi(l)} e^{\frac{1}{\beta} - \sum_{k=1}^{l}(f_k^1 - f_{\pi(k)}^2)^2}$$

$$= l! \sum_{\pi \in \Pi(l)} e^{\frac{-\|\mathbf{f}^1 - \pi(\mathbf{f}^2)\|^2}{\beta}}$$

where, $\mathbf{f}^i$ is the spectral projection vector of N_i and $\Pi(l)$ is the set of all possible permutations of l numbers.

Definition 7.4.4 *Let $N_i = \{p_1^i, \ldots, p_l^i\}$, $p_j^i = (\mathbf{x}_j^i, y_j^i)$, $\mathbf{x}_j^i \in \mathbb{R}^3$, $y_j^i \in \mathcal{Y}$ be a neighborhood, and $\mathbf{f}^i$ be the spectral projection vector corresponding (Definition 7.3.2) to N_i. The spectral kernel, K_{spec}, between neighborhoods N_i and N_j is defined as*

$$K_{\text{spec}}(N_i, N_j) = \sum_{\pi \in \Pi(l)} e^{\frac{-\|\mathbf{f}^i - \pi(\mathbf{f}^j)\|^2}{\beta}}$$

Positive semidefiniteness of this kernel follows trivially from the above discussion. Note that, computation of this kernel takes exponential time in l. However, since l is a parameter of choice, and is usually chosen to be a small value (six in our experiments), the computation time is not prohibitive. Next, we show a relation between K_{spec} and S_{spec} [Eq. (7.6)].

Theorem 7.4.1 *Let N_i and N_j be two neighborhoods with spectral projection vectors $\mathbf{f}^i$ and $\mathbf{f}^j$. Let $S_{spec}(N_i, N_j)$ be the score of alignment of N_i and N_j, obtained* *by solving problem in Eq. (7.6), for a large enough value of T such that all residues are matched.*

$$\lim_{\beta \to 0} \mathcal{K}_{\text{spec}}(N_i, N_j))^\beta = e^{-lT} e^{S_{\text{spec}}(N_i, N_j)}$$

Proof: Let π^* be the permutation that gives the optimal score $S_{\text{spec}}(N_i, N_j)$. By definition, $e^{S_{\text{spec}}(N_i, N_j)} = \max_{\pi \in \Pi(l)} e^{\sum_{k=1}^l T - (f_k^i - f_{\pi(k)}^j)^2} = e^{lT} e^{-\|\mathbf{f}^i - \pi^*(\mathbf{f}^j)\|^2}$.

$$\lim_{\beta \to 0} (K_{\text{spec}}(N_i, N_j))^\beta = \lim_{\beta \to 0} (\sum_{\pi \in \Pi(l)} e^{\frac{-\|\mathbf{f}^i - \pi(\mathbf{f}^j)\|^2}{\beta}})^\beta$$

$$= e^{-\|\mathbf{f}^i - \pi^*(\mathbf{f}^j)\|^2}$$

$$\lim_{\beta \to 0} (1 + \sum_{\pi \in \Pi(l) \setminus \{\pi^*\}} e^{\frac{-1}{\beta}(\|\mathbf{f}^i - \pi(\mathbf{f}^j)\|^2 - \|\mathbf{f}^i - \pi^*(\mathbf{f}^j)\|^2)})^\beta$$

$$= e^{-\|\mathbf{f}^i - \pi^*(\mathbf{f}^j)\|^2}$$

The last step is true since $\|\mathbf{f}^i - \pi(\mathbf{f}^j)\|^2 - \|\mathbf{f}^i - \pi^*(\mathbf{f}^j)\|^2$ is always positive, and hence $\lim_{\beta \to 0} e^{\frac{-1}{\beta}(\|\mathbf{f}^i - \pi(\mathbf{f}^j)\|^2 - \|\mathbf{f}^i - \pi^*(\mathbf{f}^j)\|^2)}$ is 0. Combining the above equations, we get the result. ☐

Pairwise Distance Substructure Kernel. The previous kernel used the spectral projection based formulation to measure the similarity between neighborhoods. However, since the size of neighborhoods are usually small, we can also capture the similarity between pairwise distances of the two neighborhoods [Eq. (7.3)]. We do this by using the convolution kernel techniques [19].

In this case, X is the set of all neighborhoods and $X_1, \ldots, X_m$ are sets of all pairwise distances d_{ij}, $i < j$ between the residues from all neighborhoods. For each neighborhood of size l, we consider all pairwise distances between residues of that neighborhood. So, $m = l(l-1)/2$. We define the *pairwise distance vector*, $\mathbf{d}$ of a neighborhood $N = \{p_1, \ldots, p_l\}$, $p_i = (\mathbf{x}_i, y_i)$ as:

$$d_{ij} = \|\mathbf{x}_i - \mathbf{x}_j\|, i, j = 1, \ldots, l, i \geq j \qquad (7.12)$$

The relation R is defined as $R(\mathbf{d}, N)$ is true iff $\mathbf{d}$ is a pariwise distance vector of N.

Definition 7.4.5 *Let* $N_i = \{p_1^i, \ldots, p_l^i\}$, $p_j^i = (\mathbf{x}_j^i, y_j^i)$, $\mathbf{x}_j^i \in \mathbb{R}^3$, $y_j^i \in \mathcal{Y}$ *be a neighborhood, and* $\mathbf{d}^i$ *be the pairwise distance vector of* N^i, *i.e.* $d_{st}^i = \|\mathbf{x}_s^i - \mathbf{x}_t^i\|$, $s, t = 1, \ldots, l, s \geq t$. *The pairwise distances kernel,* K_{pd}, *between neighborhoods* N_i *and* N_j *is defined as*

$$K_{\text{pd}}(N_i, N_j) = \frac{1}{l!} \sum_{\pi \in \Pi(l)} e^{\frac{-\|\mathbf{d}^i - \pi(\mathbf{d}^j)\|^2}{\sigma^2}}$$

where, by notation $(\pi(\mathbf{d}))_{i,j} = \|p_{\pi(i)} - p_{\pi(j)}\|$.

Under the condition that all residues from two neighborhoods N_i and N_j have a matching residue in the other neighborhood, a decreasing function of optimal distance RMSD [Eq. (7.3)] can be used as a similarity measure between the two neighborhoods. Since all residues are matching, the space of all mapping become all permutations of the residues of one neighborhood while keeping the other fixed. By using the above definition of a pairwise distance vector, we define the similarity score as

$$S_{\text{drmsd}}(N_i, N_j) = \max_{\pi \in \Pi(l)} T' - \|\mathbf{d}^i - \pi(\mathbf{d}^j)\| \tag{7.13}$$

Next, we show a relation similar to that in Theorem 1, between K_{pd} and S_{drmsd}.

Theorem 7.4.2 *Let N_i and N_j be two neighborhoods with pairwise distance vectors $\mathbf{d}^i$ and $\mathbf{d}^j$. Let $S_{drmsd}(N_i, N_j)$ be the similarity score between N_i and N_j, obtained by solving problem in Eq. (7.13).*

$$\lim_{\sigma \to 0} K_{\text{pd}}(N_i, N_j))^{\sigma^2} = e^{-T'} e^{S_{\text{drmsd}}(N_i, N_j)}$$

Proof is essentially similar to that of Theorem 1. Both Theorems 1 and 2 show that for low values of β and σ the structure kernels are related to the alignment scores between neighborhoods. This is also demonstrated in the experiments in Section 7.6.4. Next, we describe two methods for combining kernels based on sequence and structure, to get general kernels on neighborhoods.

7.4.3   Combined Sequence and Structure-Based Kernels on Neighborhoods

According to our definition, each residue in a protein structure has two components: position in 3D space that describes the structure, and a type (or attribute) that describes the sequence. This can be viewed as an *attributed pointset* ([10]), which is a set of points in an Euclidean space with an attribute attached to each point. The main difference between position and attribute is that attributes are comparable directly, while positions can be related by a rigid transformation, and hence are not comparable directly.

In [10], we proposed kernels on attributed pointsets and used them for various tasks in computer vision. Kernels capturing position and attribute similarity were combined by weighting the position kernel with the attribute kernel. Here, we begin by weighting the structure based kernels with the sequence-based kernels.

Definition 7.4.6 *Let N_i and N_j be two neighborhoods. Let K_{seq} and K_{str} be sequence- and structure-based kernels on neighborhoods. The weighting kernel, K_{wt}, on neighborhoods is defined as*

$$K_{\text{wt}}(N_i, N_j) = K_{\text{seq}}(N_i, N_j) K_{\text{str}}(N_i, N_j)$$

where K_{wt} is PSD, since it is a pointwise product of two PSD kernels. In this chapter, the choices explored for K_{seq} are K_{rep}, $K_{allpair}$, K_{diral}, and K_{perm}, while those for K_{str} are K_{spec} and K_{pd}.

Another popular method of combining information from multiple kernels, mainly popularized by multiple kernel learning literature ([38,39]), is to use a linear combination of the kernels. Following this paradigm, we define our next kernel as a convex combination of sequence- and structure-based kernels.

Definition 7.4.7 *Let N_i and N_j be two neighborhoods. Let K_{seq} and K_{str} be sequence- and structure-based kernels on neighborhoods. The convex combination kernel K_{cc} on neighborhoods is defined as*

$$K_{cc}(N_i, N_j) = \gamma K_{seq}(N_i, N_j) + (1 - \gamma)K_{str}(N_i, N_j)$$

where, $\gamma \in [0, 1]$ is a parameter. This kernel is PSD since it is a linear combination of PSD kernels with positive coefficients. The same choices for K_{seq} and K_{str} as above are explored. In Section 7.5, we combine the neighborhood kernels, K_{wt} and K_{cc}, to get kernels on entire protein structures.

7.5 KERNELS ON PROTEIN STRUCTURES

Section 7.4 defined various kernels on neighborhoods. This section describes two ways of combining these kernels to get kernels on entire protein structures. The first method uses set kernels by viewing each protein as a set of neighborhoods. We show that these kernels are related to the well-known spectrum kernels [5]. The second method uses known alignments to increase the accuracy of similarity measure.

7.5.1 Neighborhood Pair Sum Kernels

One way of combining neighborhood kernels for deriving kernels on protein structures is by viewing proteins as a set of neighborhoods. Various strategies could be used to choose the neighborhoods that describe a protein structure. For example, we could choose a minimal set of neighborhoods that cover all the residues in a protein. However, this may not have a unique solution, which may lead to a comparison of different neighborhoods of similar structures, and hence low similarity between similar structures.

For structure neighborhoods, we consider neighborhoods centered at each residue. This ensures that all residues are part of at least one neighborhood. For sequence neighborhoods, we consider neighborhoods starting at each residue except the last $l - 1$ in the protein sequence since there can not be any neighborhoods of length l starting at them.

We view a protein structure as a set of constituent neighborhoods. Thus, a protein P^A, described by n_A neighborhoods, is represented as $\hat{P}^A = \{N_1^A, \ldots, N_{n_A}^A\}$. From the set kernels described in Section 7.4.1, only the representative element kernels and all pair kernels are applicable since the number of neighborhoods in two proteins

P^A and P^B may not be the same. Considering only one neighborhood, is generally not a good representation of the entire protein structure. Thus we use the all pair sum kernel for defining kernels on protein structures.

Definition 7.5.1 *Let P^A and P^B be two proteins represented in terms of constituent neighborhoods as $\hat{P}^A = \{N_1^A, \ldots, N_{n_A}^A\}$ and $\hat{P}^B = \{N_1^B, \ldots, N_{n_B}^B\}$, and K_{nbhd} be a kernel on neighborhoods. The neighborhood pair sum kernel, K_{nps} between the two proteins is defined as*

$$K_{nps}(\hat{P}^A, \hat{P}^B) = \frac{1}{n_A n_B} \sum_{i=1}^{n_A} \sum_{j=1}^{n_B} K_{nbhd}(N_i^A, N_j^B)$$

where K_{nps} is a PSD kernel because it is of the form $\psi_A \psi_B K(A, B)$ where $K(A, B)$ is a PSD kernel and ψ_A is a function of only A. The parameter K_{nps} can be computed in $O(n_A n_B)$ time. Next, we show a relation between between K_{nps} and the spectrum kernel [5].

The spectrum kernels were designed for protein sequence classification using support vector machines. For every protein sequence s, [5] defines the k-spectrum-based feature map $\Theta_k(x)$ indexed by all k length subsequences $\mathcal{Y}^k$ as $\Theta_k(s) = (\theta_a(s))_{a \in \mathcal{Y}^k}$, where $\theta_a(s)$ is the number of occurrences of a in s. The k-spectrum kernel is defined as: $K_k^{spectrum}(s, s') = \langle \Theta_k(s), \Theta_k(s') \rangle$.

Theorem 7.5.3 *Let P and P' be two proteins with representations $\hat{P} = \{N_1, \ldots, N_n\}$ and $\hat{P}' = \{N_1', \ldots, N_{n'}'\}$, and s and s' be their sequences. Then, there is a sequence kernel on neighborhoods, K_{seq}, for which $\frac{1}{nn'} K_l^{spectrum}(s, s') = K_{nps}(\hat{P}, \hat{P}')$, where $K_{nbhd} = K_{cc}$ with $\gamma = 1$, and sequence neighborhoods of length l are used to represent P and P'.*

Proof: $K_l^{spectrum}(s, s')$ computes the number of common subsequences of length l between s and s', where each occurrence of a subsequence a is considered different. This is because $\langle \Theta_l(s), \Theta_l(s') \rangle = \sum_{a \in \mathcal{Y}^l} \theta_a(s)\theta_a(s')$, thus adding up products of counts every subsequence.

Observe that all nonzero entries in $\Theta_l(s)$ precisely correspond to sequence neighborhoods of size l in $\hat{P}$. Consider the kernel on neighborhoods $K_{seq}(N_i, N_j') = \prod_{k=1}^{l} K_I(y_k^i, y_k'^j)$, where $N_i = \{p_1^i, \ldots, p_l^i\}$, $p_k^i = (\mathbf{x}_k^i, y_k^i)$. $K_{seq}(N_i, N_j')$ is 1 if N_i and N_j' are identical, 0 otherwise. The parameter $K_{nbhd} = K_{seq}$ since $\gamma = 1$. So,

$$K_{nps}(\hat{P}, \hat{P}') = \frac{1}{nn'} \sum_{s=1}^{n} \sum_{t=1}^{n'} K_{seq}(N_s, N_t')$$

$$= \frac{1}{nn'} \sum_{a \in \mathcal{Y}^l} \theta_a(s)\theta_a(s')$$

Hence, the result. □

This result shows that when restricted to use only sequence related information, K_{nps} is essentially the length normalized version of K^{spectrum}. Note that a similar result can be derived for the mismatch kernels [5] with an appropriate choice of K_{seq}. Unfortunately, the feature map representation used to derive spectrum kernels cannot be extended directly to define kernels on structures since the feature space will be infinite. Section 7.5.2 defines kernels that use alignments generated by external structural alignment programs.

7.5.2   Alignment Kernels

Section 7.5.1 defineds kernels on protein structures that do not need any extra information. The kernels add up similarity between all pairs of neighborhoods in the two protein structures. However, any neighborhood in a protein structure is expected to be similar to only one neighborhood in the other structure. So, adding the kernels values for other pairs of neighborhoods introduces noise in the kernel value that reduces the classification accuracy.

This section alleviates this problem by utilizing alignment between residues given by a structural alignment program to compute kernels. The correspondences between residues given by a structural alignment induces correspondence between the structure neighborhoods centered at these residues. The naive structural alignment kernel adds up kernels between the corresponding neighborhoods.

Definition 7.5.2 *Let P^i and P^j be two proteins represented in terms of constituent structure neighborhoods as $\hat{P}^i = \{N_1^i, \ldots, N_{n_i}^i\}$ and $\hat{P}^j = \{N_1^j, \ldots, N_{n_j}^j\}$, and K_{nbhd} be a kernel on neighborhoods. Let ϕ_{ij} be an alignment between P^i and P^j. The naive alignment kernel, K_{nal} between the two proteins is defined as*

$$K_{nal}(P^i, P^j; \phi_{ij}) = \sum_{a \mid p_a^i \in \hat{P}^i} K_{nbhd}(N_a^i, N_{\phi_{ij}(a)}^j)$$

Note that here only structure neighborhoods can be used since some residues will not have a corresponding sequence neighborhood. Unfortunately, this kernel is not necessarily positive semidefinite. Though SVM training algorithm has no theoretical guarantees for a kernel matrix that is not PSD, they work well in practice.

While many methods have been suggested for learning with non-PSD kernels [40], most of them require computation of singular values of the kernel matrix. This may be computationally inefficient or even infeasible in many cases. Moreover, in most cases, the values of the kernel function do not remain the same as the original kernel function. Another kernel is proposed based on the alignment kernel, which while keeping the off-diagonal terms intact and only modifying the diagonal terms, is always positive semidefinite.

Definition 7.5.3 *Let $\mathcal{D} = \{P^1, \ldots, P^M\}$ be a dataset of M proteins represented in terms of constituent structure neighborhoods as $\hat{P}^i = \{N_1^i, \ldots, N_{n_i}^i\}$ and K_{nbhd} be a* *kernel on neighborhoods. Let ϕ_{ij} be an alignment between P^i and P^j, $1 \leq i, j \leq M$. The PSD alignment kernel, K_{psdal} between the two proteins P^i and P^j is defined as*

$$
K_{\text{psdal}}(P^i, P^j) = \begin{cases} \displaystyle\sum_{a \mid p_a^i \in \bar{P}^i} K_{nbhd}(N_a^i, N_{\phi_{ij}(a)}^j) & \text{if } i \neq j \\ \displaystyle\sum_{b=1}^{M} \sum_{a \mid p_a^i \in dom(\phi_{ib})} K_{nbhd}(N_a^i, N_{\phi_{ib}(a)}^i) & \text{if } i = j \end{cases}
$$

where dom(ϕ_{ib}) is the domain of function ϕ_{ib}, which is the set of all residues participating in the alignment ϕ_{ib} from structure P^i. Notice that K_{psdal} can be computed in an incremental way, which is not trivial for methods that require singular value decomposition. Next, we show that K_{psdal} is indeed PSD.

Theorem 7.5.4   *The parameter K_{psdal} is positive semidefinite if K_{nbhd} is positive valued.*

Proof: Let L_{max} be the maximum length of alignments between all pairs of proteins in the dataset $\mathcal{D}$. Consider the $M \times (\frac{M(M+1)}{2} L_{max})$ matrix H having one row for each protein in the dataset. Each row has $\frac{M(M+1)}{2}$ blocks of length L_{max} corresponding to each pairwise alignment (including alignment of every structure with itself). For rows corresponding to proteins i and j, the kth element of the block for alignment ϕ_{ij} is equal to $\sqrt{K_{nbhd}(N_k^i, N_{\phi_{ij}(k)}^j)}$. The index k runs over all the correspondences in the alignment. For alignments that have length smaller than L_{max}, put the remaining entries to be zero. It can be seen that $K_{psdal} = HH^T$. Since, each entry in K_{psdal} is a dot product between two vectors, K_{psdal} is positive semidefinite. $\square$

This theorem can also be proved using the result that diagonally dominant matrices (matrices having the property $A_{ii} \geq \sum_{j=1}^{n} |A_{ij}|$) are PSD. Note that, K_{nbhd} needs to be positive valued and not positive semidefinite. So, this method can get a kernel from any positive valued similarity measure on the neighborhoods. Unfortunately, diagonal dominance of a kernel often reduces its classification accuracy (e.g., see [41, 42]).

Computational Complexity. Time complexity of the neighborhood kernels is $O(1)$, since size of the neighborhoods is a user-defined parameter, rather than a charatheristic of data. For neighborhood size l, the time complexities of K_{rep}, K_{diral}, $K_{allpair}$, K_{perm}, K_{spec}, and K_{pd} are $O(1)$, $O(l)$, $O(l^2)$, $O(l!)$, $O(l!)$ and $O(l!)$, respectively. Since for most experiments, l was fixed at a very low value of 6, the exponential complexity of K_{perm}, K_{spec}, and K_{pd} does not pose a major problem to computational feasibility.

The time complexity of K_{nps} is $O(n_1 n_2)$, where n_1 and n_2 are the number of neighborhoods in the two proteins being compared. Time complexity of K_{nal} is $O(min(n_1, n_2))$. The parameter K_{psdal} can be implemented in amortized time complexity of $O(n)$, n being the maximum length of alignment. Memory requirements of all the kernels are $O(n_1 + n_2)$, which is necessary for storing the proteins in memory. In Section 7.6, we report results of experiments conducted for validating the kernels developed here on the task of protein structure classification.

7.6   EXPERIMENTAL RESULTS

Extensive experimentation was conducted in order to both demonstrate the practical applicability of the kernels proposed above on real protein structures, and to study properties of the proposed kernels. Section 7.6.1 describes the data set, the experimental procedure, and the quantities observed. Section 7.6.2 reports representative and average results for various types of kernels and compares them with classification performed using a popular protein structure comparison method CE [21]. Section 7.6.4 studies the effects of various parameters on the classification performance of the kernels. Section 7.6.5 describes results of experiments with spectrum kernels in order to demonstrate the difficulty of the current task.

7.6.1   Experimental Setup

The kernels proposed above were tested extensively on the well-known structural classification database called SCOP [12]. The experiments were designed so as to test utility of the proposed kernels toward the practical and difficult problem of classifying structures having very low sequence identity ($< 40\%$). The results were compared with a state of the art protein structure alignment algorithm, CE [21], which was found to be the top performer in [43].

The kernels developed were implemented in C using GCC/GNU Linux. OpenMPI over LAM was used on a cluster to speed up the computations. Eigenvalue computations were done using Lapack [44], and SVM classifications were done using Libsvm [45]. The protein structures were obtained from ASTRAL [46].

Data Set Construction. The task chosen was to classify a data set of proteins having $< 40\%$ sequence identity between any pair of proteins. This task is both difficult and relevant to computational biologists, since most standard sequence processing algorithms (e.g., BLAST [36]), cannot identify many relationships between proteins having low sequence similarity [47]. Thus, kernels utilizing the structure information to achieve accurate results on such difficult problems are highly useful. Also, the ASTRAL compendium [46] provides a 40% nonredundant data set, which is the lowest redundancy cutoff provided by ASTRAL.

We chose the classification at the superfamily level of SCOP. This level captures functional and distant evolutionary relationships, where 21 superfamilies were detected that had at least 10 proteins at 40% sequence non-redundance (in SCOP 1.69). The structural classification is performed using 21 one versus all classification problems. In order to get a balanced problem, a randomly chosen set of 10 proteins from other classes is used as the negative dataset for each class. In order to get a stable estimate of the classification accuracy, this experiment is repeated 100 times and the average is reported.

Similar tasks have been attempted by [17] and [16]. However, we concentrate on structural classification rather than functional annotation, since we are more interested in studying the properties of the proposed kernels than exploring possible diverse applications. Also, the task we have chosen is more difficult since we attempt to classify the 40% nonredundant data set, as compared to say the 90% nonredundant data set used in [16]. This allows us to concentrate on a much smaller data set (9,479 domains instead of 97,178 in SCOP 1.73), and thus allows us to use more computationally intensive algorithms.

Experimental Procedure. We use the leave-one-out cross-validation as the basic test for the classifier, due to a small number of datapoints per class. Leave-one-out cross-validation was also used in [17]. The predicted labels are used to calculate accuracies on positive and negative classes and receiver operating characterstic (ROC) curves [48]. For a group of kernels, the average results are reported in the form of area under ROC curve (AUC) [48] and average classification accuracies; and the variance around average as maximum and minimum classification accuracies. The area under ROC curve (AUC) [48] is used as the primary index for judging the quality of a classifier and AUC is also used in [16].

Each combination of the type of amino acid kernels, sequence- and structure-based kernels on neighborhoods, and method of combination of sequence and structure based kernels is called a *type* of kernel. Table 7.1 gives the types of kernels for which experiments were performed. Due to intuition from biology, all pair sum kernels were computed only for structure neighborhoods and direct alignment kernels were computed only for sequence neighborhoods. A total of 44 types of kernels were experimentally evaluated for various parameter values. Average results for each type of sequence and structure kernel are in Section 7.6.3. Due to lack of space, detailed results for each type of kernel is provided in the supplementary material.

Table 7.2 shows the values of parameters for which experimental results are reported. These parameters were found by trial and error to be appropriate for current task. Section 7.6.4 compares the performance of various kernels for these parameter values. Detailed results are reported in the supplementary material.

7.6.2   Validation of Proposed Kernels

This section validates the effectiveness of the proposed kernels on the above mentioned task. All the kernels mentioned above were used to train classifiers for the task. We report representative and average results with variances for the kernels. These results are compared with the state of the art protein structure comparison tool called CE [21]. Detailed results are available in the supplementary material.

TABLE 7.1   Types of Kernels for Which Experiments Were Performed

Seq. ker. →	Representative	All Pair
Struct. ker.	Residue Kernel	Sum Kernel

Neighborhood Pair Sum Kernels[a]

Spec. ker.	Seq. and Str. Nbhd.	Str. Nbhd.
Pair. dist. ker.	Seq. and Str. Nbhd.	Str. Nbhd.

Naive Alignment Kernels[b]

Spec. ker.	Id. and blos. ker.	Id. and blos. ker.
Pair. dist. ker.	Id. and blos. ker.	Id. and blos. ker.

Positive Semidefinite Alignment Kernels[b]

Spec. ker.	Id. and blos. ker.	Id. and blos. ker.
Pair. dist. ker.	Id. and blos. ker.	Id. and blos. ker.
Seq. ker. →	Permutation	Direct align.
Struct. ker.	Sum Kernel	Kernel

Neighborhood Pair Sum Kernels[a]

Spec. ker.	Seq. and Str. Nbhd.	Seq. Nbhd.
Pair. dist. ker.	Seq. and Str. Nbhd.	Seq. Nbhd.

Naive Alignment Kernels[b]

Spec. ker.	Id. and blos. ker.	Id. and blos. ker.
Pair. dist. ker.	Id. and blos. ker.	Id. and blos. ker.

Positive Semidefinite Alignment Kernels[b]

Spec. ker.	Id. and blos. ker.	Id. and blos. ker.
Pair. dist. ker.	Id. and blos. ker.	Id. and blos. ker.

[a] Only blosum kernels were used to compute the sequence kernels.

[b] Only structure neighborhoods were used since sequence neighborhoods are not defined for each residue, while structural alignment is a correspondence between residues.

Table 7.3 reports representative results for various kernels studied here and compares them with the results obtained from CE [21]. All the positive semidefinite alignment kernels, except the ones that use sequence information only (for $\gamma = 1$), perform comparably or better than CE. Thus, kernel based methods can be used along with SVMs to achieve performance comparable to state-of-the-art methods in computational biology.

TABLE 7.2   Values of Various Parameters for Which Experimental Results are Reported

Parameters	PSD Alignment Kernel	Naive Alignment Kernel	Neighborhood Pair Sum Kernel
α (Eq. 7.5)	10	10	10
β (Definition 7.4.4)	0.001, 0.005, 0.0001, 0.0005	0.01, 0.05 0.001, 0.005	0.001, 0.0001
σ (Definition 7.4.5)	5, 8, 9, 10	10, 11, 12, 15	8, 10, 12
γ (Definition 7.4.7)	0, 0.2, 0.5, 0.8, 1	0, 0.2, 0.5, 0.8	0.2, 0.8

TABLE 7.3 Representative Results for K_{nps} (def. 7.5.1), K_{nal} (def. 7.5.2), K_{psdal} (def. 7.5.3), and CE [21]

Kernel (γ)/ Method	Area Under ROC Curve	Positive Acc.	Negative Acc.	Area Under ROC Curve	Positive Acc.	Negative Acc.
Neighborhood Pair Sum Kernels $(K_{nps})^a$						
	Sequence Neighborhood			**Structure Neighborhood**		
K_{wt}	0.676	76.809	58.071	0.676	77.500	56.452
K_{cc} 0.2	0.625	68.619	54.309	0.626	69.761	53.571
K_{cc} 0.8	0.569	61.809	50.214	0.572	61.071	51.071
Naive Alignment Kernels $(K_{nal})^b$						
	Identity Kernel			**Blosum Kernel**		
K_{wt}	0.660	71.809	62.428	0.709	74.023	67.845
K_{cc} 0	0.700	72.666	66.071	0.696	72.702	66.309
K_{cc} 0.2	0.691	71.238	66.238	0.694	73.202	65.880
K_{cc} 0.5	0.693	72.261	66.333	0.702	73.345	67.059
K_{cc} 0.8	0.666	72.666	65.547	0.662	72.976	60.619
Positive Semidefinite Alignment Kernels $(K_{psdal})^c$						
	Identity Kernel			**Blosum Kernel**		
K_{wt}	0.803	85.071	75.904	0.802	85.309	75.238
K_{cc} 0	0.795	84.809	74.380	0.795	84.619	74.285
K_{cc} 0.2	0.790	84.309	73.357	0.789	84.166	74.523
K_{cc} 0.5	0.790	84.023	74.833	0.791	83.761	75.523
K_{cc} 0.8	0.793	83.404	74.809	0.790	83.857	75.119
K_{cc} 1	0.716	76.857	66.190	0.680	74.476	62.285
CE	0.780	96.457	60.619	0.780	96.457	60.619

[a] Results are for permutation sum sequence neighborhood kernel and spectral structure neighborhood kernel with $\alpha = 10$ and $\beta = 0.0001$.

[b] Results are for all pair sequence neighborhood kernels and pairwise distance structure neighborhood kernel with $\sigma = 12$.

[c] Results in the case of identity kernels are for all pair sequence neighborhood kernels and spectral structure neighborhood kernels with $\alpha = 10$ and $\beta = 0.0001$; and those in case of blosum kernel are for permutation sum sequence neighborhood kernel and spectral structure neighborhood kernel with $\alpha = 10$ and $\beta = 0.0001$.

The other kernels do not perform as well as positive semidefinite alignment kernels. For neighborhood pair sum kernels, this is due to inaccuracy in computing the similarity values arising out of the fact that they sum up similarities between all pairs of neighborhoods. For the naive alignment kernels, this is due to the fact that they are not necessarily positive semidefinite. Also, the naive alignment kernels perform slightly better than the neighborhood pair sum kernels, since they use the extra information provided by the structural alignment and only add up similarities between equivalent neighborhoods.

We also observe that for neighborhood pair sum (NPS) kernels, the weighting kernels perform slightly better than the linear combination kernels. However, for the alignment kernels, the performance of weighting kernels, as well as the linear combination kernels are similar. The reason is that for NPS kernels, multiplication of structure similarity component by sequence similarity leads to more effective weighing down of similarity values for the noncorresponding neighborhoods, thereby increasing the influence of similarity between corresponding neighborhoods. This principle was also used in [10] to improve the performance kernels for face recognition. This problem is not present in alignment kernels, and hence there is not much difference in accuracies of weighting and linear combination kernels.

Note that for linear combination NPS kernels there is a gradual decrease in their performance with the increase in value γ. Hence, there is an increase in component sequence similarity. This difference is not observed in the case of alignment kernels. However, there is a sharp decline in performance of alignment kernels when the component of structural similarity becomes zero (for $\gamma = 1$). From these observations, we can conclude that the structural similarity component is much more useful than sequence similarity component for the present task. This is also consistent with the biological intuition that for distantly related proteins, structural similarity is higher than sequence similarity.

Another observation is that positive classification accuracy is much higher than negative classification for all kernels. The reason is that a multi-class classification problem was posed as many binary class classification problems and the average accuracy over all problems is reported. Thus for each classification problem, the positive class is a true class while the negative class is an assortment of all other classes. This explains the asymmetry in the classification accuracies.

Figure 7.1 presents the ROC curves for the representative kernels reported above, and compares them with those from CE [21]. The NPS kernels (Figs. 7.1a and b) perform worse than CE. However, some of the naive alignment kernels (Figs. 7.1c and d) perform comparatively with CE till 30% of the false positives. After which their performance declines.

Interestingly, the positive semidefinite alignment kernels perform much better than CE for low false positive rates. For example, the positive semidefinite weighting kernel gives ∼85% true positives at 25% false positives, while CE gives only about 60% true positives at the same false positive level. However, CE performs better than the kernel based classifiers at false positive rates >35%. Overall, some kernels perform marginally better than CE (according to AUC reported in Table 7.3).

Table 7.4 reports the average results for different kernels over all types of kernels and parameter values listed in Tables 7.1 and 7.2. All the observations made with the representative results are also observed for the average results.

Variance in the performance is reported using maximum and minimum classification accuracy of the classifiers. Some classifiers obtained using K_{wt} and $K_{cc}(\gamma = 1)$ show very low minimum classification accuracy. This is due to numerical problems that arise due to the sequence-based kernel taking very low values.

It was observed that the variance in performance of the weighting kernels is much higher than the comvex combination kernels. Thus, weighting kernels are much more

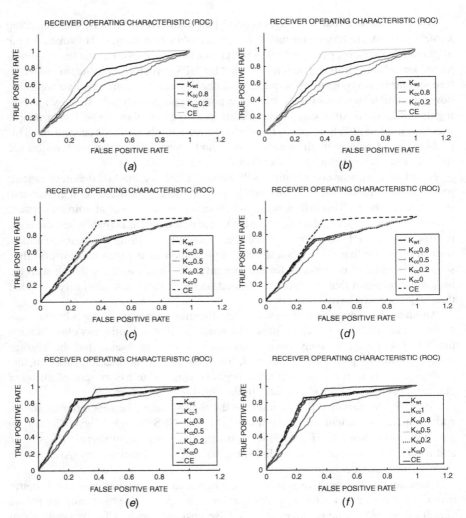

FIGURE 7.1   Representative results for K_{nps} (def. 7.5.1), K_{nal} (def. 7.5.2), K_{psdal} (def. 7.5.3), and CE [21]. Parts (a) and (b) show ROC curves for K_{nps} with sequence and structure neighborhoods, respectively. Parts (b) and (d) show ROC curves for K_{max} with identity and blosum amino acid kernels. Parts (e) and (f) show ROC curves for K_{prdal} with identity and blosum amino acid kernels.

sensitive to variation in parameters than the convex combination kernels. This can be attributed to a more profound effect of the multiplication operation.

From the above observations, we conclude that overall the kernels proposed in this chapter provide a comprehensive and effective scheme for designing classifiers for proteins having low sequence similarity. The weighting method generates more accurate albeit sensitive classifiers than convex combination. Also, in the case of

TABLE 7.4   Average Results for K_{nps} (def. 7.5.1), K_{nal} (def. 7.5.2), and K_{psdal} (def. 7.5.3)

Kernel (γ)	Area Under ROC Curve	Positive Acc.			Negative Acc.		
		Max.	Avg.	Min.	Max.	Avg.	Min.
Neighborhood Pair Sum Kernels (K_{nps})							
Sequence Neighborhood							
K_{wt}	0.611	76.547	68.242	61.547	57.595	53.539	49.952
K_{cc} 0.2	0.587	70.380	65.011	61.619	55.571	51.692	49.761
K_{cc} 0.8	0.565	65.952	62.439	56.000	52.380	50.542	47.952
Structure Neighborhood							
K_{wt}	0.608	78.000	68.357	62.666	57.333	53.571	50.404
K_{cc} 0.2	0.584	69.333	64.987	61.761	54.738	51.865	49.952
K_{cc} 0.8	0.565	65.666	62.325	55.904	53.000	50.717	46.809
Naive Alignment Kernels (K_{nal})							
Identity Kernel							
K_{wt}	0.549	74.857	59.175	45.976	62.523	52.678	44.738
K_{cc} 0	0.687	73.880	72.020	69.404	67.095	65.607	64.238
K_{cc} 0.2	0.685	73.785	72.042	69.071	67.309	65.512	63.619
K_{cc} 0.5	0.682	74.095	72.116	68.500	68.214	65.700	63.976
K_{cc} 0.8	0.652	74.857	72.210	69.190	67.904	65.430	63.333
Blosum Kernel							
K_{wt}	0.678	75.011	72.886	58.857	67.571	62.610	44.630
K_{cc} 0	0.688	73.678	72.011	69.476	67.190	65.649	64.083
K_{cc} 0.2	0.685	73.392	71.853	69.523	66.821	65.248	64.000
K_{cc} 0.5	0.682	73.583	72.197	69.666	66.630	64.454	59.059
K_{cc} 0.8	0.652	73.809	70.581	56.214	65.166	59.934	47.178
Positive Semidefinite Alignment Kernels (K_{psdal})							
Identity Kernel							
K_{wt}	0.661	85.166	68.455	5.166	76.523	63.830	11.880
K_{cc} 0	0.689	85.309	74.658	68.928	75.214	63.098	56.357
K_{cc} 0.2	0.690	84.738	74.739	69.452	74.571	63.277	56.857
K_{cc} 0.5	0.690	85.190	74.807	69.452	74.880	63.371	56.261
K_{cc} 0.8	0.690	84.571	74.657	68.357	76.119	63.223	56.166
K_{cc} 1	0.525	77.738	53.774	0.000	70.238	50.732	2.714
Blosum Kernel							
K_{wt}	0.709	85.071	76.617	70.476	74.714	65.458	58.261
K_{cc} 0	0.689	85.119	74.648	68.738	74.976	63.079	56.666
K_{cc} 0.2	0.688	83.214	74.488	68.547	74.380	63.070	56.261
K_{cc} 0.5	0.686	83.476	74.466	68.785	74.476	62.759	56.190
K_{cc} 0.8	0.677	83.380	73.866	69.071	75.047	61.819	55.761
K_{cc} 1	0.658	75.333	71.891	69.380	62.571	59.859	57.047

convex combination kernels, kernels capturing structure information turn out to be more effective for the current purpose than kernels capturing sequence similarity.

7.6.3   Comparison of Different Types of Neighborhood Kernels

This section studies the relative performance of different types of neighborhood kernels developed in this chapter. Table 7.5 reports the average results for all types of kernels, averaged over all parameter values and other types of kernels. More detailed results are reported in the supplementary material.

We observe that average performance of various types of sequence neighborhood kernels is similar for a given type of kernel on the whole protein. This can be attributed to the fact that sequence information is not very useful for the present task. Thus, different types sequence neighborhood kernels are restricted by the nature of information provided to them.

The spectral structure neighborhood kernel is performing marginally better than the pairwise distance structure neighborhood kernel. Except the naive alignment kernel, the maximum accuracies achieved by spectral neighborhood kernel-based classifiers is significantly higher than those achieved by pairwise distance neighborhood kernel-based classifiers. For naive alignment kernels, their performances are comparable. The reason that protein structures data is noisy by nature. The spectral projections are more robust to noise than pairwise distances.

The variance in accuracy was also not found to be related to the type of neighborhood kernel. Thus, we conclude that spectral kernels are slightly better than pairwise distance kernels for the current task. A characterization of the sequence neighborhood-based kernels for various kinds of tasks remains an open question.

7.6.4   Effects of Parameter Values

This section studies the effect of various parameter values on the classification accuracy of the resulting kernels. There are two parameters in for the spectral kernel K_{spec}(def. 7.4.4), α [Eq. (7.5)] and β (def. 7.4.4). The value of α is fixed at 10, which is determined to be the optimal value in previous experiments [11]. β was allowed to vary in the set indicated in Table 7.2. Table 7.6 reports average results on the different types of kernels and various values of β. The pairwise distance kernel K_{pd} (def. 7.4.5) has one parameter, σ (def. 7.4.5). The parameter σ was allowed to take values in the set provided in Table 7.2. Table 7.7 reports average results for various vales of σ. Detailed results are provided in the supplementary material.

For convex combination kernels, the parameter γ (def. 7.4.7) is varied to study the effect of sequence- and structure-based kernels on classification accuracy. This study was reported in Section 7.6.2 along with the average results. Results are presented in Table 7.4. Hence, we do not repeat it here.

From Table 7.6, we observe that in most cases, the classifier accuracy increases with decrease in value of β. This finding is in accordance with the result in Theorem 1, which says that as $\beta \to 0$, the value of K_{spec} approaches an increasing function of the spectral alignment score, which was motivated to be a good measure of structural

TABLE 7.5 Average Results for Different Types of Neighborhood Kernels

Kernel/ Method	Area Under ROC Curve	Positive Acc.			Negative Acc.		
		Max.	Avg.	Min.	Max.	Avg.	Min.
Neighborhood Pair Sum Kernels (K_{nps})							
Sequence Neighborhood							
K_{rep} [Eq. (7.9)]	0.585	75.880	65.044	55.785	55.690	51.711	48.809
K_{perm} (def. 7.4.3)	0.597	77.380	66.218	60.809	57.857	52.807	49.761
K_{diral} (def. 7.4.1)	0.582	74.857	64.874	54.857	55.833	51.485	47.238
K_{spec} (def. 7.4.4)	0.593	75.666	66.129	56.214	57.071	52.704	47.547
K_{pd} (def. 7.4.5)	0.582	71.809	64.696	60.357	54.166	51.540	49.166
Structure Neighborhood							
K_{rep} [Eq. (7.9)]	0.583	77.309	64.923	56.666	57.119	51.832	46.642
$K_{allpair}$ (def. 7.4.2)	0.584	74.500	54.876	57.428	55.380	51.907	47.714
K_{perm} (def. 7.4.3)	0.593	77.357	65.907	60.904	55.904	52.114	49.309
K_{spec} (def. 7.4.4)	0.596	76.738	66.198	56.190	57.309	52.609	48.261
K_{pd} (def. 7.4.5)	0.582	69.761	64.830	60.952	54.166	51.820	50.095
Naive Alignment Kernels (K_{nal})							
Identity Kernel							
K_{rep} [Eq. (7.9)]	0.646	73.690	68.595	48.261	66.809	62.278	47.547
$K_{allpair}$ (def. 7.4.2)	0.667	73.666	71.707	65.690	67.047	64.671	57.976
K_{perm} (def. 7.4.3)	0.678	73.904	72.014	69.142	68.904	65.715	63.380
K_{diral} (def. 7.4.1)	0.638	74.190	67.989	45.142	67.571	61.728	44.690
K_{spec} (def. 7.4.4)	0.642	74.071	68.696	45.119	68.428	62.721	46.096
K_{pd} (def. 7.4.5)	0.659	74.119	69.948	48.857	67.714	63.283	46.595
Blosum Kernel							
K_{rep} [Eq. (7.9)]	0.676	74.357	71.900	58.559	66.440	63.528	48.452
$K_{allpair}$ (def. 7.4.2)	0.681	75.345	72.202	60.047	67.654	64.310	48.297
K_{perm} (def. 7.4.3)	0.673	75.190	71.800	57.369	66.904	63.116	44.035
K_{diral} (def. 7.4.1)	0.675	74.714	71.982	58.845	66.690	63.241	48.202
K_{spec} (def. 7.4.4)	0.669	74.642	71.038	57.833	65.692	62.912	43.726
K_{pd} (def. 7.4.5)	0.685	74.345	72.930	71.059	67.595	64.225	55.702
Positive Semidefinite Alignment Kernels (K_{psdal})							
Identity Kernel							
K_{rep} [Eq. (7.9)]	0.675	84.642	71.228	61.428	74.500	63.567	56.785
$K_{allpair}$ (def. 7.4.2)	0.704	85.023	75.800	68.5	74.690	64.938	55.880
K_{perm} (def. 7.4.3)	0.648	84.952	69.375	4.880	76.261	60.275	12.166
K_{diral} (def. 7.4.1)	0.708	84.595	75.923	69.500	75.071	65.743	57.261
K_{spec} (def. 7.4.4)	0.610	84.904	74.517	4.571	75.404	65.598	13.142
K_{pd} (def. 7.4.5)	0.669	79.261	71.756	4.809	75.976	61.917	11.476
Blosum Kernel							
K_{rep} [Eq. (7.9)]	0.683	84.404	74.261	69.428	75.214	62.427	56.880
$K_{allpair}$ (def. 7.4.2)	0.678	84.785	73.847	69.309	74.523	61.905	56.642
K_{perm} (def. 7.4.3)	0.696	84.928	75.477	69.214	74.666	63.808	56.880
K_{diral} (def. 7.4.1)	0.682	85.357	74.051	69.119	74.523	62.299	57.452
K_{spec} (def. 7.4.4)	0.704	85.285	76.120	69.285	75.523	64.945	56.023
K_{pd} (def. 7.4.5)	0.664	77.928	72.706	69.500	70.142	60.503	56.357

TABLE 7.6   Average Results for the Parameter β

	Area Under	Positive Acc.			Negative Acc.		
β (def. 7.4.4)	ROC Curve	Max.	Avg.	Min.	Max.	Avg.	Min.
Neighborhood Pair Sum Kernels (K_{nps})							
Sequence Neighborhood							
0.001	0.578	67.285	63.618	60.904	55.095	51.571	49.642
0.0001	0.606	78.666	67.848	54.380	58.309	53.616	47.214
Structure Neighborhood							
0.001	0.583	67.928	64.195	60.071	54.380	52.021	49.690
0.0001	0.606	76.261	67.494	55.785	57.904	53.608	47.880
Naive Alignment Kernels (K_{nal})							
Identity Kernel							
0.05	0.655	72.880	68.511	51.857	66.214	62.536	48.023
0.01	0.656	73.404	68.670	52.785	65.357	62.281	45.642
0.005	0.655	72.642	69.251	52.428	65.571	62.051	45.571
0.001	0.605	73.796	69.348	47.119	68.095	63.694	47.428
Blosum Kernel							
0.05	0.679	74.690	71.383	69.440	66.250	64.429	60.880
0.01	0.680	75.130	71.788	69.630	65.333	64.207	61.190
0.005	0.678	74.714	72.095	71.023	65.773	63.640	61.869
0.001	0.640	72.869	69.334	56.250	65.333	58.964	43.952
Positive Semidefinite Alignment Kernels (K_{psdal})							
Identity Kernel							
0.005	0.653	77.500	70.499	58.523	69.309	60.180	56.476
0.001	0.693	79.738	74.127	58.571	71.380	64.673	62.500
0.0005	0.713	82.833	75.266	8.357	74.119	67.299	15.761
0.0001	0.744	85.785	78.595	4.380	75.833	70.448	12.238
Blosum Kernel							
0.005	0.642	75.261	70.445	69.095	63.285	58.236	56.428
0.001	0.688	78.595	74.700	70.142	68.404	63.219	57.738
0.0005	0.729	82.142	78.200	69.857	72.785	67.957	57.880
0.0001	0.755	85.380	80.809	68.857	75.500	70.411	57.571

similarity in Section 7.3.2. The decrease in average performance with a decrease in β, in the case of naive alignment kernels, is due numerical errors in some of the kernels, which is evident from the $< 50\%$ minimum classification accuracy (which is achieved by a random classifier).

We also observe that the variance in classification accuracy increases with decrease in the value of β. This results because we make the kernel more sensitive to difference in spectral projection values by the decreasing value of β. Thus, even for small noise in the spectral projections, the kernel value turns out to be zero and does not contribute toward making better classifications. Thus, even though some classifiers are very

TABLE 7.7   Average Results for the Parameter σ

σ (def. 7.4.5)	Area Under ROC Curve	Positive Acc.			Negative Acc.		
		Max.	Avg.	Min.	Max.	Avg.	Min.
Neighborhood Pair Sum Kernels (K_{nps})							
Sequence Neighborhood							
8	0.591	70.690	66.042	63.809	54.976	52.176	50.571
10	0.583	67.166	64.200	62.547	53.309	51.375	49.666
12	0.575	68.595	64.346	62.500	54.238	51.358	49.666
Structure Neighborhood							
8	0.589	69.023	66.076	64.296	53.880	52.118	50.190
10	0.583	68.357	64.648	61.880	54.476	51.460	49.333
12	0.574	68.714	63.882	62.095	53.142	51.216	48.976
Naive Alignment Kernels (K_{nal})							
Identity Kernel							
10	0.653	73.357	69.826	49.095	67.880	63.823	47.928
11	0.658	74.095	69.894	48.404	66.531	63.651	49.071
12	0.662	73.952	70.466	52.333	67.952	63.324	46.000
15	0.664	74.285	69.752	52.571	66.333	63.073	47.142
Blosum Kernel							
10	0.678	73.976	72.644	71.083	67.404	63.160	56.266
11	0.686	74.619	72.959	71.952	66.964	64.406	58.952
12	0.687	74.357	73.066	72.095	66.738	64.421	60.904
15	0.687	74.785	72.812	71.750	66.678	64.774	61.666
Positive Semidefinite Alignment Kernels (K_{psdal})							
Identity Kernel							
5	0.674	79.142	71.167	5.523	71.476	63.485	11.666
8	0.672	78.523	72.281	60.119	74.952	62.029	58.210
9	0.667	78.571	71.923	61.357	76.404	61.644	57.190
10	0.664	79.119	71.663	60.000	71.642	61.480	56.214
Blosum Kernel							
5	0.688	77.904	74.197	69.500	70.023	63.873	58.571
8	0.661	75.642	72.565	70.285	66.071	59.793	57.857
9	0.654	75.619	71.927	69.952	64.119	58.853	57.047
10	0.653	75.261	71.667	70.000	64.047	59.090	57.452

good, a lot of them are highly sensitive to the noise in data. This results in a wide variance in the classifier performance.

Table 7.7 reveals similar trends with σ as shown in Table 7.6 with β. As suggested by Theorem 2, an increase in the value of σ results in a decrease in classification performance. For naive alignment kernels, the performance does not vary much.

However, the increase in variance is not apparent for the current set of parameters. This is due to the fact that the range of parameters chosen for experimentation was not sufficiently extreme to induce numerical instability in most kernels. This is also supported by the fact that minimum classification accuracy is fairly high in most kernels.

From these observations, we conclude that in accordance with theorems described in Section 7.4.2, decreasing values of β and σ increases the classifier performance, but also makes the classifier more sensitive to noise in data.

7.6.5 Comparison with the Spectrum Kernel

Section 7.5.1 shows that the spectrum kernels [5] turn out to be a special case of our kernels, when restricted to using sequence information alone. We implemented mismatch kernels [5, 49] of which spectrum kernels are a special case and performed similar experiments on our dataset as we did for validating the kernels developed here. This was done to ascertain the difficulty of the our task, and to demonstrate that structure information is highly useful in the context such a task. This section reports results from these experiments.

The spectrum kernels are a special case of mismatch kernels for which the number of allowed mismatches is 0. We experimented with the window sizes of 4 and 5, and allowed mismatch of 0 and 1. The original authors reported that spectrum kernels performed best for window size 4 [49], which was reconfirmed in our experiments.

Table 7.8 reports the results from experiments conducted with spectrum kernels, the best result obtained used a positive semidefinite alignment kernel using sequence information only ($K_{psdal}(seq)$), overall best result obtained using positive semidefinite alignment kernel ($K_{psdal}(best)$), and CE [21]. It is clear that even the best performing spectrum kernel performs quite poorly on the current task, thereby demonstrating the difficulty of the current task and emphasizing the need to use structure information. It can also be observed that using alignment information along with only sequence based kernels ($K_{psdal}(seq)$), considerably improves the classification accuracy. Also, using the structure information in neighborhood pair sum kernels, of which spectrum kernels are a special case, improves the classification performance (AUC: 0.676 Table 7.3). Finally, both CE and $K_{psdal}(best)$ achieves reasonable accuracies on the same task.

Figure 7.2 shows ROC curves for the spectrum kernels and for other representative kernels–methods used here. The spectrum kernels perform worse than the other methods at all points of the curve. Also, the spectrum kernel with window size 4 performs better than other spectrum kernels at all points on the ROC curve, which complies with the results reported in [49]. Thus, we conclude that the current task is quite difficult for the traditional kernels and the methods developed here outperform them.

7.7 DISCUSSION AND CONCLUSION

This chapter explores construction of kernels on protein structures by combining kernels on neighborhoods. We defined two types of neighborhoods, and kernels on each type of neighborhood, utilizing both sequence and structure information.

TABLE 7.8   Results for Classification With Spectrum Kernels and Other Methods Compared Above

Kernel (Parameters)/ Method	Area Under ROC Curve	Positive Acc.	Negative Acc.
$K_{spec}4, 0$	0.621	63.285	61.595
$K_{spec}4, 1$	0.584	58.904	57.690
$K_{spec}5, 0$	0.551	57.047	54.714
$K_{spec}5, 1$	0.545	56.357	52.166
$K_{psdal}(seq)$	0.714	77.190	66.023
$K_{psdal}(best)$	0.800	85.380	74.142
CE	0.782	96.685	61.171

We also explored two different ways of combining these kernels to get kernels on neighborhoods.

The neighborhood kernels were combined in mainly two ways to form kernels on entire protein structures: by adding similarity between all pairs of neighborhoods (K_{nps}), and adding similarity between equivalent pairs of neighborhoods (K_{nal} and $_{psdal}$). The NPS kernels do not require any structural alignment information while the other kernels require structural alignment.

Experiments conducted on the well-known structural classification benchmark SCOP [12] show that the alignment kernels perform reasonably accurately on the difficult task of classifying 40% sequence nonredundant data set. Some of them also outperformed the well known structural alignment program CE [21]. Thus, the kernels developed here can be useful for real-life bioinformatics applications.

Various experiments with the kernels confirmed that they behave predictably with respect to various parameters. For example, in Section 7.4.2, it was predicted that

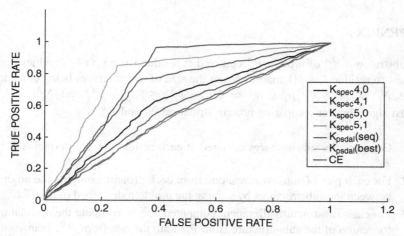

FIGURE 7.2 Results for spectrum kernels and other kernels–methods reported above.

decreasing the values of β and σ will increase the classification accuracy to a point where numerical errors start reducing them. It was validated by experimental results in Section 7.6.4. Also, as expected, structural information was found to be more effective for the current task than sequence information.

The NPS kernels are designed from basic principles to capture structure and sequence information in proteins, and do not require any structural alignment. This approach is in contrast with the approach taken in [16], which essentially tries to make a positive semidefinite kernel out of the MAMMOTH similarity score. In spite of these advantages, NPS kernels have high computational complexity and are not very accurate. An interesting problem is to improve the accuracy of such kernels without increasing the time complexity. Another interesting approach could be to train a probabilistic model for protein structures and define fisher kernels [6] on the same.

The K_{nps} were shown to be analogous to the spectrum kernels in the sense that when restricted to use only sequence information, they turned out to be the normalized versions of the spectrum kernels. However, while the neighborhood pair sum kernels do not perform as well as the structure alignment algorithms (CE), the spectrum kernel is reported to be performing comparably with the sequence alignment algorithms (e.g., BLAST or Smith–Waterman [49]).

We have defined various sequence based kernels on neighborhoods, following various interpretations of the sequence neighborhoods (e.g., sets, strings, structures, etc.). However, not much variation was observed in performance of each of these types of kernels. The reason for this is that sequence information is not sufficient for achieving good accuracy on the current task. It will be interesting to see how these sequence based kernels on neighborhoods fare on different types of sequence processing tasks, when combined in a manner analogous to the ones described in this chapter.

In summary, we have described neighborhood based kernels, which form a reasonably broad class of kernels. Even though the kernels described here were designed for protein structures, we believe the same design principles can be applied to design kernels on general attributed pointsets [10].

APPENDIX A

A substructure N_i^A of protein P^A centered at residue i is a set of l residues that are closest to residue i in 3D space, l being the size of substructures being considered. Thus, $N_i^A = \{p_j^A \in P^A | p_k^A \notin N_i^A \Rightarrow \|p_j^A - p_i^A\| \le \|p_k^A - p_i^A\|$ and $|N_i^A| = l\}$. The robust algorithm for comparing protein structures P^A and P^B is

1. Compute the substructures centered at each residue for both proteins P^A and P^B.
2. For each pair of substructures, one from each protein, compute the alignment between the substructures by solving the problem described in Eq. (7.6).
3. For each substructure alignment computed above, compute the optimal transformation of the sub-structure from P^A onto the one from P^B. Transform the

whole of P^A onto P^B using the computed transformation, and compute the similarity score between residues of P^A and P^B.

4. Compute the optimal alignment between P^A and P^B by solving the assignment problem using the similarity score computed above.

5. Report the best alignment of all the alignments computed in the above step as the optimal one.

The substructure-based algorithm relies on the assumption that the optimal structural alignment between two protein structures contains at least one pair of optimally and fully aligned sub-structures, one from each of the proteins. For each substructure alignment computed in step 2 above, the optimal transformation superposing the corresponding residues is calculated using the method described in [31]. The "best" alignment mentioned in step 5 is decided on the basis of both RMSD and the length of alignment. A detailed description and benchmarking of the method will be presented elsewhere.

REFERENCES

1. J. Shawe-Taylor and N. Cristianini (2004), *Kernel Methods for Pattern Analysis.* Cambridge University Press.

2. L. Wolf and A. Shashua (2003), Learning over sets using kernel principal angles. *J. Mach. Learning Res.*, (4):913–931.

3. R. Kondor and T. Jebara (2003), A kernel between sets of vectors. Tom Fawcett, Nina Mishra, Tom Fawcett, and Nina Mishra (Eds.), *ICML*, AAAI Press, pp. 361–368.

4. A. Shashua and T. Hazan (2005), Algebraic set kernels with application to inference over local image representations. Lawrence K. Saul, Yair Weiss, and Léon Bottou (Eds.), *Advances in Neural Information Processing Systems 17*, MIT Press, Cambridge, MA, pp. 1257–1264.

5. C. Leslie and R. Kwang (2004), Fast string kernels using inexact matching for protein sequences, *J. Mach. Learning Res.*, 5:1435–1455.

6. T. Jaakkola, M. Diekhaus, and D. Haussler (1999), Using the fisher kernel method to detect remote protein homologies. *7th Intell. Sys. Mol. Biol.*, pp. 149–158.

7. L. Holm and C. Sander (1996), Mapping the protein universe. *Science*, 273(5275):595–602.

8. I. Eidhammer, I. Jonassen, and W. R. Taylor (2000), Structure comparison and structure patterns. *J. Computat. Biol.*, 7(5):685–716.

9. H. J. Wolfson and I. Rigoutsos (1997), Geometric hashing: An overview. *IEEE Comput. Sci. Eng.*, 4(4):10–21.

10. M. Parsana, S. Bhattacharya, C. Bhattacharyya, and K.R. Ramakrishnan (2008), Kernels on attributed pointsets with applications. In J.C. Platt, D. Koller, Y. Singer, and S. Roweis (Eds.), *Advances in Neural Information Processing Systems 20*, Cambridge, MA, MIT Press, pp. 1129–1136.

11. S. Bhattacharya, C. Bhattacharyya, and N. Chandra (2007), Comparison of protein structures by growing neighborhood alignments. *BMC Bioinformat.*, 8(77).

12. A. G. Murzin, S. E. Brenner, T. Hubbard, and C. Chothia (1995), Scop: a structural classification of proteins database for the investigation of sequences and structures. *J. Mol. Biol.*, 247:536–540.

13. C. A. Orengo, A. D. Michie, S. Jones, D. T.-Jones, M. B. Swindells, and J. M Thornton (1997), Cath- a hierarchic classification of protein domain structures. *Structure*, 5(8):1093–1108.

14. J.-P. Vert, H. Saigo and T. Akutsu (2004), *Kernel Methods in Computational Biology*, chapter Local alignment kernels for biological sequences, MIT Press, MA, pp. 131–154.

15. K. M. Borgwardt, C. S. Ong, S. Schauer, S. V. N. Vishwanathan, A. J. Smola, and H.-P. Kriegel (2005), Protein function prediction via graph kernels. *Bioinformatics*, 21 Suppl. 1:47–56.

16. J. Qiu, M. Hue, A. Ben.-Hur J. P. Vert, and W. S. Noble (2007), A structural alignment kernel for protein structures. *Bioinformatics*, 23:1090–1098.

17. C. Wang and S. D. Scott (2005), New kernels for protein structural notif discovery and function classification. *International Conference on Machine Learning*.

18. S. Bhattacharya, C. Bhattacharyya, and N.R. Chandra. Structural alignment based kernels for protein structure classification, *24th International Conference on Machine Learning (ICML)*, 2007.

19. D. Haussler (1999), Convolution kernels on discrete structures. Technical report, University of California, Santa Cruz.

20. S. Bhattacharya, C. Bhattacharyya, and N. Chandra (2006), Projections for fast protein structure retrieval. *BMC Bioinformat.*, 7 Suppl.:5S–S5.

21. P. E. Bourne and I. N. Shindyalov (1998), Protein structure alignment by incremental combinatorial extension of optimal path. *Protein Eng.*, 11(9):739–747.

22. B. Scholkopf and A.J. Smola (2002), *Learning with Kernels*. MIT Press, MA.

23. T. Hofmann, B. Scholkopf, and A. J. Smola (2007), Kernel methods in machine learning. Technical report, arXiv, Avialble at ⟨http://arxiv.org/abs/math/0701907v1⟩.

24. M. Collins and N. Duffy (2001), Convolution kernels for natural language. *Advances in Neural Information Processing Systems*, MIT Press, Cambridge, MA. pp. 625–632.

25. S. V. N. Vishwanathan and A. Smola (2005), Binet-cauchy kernels. In Lawrence K. Saul, Yair Weiss, and Léon Bottou, editors, *Advances in Neural Information Processing Systems 17*, MIT Press, Cambridge, MA, pp. 144–448.

26. C. Cortes, P. Haffner, and M. Mohri (2004), Rational kernels: Theory and algorithms. *J. Mach. Learning Res.*, (5):1035–1062.

27. R. Kondor and J. Lafferty (2002), Diffusion kernels on graphs and other discrete structures. *Proceedings of International Conference on Machine Learning (ICML)*.

28. H. Kashima, K. Tsuda, and A. Inokuchi (2003), Marginalized kernels between labeled graphs. *Proceeding of the Twentieth International Conference on Machine Learning*, AAAI Press, pp. 321–328.

29. K. M. Borgwardt and H.-P. Kriegel (2005), Shortest-path kernels on graphs. In *ICDM '05: Proceedings of the Fifth IEEE International Conference on Data Mining*, Washington, DC, 2005. IEEE Computer Society, pp. 74–81.

30. T. Horváth, T. Gärtner, and S. Wrobel (2004), Cyclic pattern kernels for predictive graph mining. *KDD '04: Proceedings of the tenth ACM SIGKDD international conference on Knowledge discovery and data mining*, ACM, NY, pp. 158–167.

31. B. K. P. Horn (1987), Closed form solution of absolute orientation using unit quaternions. *J. Opt. Soc. Am.*, 4(4):629–642.

32. L. Holm and C. Sander (1993), Protein structure comparison by alignment of distance matrices, *J. Mol. Biol.*, 233:123–138.

33. S. Umeyama (1988), An eigendecomposition approach to weighted graph matching problems. *IEEE Trans. Pattern Anal. Mach. Intell.*, 10(5):695–703.

34. D. Bertsimas and J. Tsitsiklis (1997), *Introduction to Linear Optimization*. Athena Scientific.

35. J. Shapiro and D. Brutlag (2004), Foldminer: Structural motif discovery using an improved superposition algorithm. *Protein Sci.*, 13:278–294.

36. S. F. Altschul W. Gish, W. Miller, E. W. Myers, D. J. Lipman (1990), Basic local alignment search tool. *J. Mol. Biol.*, 215(3):403–410.

37. S. Henikoff and J.G. Henikoff (1992), Amino acid substitution matrices from protein blocks. *Proc. Natt. Acad. Sci.*, 89:10915–10919.

38. G. R. G. Lanckriet, N. Cristianini, P. Bartlett, L. El Ghaoui, and M. I. Jordan (2004), Learning the kernel matrix with semidefinite programming. *J. Mach. Learning Res.*, 5:27–72.

39. F. R. Bach, G. R. G. Lanckriet, and M. I. Jordan (2004), Multiple kernel learning, conic duality, and the smo algorithm. *ICML '04: Proceedings of the twenty-first international conference on Machine learning* p. 6, ACM. New York, NY.

40. K. Tsuda (1999), Support vector classifier with asymmetric kernel functions. *European Symposium on Artificial Neural Networks (ESANN)*, pp. 183–188.

41. B. Schölkopf, J. Weston, E. Eskin, C. S. Leslie, and W. S. Noble (2002), A kernel approach for learning from almost orthogonal patterns. *ECML*, 511–528.

42. D. Greene and P. Cunningham (2006), Practical solutions to the problem of diagonal dominance in kernel document clustering. *ICML' 06: Proceedings of the 23rd international conference on Machine learning*, ACM, NY. pp. 377–384.

43. M. Novotny, D. Madsen, and G. J. Kleywegt (2004), Evaluation of protein fold comparison servers. *PROTEINS: Struct., Function, and Bioinformat.*, 54:260–270.

44. E. Anderson, Z. Bai, C. Bischof, S. Blackford, J. Demmel, J. Dongarra, J. Du Croz, A. Greenbaum, S. Hammarling, A. McKenney, and D. Sorensen (1999), *LAPACK Users' Guide*. Society for Industrial and Applied Mathematics, 3rd ed., Philadelphia, PA.

45. C.-C. Chang and C.-J. Lin (2001), *LIBSVM: a library for support vector machines*, Available at http://www.csie.ntu.edu.tw/~cjlin/libsvm.

46. J. M. Chandonia, G. Hon, N. S. Walker, L. Lo Conte, P. Koehl, M. Levitt, and S. E. Brenner (2004), The astral compendium in 2004. *Nucleic Acids Res.*, 32:D189–D192.

47. G. Wang and R. L. Dunbrack (2003), Pisces: a protein sequence culling server. *Bioinformatics*, 19(12):1589–1591.

48. F. J. Provost and T. Fawcett (2001), Robust classification for imprecise environments. *Mach. Learning*, 42(3):203–231.

49. C. S. Leslie, E. Eskin, A. Cohen J. Weston, and W. S. Noble (2004), Mismatch string kernels for discriminative protein classification, *Bioinformatics*, 4:467–476.

8

CHARACTERIZATION OF CONFORMATIONAL PATTERNS IN ACTIVE AND INACTIVE FORMS OF KINASES USING PROTEIN BLOCKS APPROACH

G. Agarwal, D. C. Dinesh, N. Srinivasan, and Alexandre G. de Brevern

8.1 INTRODUCTION

The three-dimensional (3D) structure, which is critical for the function of a protein is usually conserved during evolution. It holds a wealth of information that can be harnessed to understand various aspects of proteins including sequence–structure–function–evolutionary relationships. The understanding of these complex relationships is facilitated by a simplistic one-dimensional (1D) representation of the tertiary structure like a string of letters. The advantage is an easier visualization without losing much of the vital information due to dimension reduction. Using various methodologies, local structural patterns that can be combined to generate the desired backbone conformation have been identified that use atomic coordinates characterising 3D structures of proteins. Protein blocks (PBs) is a set of 16 such local structural descriptors, denoted by letters $a \ldots p$ that have been derived using unsupervised machine learning algorithms and can approximate the 3D space of proteins. Each letter corresponds to a pentapeptide with distinct values of eight dihedral angles (Φ, Ψ).

We demonstrate the use of PBs to characterize structural variations in enzymes using kinases as the case study. A protein kinase undergoes structural alterations

Computational Intelligence and Pattern Analysis in Biological Informatics, Edited by Ujjwal Maulik, Sanghamitra Bandyopadhyay, and Jason T. L. Wang
Copyright © 2010 John Wiley & Sons, Inc.

as it switches to its active conformation from its inactive form. Crystal structures of several protein kinases are available in different enzymatic states. First, we have applied the PBs approach in distinguishing between conformation changes and rigid-body displacements between the structures of active and inactive forms of a kinase. Second, we have performed a comparison of conformational patterns of active forms of a kinase with the active and inactive forms of a closely related kinase. Third, we have studied the structural differences in the active states of homologous kinases. Such studies might help in understanding the structural differences among these enzymes at a different level, as well as guide in making drug targets for a specific kinase.

Section 8.1.1 and Section 8.1.2 give a brief introduction on PBs and protein kinases, respectively, followed by the analyses on conformational plasticity in kinases using PBs in the subsequent sections.

8.1.1 An Introduction to Protein Blocks

The tertiary structure of a protein is complex and is formed by a specific arrangement of regular secondary structures, namely, helices and strands connected by less regular coils. Combinations of secondary structures in specific arrangements, called motifs, are frequently observed in proteins and are associated with specific functions; EF hand and helix–turn–helix motifs are some of the examples. These motifs are patterns that can act as functional signatures. Although the three-state representation (α-helix, β-strand, and coil) has been used for various structural analyses, it suffers from certain limitations. The description lacks the detailed information on relative orientation of secondary structures and ambiguity in assigning their beginning and end and precise definition of distinct conformations that are collectively classified as coils. Thus, it fails to capture the subtle variations in structures of closely related proteins. In addition, it lacks the information required to reconstruct the backbone of a protein structure. The depth of knowledge gained through the analysis of 3D structures is partly dependant on the details and accuracy of the representation. The description of protein structures as secondary structural elements is an oversimplification. Therefore, elaborate local structures that can describe a protein structure more precisely have been derived without using any *a priori* information on 3D structures. The more detailed descriptors were to serve two purposes. First, a combination of these fragments, like building blocks, would be able to approximate the backbone conformation of known structures. The higher the number of these fragments in a library, the more precise is the description. Second, they would be useful in understanding sequence–structure relationships and in predicting a fold solely from its sequence. However, fewer fragments would be better for adequate prediction of such relationships. The number of fragments in a library is a compromise between the two requirements.

Many groups have derived libraries of short protein structures called structural alphabets [1]. These libraries differ in the methodologies used to derive fragments and in the parameters used to describe these fragments [2–11]. The description parameters include the Cα coordinates, Cα distances, and dihedral angles that are used by methods like hierarchical clustering, empirical function, artificial neural network, hidden Markov model, and Kohonen maps for classification. These libraries differ in length of the fragments and the number of prototypes used to describe them.

One such library of local structural descriptors are PBs, which are highly informative and have proved to be useful in various applications. It is a set of 16 structural
prototypes named as *a* to *p*, each describing a five residue peptide [8]. Thus, each of
the 16 prototypes is defined by a set of 8 dihedral angles. The PBs *d* and *m* roughly
represent the backbone of strand and helix, respectively. The prototypes *a* to *c* are
associated with the N-caps of the β strand and *e* to *f* to its C-caps. The PBs *k* to *l* and
n to *p*, respectively, describes the N- and C-caps of α helix and *g* to *j* represent PBs,
which can be associated with coils. These have been identified using unsupervised
machine learning algorithm [8]. The dihedral angles were calculated for each of the
overlapping fragment, five residues long, extracted from a nonredundant set of protein structures. The difference in the values of the angles among these fragments was
scored using root-mean-square deviation on angular (RMSDA [7]) values. An unsupervised approach related to self-organizing map (SOM [12]) was trained to learn
the difference in structural fragments using RMSDA as the distance metric and also
the transition probabilities between fragments in a sequence. The process resulted
in generation of 16 prototypes. It can approximate the local backbone conformation
with an RMSD of 0.42 Å [13]. Figure 8.1 shows the 3D structure of ubiquitin conjugating enzyme [14] transformed into a 1D PB sequence. The PBs approach has
proved useful in various kinds of analyses as described below, and at present it is the
most widely used structural alphabet.

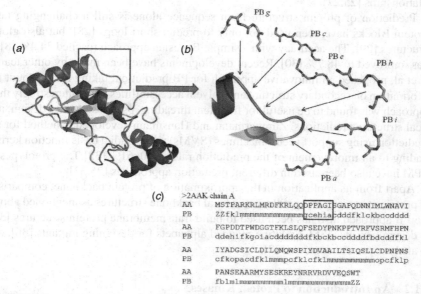

FIGURE 8.1 Transformation of a 3D structure of ubiquitin conjugating enzyme (PDB code
2AAKv [14]) to its 1D PBs sequence. (*a*) A 3D representation of 2AAK. (*b*) Focuses on the
loop region and correspondence in terms of PBs, with PBs *gcehia*. (*c*) The complete structure
encoded in terms of PBs, the loop region in (*b*) is boxed. This figure and Figures 8.2, 8.5, and
8.8 have been generated using PyMOL [15].

While the superposition of 3D structures is complex, two structures encoded as a string of PBs can be aligned through a simple dynamic programming algorithm. The PB-ALIGN algorithm, which uses dynamic programming and PB-specific substitution table to align two PB sequences, has been developed [16,17]. A substitution matrix specific to blocks, which contains the probability of substitution of a PB by any of the 16 PBs, has been generated. The PALI database [18], containing structure-based sequence alignment of homologous protein structures in every SCOP family, was used to generate the matrix. The frequency of substitution for every PB was calculated for all topologically equivalent regions and normalized by the occurrence of blocks in the database. Apart from aligning two structures (see Fig. 8.2), the PB-ALIGN algorithm has also been used successfully in database mining to identify proteins of similar structure [21]. The PB approach also has been applied in identifying Mg^{2+} binding sites in proteins [22].

Protein Blocks are five residue long fragments. To assess the structural stability of these short fragments, we identified the most frequent series of five consecutive PBs. They proved their capabilities to describe long length fragments [23]. A novel approach named the hybrid protein model (HPM) was developed [24,25]. This innovative approach made it possible to create longer prototypes that are 10–13 residues in length. Alongside, the number of prototypes has increased significantly to take into account structural variability for these longer fragments (e.g., 100–130 prototypes). These longer fragments were used to perform simple structural superimposition [26], methodological optimization [24], and analysis of sequence–structure relationships [25,27].

Prediction of protein structure from sequence alone is still a challenging task. Protein Blocks have been used not only to predict short loops [28], but also global structures [29]. The accuracy with a simple Bayesian approach reached 34.4% [8]; it was improved to 48.7% [30]. Recent developments have been made by other teams. Li et al. proposed an innovative approach for PB prediction, taking into account the information on secondary structure and solvent accessibilities [31]. Interestingly their approach was found to be useful for fragment threading, pseudosequence design, and local structure predictions. Zimmermann and Hansmann developed a method for PB prediction using support vector machines (SVMs) with a radial basis function kernel, leading to an improvement of the prediction rate of 60–61% [32]. The prototypes of HPM have also been used in different prediction approaches [25,33].

Apart from its application in the approximation of protein backbone, comparison of protein structures and prediction of local backbone structures as mentioned above, the PB approach also has been used to build transmembrane protein structures [34], to design peptides [35], to define reduced alphabets for designing mutants [36], and to analyze protein contacts [37].

8.1.2 An Introduction to Protein Kinases

Protein phosphorylation is an important regulatory mechanism used by cells to respond to external stimuli (e.g., neurotransmitters, hormones, or stress signals). Protein kinases are enzymes that phosphorylate the target protein by transfer of γ phosphate

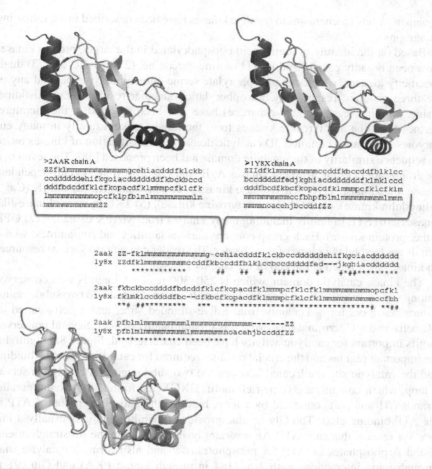

FIGURE 8.2 Protein structure superimposition using PB-ALIGN [17]. First, the protein structures are encoded in terms of PBs. In this example, the two proteins are the ubiquitin conjugating enzyme (cf. Fig. 8.1) and a ubiquitin protein ligase (PDB code 1Y8X [19]). Then, using global and / or local alignment, in a similar way to CLUSTALW [20], the two PB sequences are aligned. Identical (*) and similar (#) PBs have been underlined. The protein structures are easily superimposed from this PB sequence alignment.

of an adenosine triphosphate (ATP) molecule. The target proteins include enzymes (e.g., glycogen synthase and other kinases); transcription factors (e.g., c-Jun) and non-enzymatic proteins (e.g., histones) that are involved in distinct signaling pathways linked to metabolism, gene expression, cell motility, cell division, cell differentiation, and apoptosis. Phosphorylation of target protein alters its subcellular localization, activity levels or its association with other proteins, affecting the downstream processes in the signaling pathway. Since kinases are key players in the regulation of these processes, a tight regulation of their activity is crucial for normal functioning of an organism. A few mechanisms to regulate kinases have been described in the following paragraphs.

Based on the identity of amino acid phosphorylated in the target, protein kinases have been broadly categorized into (1) serine–threonine, (2) tyrosine, and (3) dual-specificity kinases, which can phosphorylate serine–threonine, tyrosine, and any of the three residues, respectively. Phosphorylation at other residues (e.g., histidine, lysine, arginine, cysteine, and aspartate) have also been reported in the literature. Serine–threonine and tyrosine kinases form the largest protein family in many eukaryotes and share a common 3D catalytic domain. A classification of kinases based on sequence similarity of the catalytic domain has been proposed [38]. The seven major groups are (1) AGC (protein kinases A, B, and C), (2) CMGC (cyclin-dependant kinase, map kinase, glycogen synthase kinase 3, casein kinase II), (3) CaMK (Ca^{2+}, calmodulin kinase), (4) PTK (protein tyrosine kinase), (5) TKL (tyrosine kinase-like kinases), (6) STE (a family including many kinases from MAPK cascade), (7) OPK (other protein kinase). Each group contains various families and subfamilies, whose details are beyond the scope of this chapter. The reader can refer to various resources on kinases mentioned at the end of the chapter [39,40].

The kinase catalytic domain, which is 250–300 residues long, is well conserved among serine–threonine and tyrosine kinases. It can be divided into two subdomains: N-terminal lobe, formed mainly from a five-stranded sheet and a helix called an αC helix and a C terminal lobe, which is predominantly helical. Several conserved motifs important for catalytic activity have been characterized. Figure 8.3 highlights the important regions and the crucial residues required for catalysis. The ATP binding and the catalytic site are located between the two subdomains. A highly conserved P loop, which contains a glycine-rich motif, GXGXφG, formed by two antiparallel strands (β1 and β2) connected by a loop, binds to the phosphate group of ATP in the ATP binding cleft. The Gly residue provides flexibility and φ is usually a Phe or a Tyr residue that caps ATP. An invariant lysine, located in the β3 strand, orients α and β phosphates of ATP for phosphotransfer and also forms a catalytic triad through ionic interactions with Asp (184 in protein kinase PKA) and Glu (91 in PKA) that are located in the αC helix. These interactions are important to maintain kinase in its active state. Catalytic loop, part of the C-terminal lobe, contains an Asp residue that acts as a base and phosphorylates the OH group of the substrate. The activation loop present in the C-terminal lobe is phosphorylated when a kinase is in an active state. This causes stabilization of the loop conformation allowing the binding of substrate. The DFG motif in a typical kinase structure lies N-terminal to the activation loop, D in this motif interacts with the Mg^{2+} ion. The C-terminal end of the activation loop is marked by a conserved APE motif. The Glu forms electrostatic interactions with a conserved Arg residue. Another important interaction responsible for stabilization of the catalytic loop is formed between the Tyr and Arg residues. The placement of the DFG motif and phosphorylation sites vary among different kinases. The phosphorylation site and the nearby residues form a signature, specific for each kinase, that acts as a peptide positioning region.

The fact that protein kinases regulate important cellular processes necessitates a tight regulation of activation in these proteins. The enzymes are usually kept

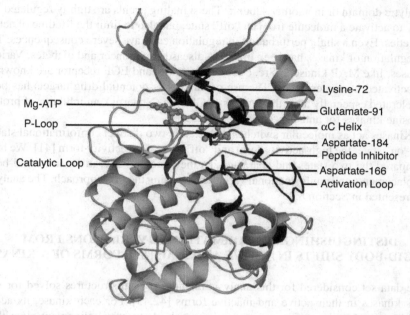

Lysine-72

Mg-ATP

Glutamate-91

P-Loop

αC Helix

Aspartate-184

Peptide Inhibitor

Catalytic Loop

Aspartate-166

Activation Loop

FIGURE 8.3 The catalytic domain of kinase. The motifs important for ligand binding and catalysis have been marked. The key residues important for function are shown as sticks. Mg-ATP is shown as spheres.

"off" and the activation is under multiple layers of control. Few important modes of regulation of these enzymes are described [39]. (a) The binding of extracellular ligands to receptors–ion channels leads to a change in the concentration of secondary messengers including small molecules: adenosine $3'$: $5'$-cyclic monophosphate (cAMP), guanosine $3'$: $5'$-cyclic monophosphate (cGMP); lipid secondary messengers: diacylglycerol, phosphatidylinostiol, 3,4,5-triphosphate, and Ca^{2+}. Most secondary messengers such as cAMP, for example; exert their effect through allosteric binding to additional domains–subunits in kinases as in PKA and Ca^{2+}–calmodulin activation as in CaMK. The secondary messengers-dependant kinases, in the absence of secondary messengers, are kept in the inactive state by association with autoinhibitory regions. (b) The catalytic subunits in cyclin-dependant kinases, for example, are activated only after their association with regulatory subunits (e.g., cyclins) whose level of expression varies depending on the functional state of the cell. (c) In Src kinases, for example, additional domains (e.g., SH2 and SH3) target the enzyme to different subcellular localization. (d) In receptor kinases, the external signal induces oligomerization of receptors leading to autophosphorylation of intracellular domains. The autophosphorylated site may serve as a docking site for accessory proteins leading to the activation of downstream processes in the signaling cascade. (e) Many protein kinases are activated by phosphorylation in sites located mainly in the activation loop of the catalytic domain or sometimes in regions beyond the catalytic domain or in another subunit. The signaling events are tightly regulated not only to activate a molecule from an "off" state, but also to limit the lifetime of active moieties. Even a slight perturbation in regulation can have severe consequences. The deregulation of kinases has been linked to diseases like cancer and diabetes. Various kinases, like MAP kinase, c-Src, c-Abl, PI3 kinase, and EGF receptor are known to be activated in cancer genes. The use of kinases as potential drug targets has been accelerated especially after the success of Gleevac (Novartis), an inhibitor of protein tyrosine kinases for anti-cancer therapy.

Kinases act as molecular switches and exist in two distinct conformational states: the "on" state, the high-activity form and "off" state, low-activity form [41]. We have compared the two states and characterized the structural alterations into rigid-body displacements and conformational variations by using the PBs approach. The analysis is presented in Section 8.2.

8.2 DISTINGUISHING CONFORMATIONAL VARIATIONS FROM RIGID-BODY SHIFTS IN ACTIVE AND INACTIVE FORMS OF A KINASE

The data set considered for this analysis includes crystal structures solved for various kinases in their active and inactive forms [42,43]. For each kinase, its active and inactive forms were superposed using a robust structural alignment algorithm, MUSTANG [44]. The regions that correspond to high deviation in their $C\alpha$ position were identified by calculating $C\alpha$–$C\alpha$ deviation values for every pair of equivalent residues in the two aligned protein structures. Also, each of the two structures was encoded as a string of PBs. The two PB sequences were then mapped onto the structural alignment previously generated using MUSTANG. A score was assigned to all positions where the deviation in $C\alpha$ positions is high, by using the substitution table for PBs [16]. The variable regions, which have undergone only rigid-body movements, will be reflected as high PB scores. Since the local structure has remained the same and has only shifted, the corresponding PBs would be identical or highly similar giving a positive score for the alignment region. On the contrary, a low PB score would indicate differences in the properties of aligned PBs indicating a conformation change at the structurally variable region. This approach was applied to analyze the structural differences in the two forms of various kinases and the results for individual cases are discussed below.

8.2.1 Insulin Receptor Kinase

Insulin receptor kinase is a transmembrane protein tyrosine kinase receptor that regulates pathways involved in cell metabolism and growth. A switch from its inactive to active form requires binding of insulin in the extracellular domain. The signal of ligand binding is transmitted to the catalytic domain located in the cytosolic side. The response to the signal includes autophosphorylation of tyrosine residues in the activation loop of the kinase domain. Phosphorylation of insulin response substrates by activated kinases leads to the activation of downstream molecules in the signaling

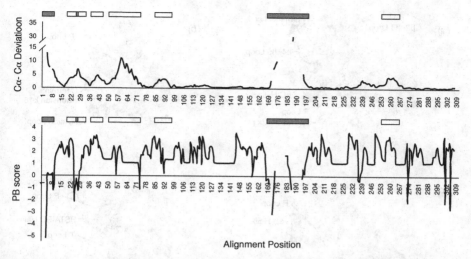

FIGURE 8.4 A plot of Cα–Cα deviation and PB score versus the alignment position for the aligned structures of distinct states of insulin receptor kinase (IRK). The regions corresponding to conformational variations and rigid-body shifts are indicated as filled and open boxes, respectively.

pathway. Crystal structures of human IRK in both the active (PDB code 1IRK, [43]) and inactive forms (1IR3,[46]) have been reported. Figure 8.4 shows a plot of Cα–Cα deviation values and PB scores corresponding to each position in the alignment of the active and inactive forms of kinases. The regions with high deviation of Cα positions and high PB scores that correspond to rigid-body shifts are indicated in open rectangles. The regions with high deviation and low scores that correspond to conformational differences are indicated in filled rectangles. The regions of structural variations in the two forms of IRK have also been marked in Figure 8.5(a). The rigid-body shifts are shown in dark gray and conformational variations are in black. These observations are consistent with structural variations in IRK reported in the literature. In the inactive form, the activation loop is in an autoinhibitory conformation preventing the binding of substrate and restricting the access of an ATP molecule. Phosphorylation of three tyrosine residues in the activation loop of the protein results in a large displacement in the loop that is as high as 30 Å. Overall, there is a rigid-body shift in the N-terminal domain that is prominent in β1 and β2 strands, P loop connected to the strands, and αC helix [Fig. 8.5(a)]. The residues in nucleotide binding (P loop) form contacts with phosphates of ATP bound at the active site. A small region in P loop motif undergoes slight conformational change as reflected from the scores in the blocks alignment. The movement of helix brings a conserved Glu in close proximity to Lys in the ATP binding site [45]. These structural alterations together result in the alignment of residues for optimal interactions that are required for catalysis.

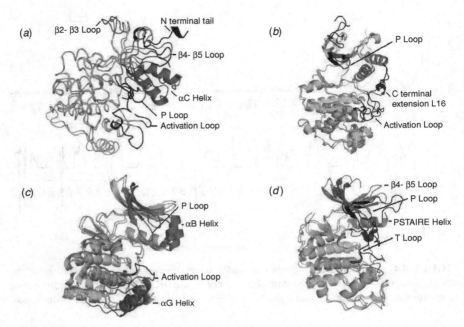

FIGURE 8.5 Superpositions of active and inactive states of various kinases. (*a*) Insulin receptor kinase, (*b*) mitogen activated protein kinase (MAPK), (*c*) protein kinase A, (*d*) cyclin-dependant protein kinase. The regions undergoing marked structural alterations have been labeled.

8.2.2 Mitogen-Activated Protein Kinase

Mitogen-Activated Protein Kinase are serine–threonine specific kinases that control embyogenesis, cell transformation, cell proliferation, cell differentiation, and apoptosis. The members of the MAPK family include ERKs, JNKs, and P38 kinases. The ERKs are activated by mitogen and growth factors, while JNK and P38 are activated in response to inflammatory cytokines, growth factors, and cellular stress. The dual phosphorylation at Thr and Tyr in the TXY motif located in the activation loop causes the switching of kinase to its active form. The activated kinases phosphorylate various transcription factors, cytoskeletal elements, other protein kinases, and enzymes. Since these enzymes mediate key events throughout the cell, they are drug targets for a wide range of diseases including cancer and Alzheimer. The superposition of the structures of active ERK2 (2ERK, [47]) and inactive state (1ERK, [48]) of the enzyme are shown in Figure 8.5(*b*). Although, no marked rigid-body displacements were observed, conformational variations were seen in nucleotide binding loop (P loop), activation loop, and a C-terminal extension L16, a region specific to MAPK. The N-terminal regions are disordered in both the protein structures. The activation loop is the central regulator. Conformational change in the activation loop brings the phosphorylated Ser and Tyr residues closer to an Arg that provides charge stabilization. One of the phosphorylated residues now sits between the two domains facilitating domain closure while the other phosphorylated residue on the surface forms the P+1 specificity site. A small loop region in inactive kinase in L16 changes to a 3_{10} helix in the active form. This conformation change was also captured by a change in PBs between the active and inactive form that corresponds to loops and helices, respectively. The conversion to helical structure brings a previously buried Phe on the surface that now forms stacking interactions with a His in the activation loop. The 3_{10} helix promotes tighter interactions between the two domains. Also, the exposure of previously buried Leu residues to solvent creates a hydrophobic patch that facilitates homodimerization, known to be important for nuclear localization of the enzyme. The MAPK insertion region does not undergo significant change. The interaction of the phosphorylated region in the activation loop with the N-terminal lobe and L16 orients the N- and C-terminal lobe.

8.2.3   Protein Kinase A

Protein Kinase A is a cAMP dependant protein kinase and plays a key role in cellular response to this secondary messenger. The enzyme is a heterotetramer of two regulatory and two catalytic subunits. Activation of the kinase is mediated by binding of cAMP to the regulatory subunits with subsequent release of catalytic subunits. The tertiary structures of active (1ATP, [49]) and inactive forms (1J3H, [50]) were superposed. The comparison of the alignment of the two structures revealed structural alterations in the nucleotide binding loop, the αB helix, the αG helix, and the activation loop [Fig. 8.5(c)]. The phosphorylation of the residues in activation loop switches the enzyme to its active form. The conformational change in the activation loop is linked to adjustments in the rest of the structure to realign the catalytically important residues for efficient phosphotransfer. The rigid-body shift in the P loop brings the residues of this loop closer to ATP allowing the interactions with α and β phosphate groups to form. The loop connecting the helices F and G is the peptide-binding loop. Due to a shift in this loop and in the G helix, the residues in this region can now extend the network of interactions from the substrate-binding region to the active site allowing a communication between the distant regions promoting catalysis.

8.2.4   Cyclin-Dependant Kinase

Cyclin-Dependant Kinase 2 (CDK2) is a serine–threonine specific kinase that coordinates the events in eukaryotic cell cycle. The activation of the kinase requires binding to cognate cyclin and phosphorylation in the activation segment in a two-step process. The structure of phosphorylated CDK2 in complex with cyclin A and ATPγ S, the fully active form (1JST [51]), was compared with the unphosphorylated, apo form (1B38 [52]). Based on the PB scores, marked conformation changes were observed in the T loop that contains the phosphorylation site analogous to the activation loop in PKA. Other regions that undergo variations include the nucleotide-binding loop and the loop connecting β3 to PSTAIRE helix [Fig. 8.5(d)]. High PB scores that correspond to rigid-body shifts were observed for $\beta 1$ and $\beta 2$ strands and β hairpin connected to the PSTAIRE helix. Binding of cyclin results in variation in the activation segment and the PSTAIRE helix. The additional interactions formed by the phosphorylated T segment with cyclin compared to the unphosphorylated segment cause further stabilization of the complex. Binding of cyclin restores the interaction between Lys in the $\beta 3$ strand and Glu in the PSTAIRE helix. The PSTAIRE helix seems to play a key role in regulation. The residues in this helix interacts with cyclin and help in neutralization of charge at the phosphorylated site. Although an arginine from the catalytic loop also helps in charge neutralization, no significant structural alterations were observed in this region.

The above analyses indicate that different protein kinases share regions that undergo structural variations to switch to their active forms. However, the nature of structural alterations is not similar.

8.3   CROSS COMPARISON OF ACTIVE AND INACTIVE FORMS OF CLOSELY RELATED KINASES

This section describes the analyses on comparison of active forms of a kinase with the active and inactive forms of a closely related kinase. We show the results for two closely related pairs: (1) PKA [active, 1ATP[49] and inactive, 1J3H [50]], protein kinase B (PKB) [active, 1O6L [53] and inactive, 1MRV[54]]; (2) IRK [active, 1IRK [45] and inactive, 1IR3 [46]], insulin-like growth factor receptor kinase (ILGFRK) [active, 1K3A [55] and inactive, 1JQH [56]].

For each pair of closely related kinases, the active forms were aligned using MUSTANG [44]. The structures of the active forms of kinases were also superposed on the inactive form of a closely related kinase. The structures of each kinase were transformed as PBs and mapped on the structure-based sequence alignments. For all alignment positions where residues were aligned, the PB scores were calculated using the PB substitution matrix. A normalized PB score was calculated after adding values over the entire alignment and dividing by the number of residue–residue alignment positions. The analysis revealed a high PB score for an alignment of the active forms compared to the cross-comparison of the active and inactive forms for each pair of closely related kinases. Additionally, the alignment of active and inactive forms of the same enzyme scored lower than the pair of active kinases. The results are presented in Figure 8.6.

The analysis indicates a higher global similarity in the active forms of closely related kinases as compared to the active and inactive forms. This preliminary study suggests a possibility of identifying the functional state of a kinase based on the PB score obtained after its comparison with the other known states of the same enzyme or its close homologs.

8.4   COMPARISON OF THE ACTIVE STATES OF HOMOLOGOUS KINASES

In this analysis, the structures of the active forms of PKA, IRK, CDK2, and MAPK have been compared. Although, the proteins share only 14% similarity in sequence,

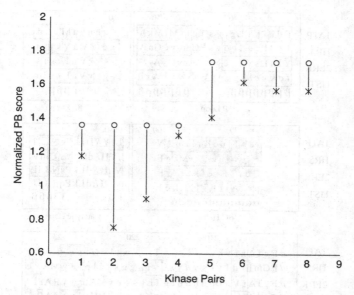

FIGURE 8.6 The plot highlights the difference in PBs score obtained after alignment of active pairs and active–inactive pairs in closely related kinases. The positions in the plot that refer to PB scores for active pairs are shown as dots and active–inactive pairs are indicated as crosses. The notation for kinase pairs is as follows: (1) PKA active–PKB active compared to PKA active–PKB inactive, (2) PKA active–PKB active compared to PKB active–PKA inactive, (3) PKA active–PKB active compared to PKA active–PKA inactive, (4) PKA active–PKB active compared to PKB active–PKB inactive, (5) IRK active–ILGFRK active compared to IRK active–ILGFRK inactive, (6) IRK active–ILGFRK active compared to ILGFRK active–IRK inactive, (7) IRK active–ILGFRK active compared to IRK active–IRK inactive, (8) IRK active–ILGFRK active compared to ILGFRK active–ILGFRK inactive.

the structures of the active kinases share remarkable similarity. Figure 8.7 shows a block of structure-based sequence alignment generated after simultaneous superposition of the structures of above mentioned kinases using MUSTANG [44] algorithm and represented in JOY [57] format. As shown in Figure 8.7, the residues that play an important role either in catalysis or in ligand binding are conserved: Gly-rich motif in P loop; Lys in $\beta 3$ strand that positions α and β phosphates of ATP for catalysis; Glu in αC helix that forms ion-pair with Lys and is important for catalysis; catalytic Asp, His, and Arg residues in the catalytic loop; conserved Asp in F helix (not shown in the figure), and DFG and APE motifs in the activation loop. Although important residues are aligned, certain regions holding these residues show high Cα–Cα deviation with respect to equivalent regions in other kinases (see Fig. 8.8). The P loop in PKA is shifted away compared to the loop in other kinases, which overlap better. The representation as PBs shows dissimilarity in the properties of PBs corresponding to this region suggesting a variation in local structure. There is a rigid-body shift in the αC helix of IRK. The helix movement is known to be coupled to nucleotide binding at the active site of the enzyme. The N-terminal DFG motif in IRK shows slight

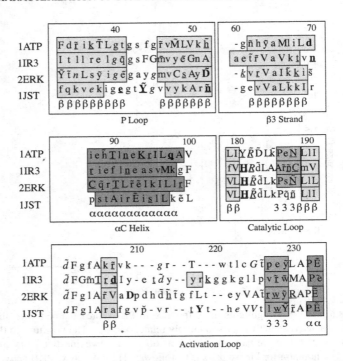

FIGURE 8.7 A multiple alignment of the structures of active kinases. The alignment has been labeled for various regions. Secondary structures are marked in the figure; α corresponds to α-helix, β refers to β-strand and 3 to 3_{10} helix. The solvent inaccessible regions are shown in upper case while buried regions are in lower case.

deviation compared to other kinases. This deviation corresponds to a conformational variation. The activation segment differs in length and is conformationally distinct among these kinases. The primary phosphorylation sites in these kinases do not lie at topologically equivalent regions. The helices F and G are conserved.

The above analysis highlights the similarities and differences in the structures of active forms of kinases through identification of regions of high $C\alpha$–$C\alpha$ deviation and their representation as PBs.

8.5 CONCLUSIONS

Protein blocks are a higher level abstraction of protein structures as compared to the standard three-state description as helix, strand, and coil.

The PBs approach can be used successfully in distinguishing rigid-body shifts from conformational variations, as has been exemplified for kinases, which have distinct 3D structures in their active and inactive states. The regions with high deviation in $C\alpha$ positions and low PB scores correspond to conformational variations. On the

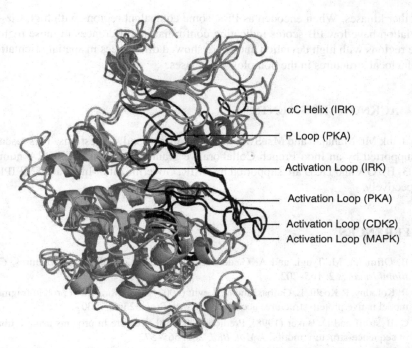

FIGURE 8.8   The superposition of PKA, IRK, MAPK, and CDK structures in their active state is shown. The structurally variable regions are shown in black.

contrary, a high PB score for regions with high deviation indicates a similarity in local structure with gross reorganization of the local region on the 3D structure. Under such circumstances, a large value of $C\alpha$–$C\alpha$ deviation is a consequence of displacement of the region. Based on our analyses using this approach, we find that the regions in inactive protein kinases that undergo structural alterations while switching to their active states are generally common among these kinases; however, the nature of variations is different. The study can be extended to analyze structural variations in proteins at various levels. Examples include the study of homologous proteins to understand structural differences, analyses of structural changes induced in proteins on binding to different ligand–effector molecules, and study of structural alterations at protein–protein interfaces because of binding to its interacting partner.

A cross-comparison of active and inactive states of closely related kinases indicates a higher global similarity in the structure of active states of the kinases as reflected from their PB scores compared to the active and inactive forms. This kind of study might be useful in estimating the activity levels(state) of kinases based on their PB score.

Even though the active states of various kinases are structurally quite similar, differences do exist. We have compared the active forms of four different kinases and identified the regions, which deviate from the topologically equivalent regions in other kinases. When encoded as PBs, some equivalent regions with high $C\alpha$–$C\alpha$ deviation have low PB scores indicating conformation differences in those regions. The regions with high deviation and score showed differences in spatial orientations of the local structures in the homologous kinases.

8.6   ACKNOWLEDGMENTS

We thank Mr. Mahajan and Ms. Swapna for comments and suggestions. This research is supported by an Indo-French Collaborative grant (grant from CEFIPRA number 3903- E). GA and DCD are supported by CSIR, Government of India and CEFIPRA, respectively.

REFERENCES

1. B. Offmann, M. Tyagi, and A. G. de Brevern (2007), Local Protein Structures, *Curr. Bioinformatics* 2: 165–202.
2. R. Kolodny, P. Koehl, L. Guibas, and M. Levitt (2002) Small libraries of protein fragments model native protein structures accurately, *J. Mol. Biol.* 323: 297–307.
3. C. Bystroff and D. Baker (1998), Prediction of local structure in proteins using a library of sequence-structure motifs, *J. Mol. Biol.* 281: 565–577.
4. R. Unger and J. L. Sussman (1993), The importance of short structural motifs in protein structure analysis, *J. Comput. Aided. Mol. Des.* 7: 457–472.
5. M. J. Rooman, J. Rodriguez, and S. J. Wodak (1990), Automatic definition of recurrent local structure motifs in proteins, *J. Mol. Biol.* 213: 327–336.
6. A. C. Camproux, P. Tuffery, J. P. Chevrolat, J. F. Boisvieux, and S. Hazout (1999), Hidden Markov model approach for identifying the modular framework of the protein backbone, *Protein Eng.* 12: 1063–1073.
7. J. Schuchhardt, G. Schneider, J. Reichelt, D. Schomburg, and P. Wrede (1996), Local structural motifs of protein backbones are classified by self-organizing neural networks, *Protein Eng.* 9: 833–842.
8. A. G. de Brevern, C. Etchebest, and S. Hazout (2000), Bayesian probabilistic approach for predicting backbone structures in terms of protein blocks, *Proteins* 41: 271–287.
9. S. J. Prestrelski, D. M Byler, and M. N Liebman (1992), Generation of a substructure library for the description and classification of protein secondary structure. II. Application to spectra-structure correlations in Fourier transform infrared spectroscopy, *Proteins* 14: 440–450.
10. S. Y. Ku and Y. J. Hu (2008), Protein structure search and local structure characterization, *BMC Bioinformatics* 9: 349.
11. J. S. Fetrow, M. J Palumbo, and G. Berg (1997), Patterns, structures, and amino acid frequencies in structural building blocks, a protein secondary structure classification scheme, *Proteins* 27: 249–271.
12. T. Kohonen (1982), Self-organized formation of topologically correct feature maps, *Biol. Cybernetics* 43: 59–69.

13. A. G. de Brevern (2005), New assessment of a structural alphabet, *In Silico Biol.* 5: 283–289.

14. W. J. Cook, L. C. Jeffrey, M. L. Sullivan, and R. D Vierstra (1992), Three-dimensional structure of a ubiquitin-conjugating enzyme (E2), *J. Biol. Chem.* 267: 15116–15121.

15. W. L. DeLano (2002), *The PyMOL Molecular Graphics System*. USA: Delano Scientific, San Carlos, CA.

16. M. Tyagi, V. S. Gowri, N. Srinivasan, A. G. de Brevern, and B. Offmann (2006), A substitution matrix for structural alphabet based on structural alignment of homologous proteins and its applications, *Proteins* 65: 32–39.

17. M. Tyagi, et al. (2006), Protein Block Expert (PBE): a web-based protein structure analysis server using a structural alphabet, *Nucleic Acids Res.* 34: W119–123.

18. S. Balaji and N. Srinivasan (2001), Use of a database of structural alignments and phylogenetic trees in investigating the relationship between sequence and structural variability among homologous proteins, *Protein Eng.* 14: 219–226.

19. D. T. Huang, A. Paydar, M. Zhuang, M. B. Waddell, and J. M. Holton et al (2005), Structural basis for recruitment of Ubc12 by an E2 binding domain in NEDD8s E1, *Mol. Cell* 17: 341–350.

20. J. D. Thompson, D. G. Higgins, and T. J. Gibson (1994), CLUSTAL W: improving the sensitivity of progressive multiple sequence alignment through sequence weighting, position-specific gap penalties and weight matrix choice, *Nucleic Acids Res.* 22: 4673–4680.

21. M. Tyagi, A. G. de Brevern, N. Srinivasan, and B. Offmann (2008), Protein structure mining using a structural alphabet, *Proteins* 71: 920–937.

22. M. Dudev and C. Lim (2007), Discovering structural motifs using a structural alphabet: application to magnesium-binding sites, *BMC Bioinformatics* 8: 106.

23. A. G. de Brevern, H. Valadie, S. Hazout, and C. Etchebest (2002), Extension of a local backbone description using a structural alphabet: a new approach to the sequence-structure relationship, *Protein Sci.* 11: 2871–2886.

24. A. G. de Brevern and S. Hazout (2003), Hybrid protein model for optimally defining 3D protein structure fragments, *Bioinformatics* 19: 345–353.

25. C. Benros, A. G. de Brevern, C. Etchebest, and S. Hazout (2006), Assessing a novel approach for predicting local 3D protein structures from sequence, *Proteins* 62: 865–880.

26. A. G. de Brevern and S. Hazout (2001), Compacting local protein folds by a Hybrid Protein Model, *Theor. Chem. Acc.* 106: 36–49.

27. C. Benros, A. G. de Brevern, and S. Hazout (2009), Analyzing the sequence-structure relationship of a library of local structural prototypes, *J. Theor. Biol.* 256: 215–226.

28. L. Fourrier, C. Benros, and A. G. de Brevern (2004), Use of a structural alphabet for analysis of short loops connecting repetitive structures, *BMC Bioinformatics* 5: 58.

29. Q. W. Dong, X. L. Wang, and L. Lin (2007), Methods for optimizing the structure alphabet sequences of proteins, *Comput. Biol. Med.* 37: 1610–1616.

30. C. Etchebest, C. Benros, S. Hazout, and A. G. de Brevern (2005), A structural alphabet for local protein structures: improved prediction methods, *Proteins* 59: 810–827.

31. Q. Li, C. Zhou, and H. Liu (2009), Fragment-based local statistical potentials derived by combining an alphabet of protein local structures with secondary structures and solvent accessibilities, *Proteins* 74: 820–836.

32. O. Zimmermann and U. H. Hansmann (2008), LOCUSTRA: accurate prediction of local protein structure using a two-layer support vector machine approach, *J. Chem. Inf. Model.* 48: 1903–1908.

33. A. Bornot, C. Etchebest, and A. G. de Brevern (2009), A new prediction strategy for long local protein structures using an original description, *Proteins* 76: 570–587.

34. A. G. de Brevern et al. (2005), A structural model of a seven-transmembrane helix receptor: the Duffy antigen/receptor for chemokine (DARC), *Biochim. Biophys. Acta.* 1724: 288–306.

35. A. Thomas et al. (2006), Prediction of peptide structure: how far are we? *Proteins* 65: 889–897.

36. C. Etchebest, C. Benros, A. Bornot, A. C. Camproux, and A. G. de Brevern (2007), A reduced amino acid alphabet for understanding and designing protein adaptation to mutation, *Eur. Biophys. J.* 36: 1059–1069.

37. G. Faure, A. Bornot, and A. G. de Brevern (2009), Analysis of protein contacts into Protein Units, *Biochimie* 91: 876–887

38. S. K. Hanks and T. Hunter (1995), Protein kinases 6. The eukaryotic protein kinase superfamily: kinase (catalytic) domain structure and classification, *Faseb J.* 9: 576–596.

39. G. D. Hardie and S. Hanks (1995), *The Protein Kinase Facts Book* Vol.1, Set : Protein–Serine Kinases, London, Academic Press Inc. Ltd.

40. G. D. Hardie and S. Hanks (1995), The Protein Kinase Facts Book Vol.2, Set : Protein–Tyrosine Kinases, London, Academic Press Inc. Ltd.

41. M. Huse and J. Kuriyan (2002), The conformational plasticity of protein kinases, *Cell* 109: 275–282.

42. A. Krupa, G. Preethi, and N. Srinivasan (2004), Structural modes of stabilization of permissive phosphorylation sites in protein kinases: distinct strategies in Ser/Thr and Tyr kinases, *J. Mol. Biol.* 339: 1025–1039.

43. E. J. Goldsmith, R. Akella, X. Min, T. Zhou, and J. M. Humphreys (2007), Substrate and docking interactions in serine/threonine protein kinases, *Chem Rev* 107: 5065–5081.

44. A. S. Konagurthu, J. C. Whisstock, P. J. Stuckey, and A. M. Lesk (2006), MUSTANG: a multiple structural alignment algorithm, *Proteins* 64: 559–574.

45. S. R. Hubbard (1997), Crystal structure of the activated insulin receptor tyrosine kinase in complex with peptide substrate and ATP analog, *Embo. J.* 16: 5572–5581.

46. S. R. Hubbard, L. Wei, L Ellis, and W. A. Hendrickson (1994), Crystal structure of the tyrosine kinase domain of the human insulin receptor, *Nature (London)*, 372: 746–754.

47. B. J. Canagarajah, A. Khokhlatchev, M. H. Cobb, and E. J. Goldsmith (1997), Activation mechanism of the MAP kinase ERK2 by dual phosphorylation, *Cell* 90: 859–869.

48. F. Zhang, A. Strand, D. Robbins, M. H. Cobb, and E. J. Goldsmith (1994), Atomic structure of the MAP kinase ERK2 at 2.3 Å resolution, *Nature (London)*, 367: 704–711.

49. J. Zheng et al. (1993), 2.2 Å refined crystal structure of the catalytic subunit of cAMP-dependent protein kinase complexed with MnATP and a peptide inhibitor, *Acta Crystallogr. D Biol. Crystallogr* 49: 362–365.

50. P. Akamine et al. (2003), Dynamic features of cAMP-dependent protein kinase revealed by apoenzyme crystal structure, *J. Mol. Biol.* 327: 159–171.

51. A. A. Russo, P. D. Jeffrey, and N. P. Pavletich (1996), Structural basis of cyclin-dependent kinase activation by phosphorylation, *Nat. Struct. Biol.* 3: 696–700.

52. N. R. Brown et al. (1999), Effects of phosphorylation of threonine 160 on cyclin-dependent kinase 2 structure and activity, *J. Biol. Chem.* 274: 8746–8756.

53. J. Yang et al. (2002), Crystal structure of an activated Akt/protein kinase B ternary complex with GSK3-peptide and AMP-PNP, *Nat. Struct. Biol.* 9: 940–944.

54. X. Huang et al. (2003), Crystal structure of an inactive Akt2 kinase domain, *Structure* 11: 21–30.

55. S. Favelyukis, J. H. Till, S. R. Hubbard, and W. T. Miller (2001), Structure and autoregulation of the insulin-like growth factor 1 receptor kinase, *Nat. Struct. Biol.* 8: 1058–1063.

56. A. Pautsch et al. (2001), Crystal structure of bisphosphorylated IGF-1 receptor kinase: insight into domain movements upon kinase activation, *Structure* 9: 955–965.

57. K. Mizuguchi, C. M. Deane, T. L. Blundell, M. S. Johnson, and J. P. Overington (1998), JOY: protein sequence-structure representation and analysis, *Bioinformatics* 14: 617–623.

9

KERNEL FUNCTION APPLICATIONS IN CHEMINFORMATICS

AARON SMALTER AND JUN HUAN

9.1 INTRODUCTION

The fast accumulation of data describing chemical compound structures and biological activity calls for the development of efficient informatics tools. *Cheminformatics* is a rapidly emerging research discipline that employs a wide array of statistical, data mining, and machine learning techniques with the goal of establishing robust relationships between chemical structures and their biological properties. Hence, cheminformatics is an important component on the application side of applying informatics approach to life science problems. It has a broad range of applications in chemistry and biology; arguably the most commonly known roles are in the area of drug discovery where cheminformatics tools play a central role in the analysis and interpretation of structure–activity data collected by various means of modern high throughput screening technology. Traditionally, the analysis of large chemical structure–activity databases was done only within pharmaceutical companies, and up until recently the academic community has had only limited access to such databases. This situation, however, has changed dramatically in very recent years.

In 2002, the National Cancer Institute created the Initiative for Chemical Genetics (ICG) with the goal of offering to the academic research community a large database of chemicals with their roles in cancer research [1]. Two years later, the National Health Institute (NIH) launched a Molecular Libraries Initiative (MLI) that included the formation of the national Molecular Library Screening Centers Network (MLSCN). MLSCN is a consortium of 10 high-throughput screening centers for screening large chemical libraries [2]. Collectively, ICG and MLSCN aim to offer to

Computational Intelligence and Pattern Analysis in Biological Informatics, Edited by Ujjwal Maulik, Sanghamitra Bandyopadhyay, and Jason T. L. Wang
Copyright © 2010 John Wiley & Sons, Inc.

the academic research community the results of testing about a million compounds against hundreds of biological targets. To organize this data and to provide public access to the results, the PubChem and Chembank database have been developed as the central repository for chemical structure–activity data. These databases currently contain >18 million chemical compound records, >1000 bioassay results, and links from chemicals to bioassay description, literature, references, and assay data for each entry.

Many machine learning and data mining algorithms have been applied to study the structure–activity relationship of chemicals. For example, Xue et al. reported promising results of applying five different machine learning algorithms: logistic regression, C4.5 decision tree, k-nearest neighbor, probabilistic neural network, and support vector machines, to predicting the toxicity of chemicals against an organism of Tetrahymena pyriformis [3]. Advanced techniques, [e.g., random forest and MARS (multivariate adaptive regression splines)] have also been applied to cheminformatics applications [4, 5].

This chapter, addresses as the problem of graph classification through study of kernel functions and the application of graph classification in chemical quantitative structure–activity relationship (QSAR) study. Graphs, especially the connectivity maps, have been used for modeling chemical structure for decades. In a connectivity map, nodes represent atoms and edges represent chemical bounds between atoms.

Recently, support vector machines (SVM) have gained popularity in drug design and cheminformatics. A key insight of SVM is the utilization of kernel functions (i.e., inner product of two points in a Hilbert space) to transform a nonlinear classification problem into a linear one. Design of a good kernel function for graphs is therefore a critical issue. The initial effort to define kernels for semistructured data was done by Haussler in his work on the *R-Convolution* kernel, which provided a framework that many current graph kernel functions follow [6].

While kernel functions and classifier (e.g., SVMs) for graphs have received a great deal of attention recently, most approaches are stymied by graph complexity. Precise comparisons are slow to compute, but simpler methods do not capture enough information about graph topology and structure. The focus of this work is to augment simple graph representations with structure information, allowing the use of fast kernel functions while recognizing important topological similarities. This work draws from several studies: incorporating structure feature graphs into kernel functions [7], extensions for approximate matching of such structure features [8], set-based matching kernels with structure features [9], and an application of wavelets for simplified topology comparison in graph kernels [10].

The material presented here explores some graph kernel functions that improve on existing methods with respect to both classification accuracy and kernel computation time. The following key insights are explored. First, problem relevant structure features can be used to annotate graph vertices in an alignment-based kernel function, raising model accuracy and adding explanatory capability [7]. Second, extensions for matching approximate structure features [8], as well as a faster, simpler kernel function [9], lead to gains in accuracy, as well as faster computation time. Finally, wavelet functions can be applied to graphs in order to summarize feature information in local graph topology, greatly reducing the kernel computation time [10]. We demonstrate a comprehensive experimental study, in the context of QSAR study in cheminformatics, for graph-based modeling and classification.

9.2 BACKGROUND

Before proceeding to algorithmic details, this chapter presents some general background material from a variety of directions. The work of this chapter draws from techniques in data mining, as well as machine learning and chemical property prediction. This chapter will address the following topics: chemical structures as graphs, graph classification, kernel functions, graph mining, and wavelet analysis for graphs.

9.2.1 Chemical Structure

Chemical compounds are organic molecules that are easily modeled by a graph representation. In this approach, *nodes* in a graph model *atoms* in a chemical structure and *edges* in the graph to model chemical *bonds* in the chemical structure. In this representation, nodes are labeled with the atom element type, and edges are labeled with the bond type (single, double, and aromatic bond). The edges in the graph are undirected, since there is no directionality associated with chemical bonds. Figure 9.1 shows an example chemical structure, where unlabeled vertices are assumed to be carbon (C).

Figure 9.2 shows two sample chemical structures on the left, and their graph representation on the right.

9.2.2 Graph Classification

Many classifiers exist for classification of objects as feature vectors. The feature vector embeds objects as points in a space where the data is modeled. Recently, an important linear classifier has gained a great deal of attention, the SVM. It is not only fast to train with great model generalization power, but it is also a kernel classifier giving it additional advantages over established vector space classifiers. These issues will be addressed in Section 9.2.3 on kernel functions.

The SVM builds a classification model by finding a linear hyperplane that best separates the classes of data objects. The *optimal separating hyperplane* (OSH) is chosen by maximizing the margin between the hyperplane and the nearest data points (termed support vectors).

When data are not linearly separable, called the soft-margin case, the SVM finds a hyperplane that optimizes an additional constraint. Often this constraint is a penalty for misclassified samples expressed in various ways.

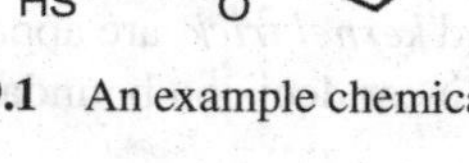

FIGURE 9.1   An example chemical structure.

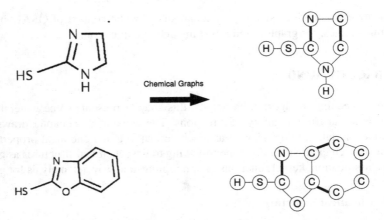

FIGURE 9.2   Graph representations of chemicals.

The problem of finding an OSH is formulated as a convex optimization problem. Hence, it can leverage very powerful algorithms for exactly finding the OSH. Once a OSH has been found, classification of additional objects is easily determined by finding which side of the hyperplane the object resides on. The efficiency of these operations makes SVM an extremely fast classifier. Since the SVM model ideally depends only on a small number of support vectors, it generalizes well and is compact to store.

Crucially, the SVM problem can be formulated such that it represents objects using only the dot products between their vectors. This modification allows the dot products to be replaced with a kernel function between objects, the use of which is discussed further in Section 9.2.3.

9.2.3   Kernel Functions

A kernel function K is a mapping between a pair of graphs into a real number, $K : GxG \rightarrow \mathbb{R}$. This function defines an inner product between two graphs and must satisfy the following properties:

Positive semidefinite. $\sum_i \sum_j K(g_i, g_j)c_i c_j \geq 0, \forall g \in G, \forall c \in \mathbb{R}$.
Symmetric. $K(g_i, g_j) = K(g_j, g_i), \forall g \in G$.

Such a function embeds graphs or any other objects into a Hilbert space, and is termed a Mercer kernel from Mercer's theorem.

Kernel functions can enhance classification in two ways: first, by mapping vector objects into higher dimensional spaces; second, by embedding nonvector objects in an implicitly defined space. The advantages of mapping objects into a higher dimensional space, the so-called *kernel trick*, are apparent in a variety of cases where objects are not separable by a linear decision boundary.

This implicit embedding is not only useful for nonlinear mappings, but also serves to decouple the object representation from the spatial embedding. A kernel function need only be defined between data objects in order to apply SVM classification. Therefore SVM can be used for classification of graph objects by defining a kernel function between graphs, without explicitly defining any set of graph features.

9.2.4   Graph Database Mining

This section discusses a few important definitions for graph database mining: labeled graphs, subgraph isomorphic relation, and graph classification.

Definition 9.2.1   *A **labeled graph** G is a quadruple $G = (V, E, \Sigma, \lambda)$ where V is a set of vertices or nodes and $E \subseteq V \times V$ is a set of undirected edges. A set of (disjoint) vertex and edge labels Σ, and $\lambda: V \cup E \rightarrow \Sigma$ is a function that assigns labels to vertices and edges. Assume that a total ordering is defined on the labels in Σ.*

A *graph database* is a set of labeled graphs.

Definition 9.2.2   *A graph $G' = (V', E', \Sigma', \lambda')$ is **subgraph isomorphic** to $G = (V, E, \Sigma, \lambda)$, denoted by $G' \subseteq G$, if there exists a 1-1 mapping $f : V' \rightarrow V$ such that*

$$\forall v \in V', \lambda'(v) = \lambda(f(v))$$

$$\forall (u, v) \in E', (f(u), f(v)) \in E,$$

and

$$\forall (u, v) \in E', \lambda'(u, v) = \lambda(f(u), f(v))$$

The function f is a *subgraph isomorphism* from graph G' to graph G. It is said G' *occurs* in G if $G' \subseteq G$. Given a subgraph isomorphism f, the image of the domain V' $(f(V'))$ is an *embedding* of G' in G.

Example 9.1   Figure 9.3 shows a graph database of three labeled graphs. The mapping (isomorphism) $q_1 \rightarrow p_3$, $q_2 \rightarrow p_1$, and $q_3 \rightarrow p_2$ demonstrates that graph Q is subgraph isomorphic to P, and hence Q *occurs* in P. Set $\{p_1, p_2, p_3\}$ is an embedding of Q in P. Similarly, graph S occurs in graph P, but not Q.

Problem Statement: Given a graph space G^*, a set of n graphs sampled from G^* and the related target values of these graphs $D = \{(G_i, T_i,)\}_{i=1}^n$, the **graph classification problem** is to estimate a function $F : G^* \rightarrow T$ that accurately map graphs to their target value.

By *classification*, all target values are assumed to be discrete values, otherwise it is a *regression* problem. Below, several algorithms are reviewed for graph classification that work within a common framework called a kernel function. The term *kernel function* refers to an operation of computing the inner product between two points in a Hilbert space. Kernel functions are widely used in classification of data in a high-dimensional feature space.

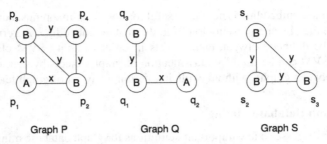

FIGURE 9.3   A database of three labeled graphs.

9.2.5 Wavelet Analysis for Graphs

Wavelet functions are commonly used as a means for decomposing and representing a function or signal as its constituent parts, across various resolutions or scales. Wavelets are usually applied to numerically valued data (e.g., communication signals or mathematical functions), as well as to some regularly structured numeric data (e.g., matrices and images).

Graphs, however, are arbitrarily structured and may represent many relationships and topologies between data elements. Recent work has established the successful application of wavelet functions to graphs for multiresolution analysis [11]. The use of wavelets in this capacity is different than the use of wavelets for signal and image compression (e.g., in [12]). The complex graph topology must be projected into a Euclidean space, and wavelets are used to summarize the information in the local topology around graph nodes.

Given a vertex v in graph G, define the h-hop neighbors of v as the set of other nodes in G whose shortest path to v is h nodes. The sets of h-hop neighbors then lead to the notion of hop distance, which suitably projects the nodes of a graph into Euclidean space.

Wavelets are then used to summarize feature information in the local topology around vertices in a graph. Since regions near the origin in a wavelet function are strongly positive, while the regions farther away are strongly negative, the distant regions are neutral. By using a wavelet function to compute a weighted sum over vertex features arranged according to hop distance corresponds to a comparison of vertex features in the local neighborhood to those in the distant neighborhood.

9.3 RELATED WORKS

Given that graphs are such powerful and interesting structures, their classification has been extensively studied. This chapter reviews the related work covering pattern mining, kernel functions, and wavelets for graph analysis.

This section surveys work related to graph classification methods by dividing them into two categories. The first category explicitly collects a set of *features* from the graphs. The possible features included are both structural and chemical. Structural features are graph fragments of different types. Examples are paths, cycles, trees, and general subgraphs [13]. Chemical descriptors, as they are called in QSAR work, are properties describing a molecule overall (e.g., as weight and charge).

Once a set of features is determined, a graph is described by a feature vector, and any existing classification methods (e.g., CBA [14] and decision tree [15]) that work in an n-dimensional Euclidian space, may be applied for graph classification.

The second classification approach is to implicitly collect a (possibly infinite) set of features from graphs. Rather than computing the features, this approach computes the similarity of graphs, using the framework of *kernel functions* [16]. The advantage of a kernel method is that it has a lower chance of over fitting, which is a serious concern in high-dimensional space with low sample size.

The following sections summarize recent work related to pattern mining and structural features, as well as vector-based classification , kernel functions for classification, and wavelets for graphs.

9.3.1   Pattern Mining

Algorithms that search for frequent patterns (e.g., trees, paths, and cyclic graphs) in graphs can be roughly divided into three groups.

The first group uses a level-wise search strategy, including AGM [17] and FSG [18]. The second category takes a depth-first search strategy, including gSpan [19] and FFSM [20]. Different from level-wise search algorithms AGM and FSG, the depth-first search strategy utilizes a back-track algorithm to mine frequent subgraphs. The advantage of a depth-first search is a better memory utilization, since depth-first search keeps one frequent subgraph in memory and enumerates its supergraphs, in contrast to keeping all k-edge frequent subgraph in memory.

The third category of frequent subgraph mining algorithms does not work directly on a graph space to identify frequent patterns. Instead, algorithms in this category first project a graph space to another space (e.g., that of trees), then identify frequent patterns in the projected space, and finally reconstruct all frequent patterns in the graph space. This strategy is called *progressive mining*. Algorithms in this category includes SPIN [21] and GASTON [22].

9.3.1.1 Frequent Subgraphs Frequent subgraph mining is a technique used to enumerate graph substructures that occur in a graph database with at least some specified frequency. This minimum frequency threshold is termed the *support threshold* by the data mining community. After limiting returned subgraphs by frequency, types found can be further constrained by setting upper and lower limits on the number of vertices they can contain. In much of this articles work, the FFSM algorithm [23] is used for fast computation of frequent subgraphs. Figure 9.4, shows an example of this frequent subgraph enumeration. Some work has been done by Deshpande et al. [24] toward the use of these frequent substructures in the classification of chemical compounds with promising results.

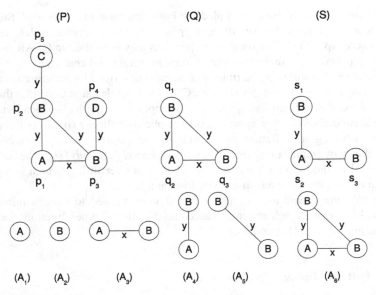

FIGURE 9.4   Example graphs and frequent subgraphs (support $= 2/3$).

9.3.1.2 Chemical Properties and Target Prediction

9.3.1.2 Chemical Properties and Target Prediction   A *target property* of the chemical compound is a measurable quantity of the compound. There are two categories of target properties: continuous (e.g., binding affinities to a protein) and discrete target properties (e.g., active compounds vs inactive compounds).

The relationship between a chemical compound and its target property is typically investigated through a quantitative structure–property relationship (QSPR). (Such a study a also known as a quantitative structure–activity relationship (QSAR), but *property* refers to a broader range of applications than activity.) Abstractly, any QSPR method generally may be defined as a function that maps a chemical space to a property space in the form of

$$P = \hat{k}(D) \tag{9.1}$$

Here, D is a chemical structure, P is a property, and the function $\hat{k}$ is an estimated mapping from a chemical to a property space.

Different QSPR methodologies can be understood in terms of the types of target property values (continuous or discrete), types of features, and algorithms that map descriptors to target properties.

9.3.2   Vector-Based Classification

Several classification algorithms based on explicitly collected features exist for graph classification in a variety of applications. What follows is a brief survey of popular methods for some pertinent applications

Recent methods applied to QSAR and chemical activity prediction include decision trees, classification based on association [14], and random forest among many others. Decision trees use a collection of simple learners organized in a hierarchical tree structure to classify a object. Nonleaf nodes make decisions about an object based on one of it's properties and send it to one of the children. Leaf nodes of the tree correspond to classification categories. Random forest uses a collection of randomly generated decision trees and typically classify an object according to the mode of the classes returned by all trees.

Classification based on association (CBA) is somewhat different than these other methods. It seeks to find a set of association rules of the form $A \rightarrow c_i$, where A is some set of properties and c_i is a class label. The XRules [13] are similar to CBA and utilize frequent tree patterns to build a rule-based classifier for XML data. Specifically, XRules first identifies a set of frequent tree patterns. An association rule: $G \rightarrow c_i$ is then formed where G is a tree pattern and c_i is a class label. The *confidence* of the rule is the conditional probability $p(c_i|G)$ estimated from the training data. The XRules carefully selects a subset of rules with high confidence values and uses those rules for classification.

Graph boosting [25] also utilizes substructures toward graph classification. Similar to XRules, graph boosting uses rules with the format of $G \rightarrow c_i$. Different from XRules, it uses the boosting technique to assign weights to different rules. The final classification result is computed as the weighted majority.

9.3.3   Kernel Functions for Graph Classification

The term kernel function refers to an operation for computing the inner product between two vectors in a feature space, thus avoiding the explicit computation of coordinates in that feature space. Graph kernel functions are simply kernel functions that have been defined to compute the similarity between two graph structures. In recent years, a variety of graph kernel functions have been developed, with promising results as described by Ralaivola et al. [26].

Graph kernel functions can be roughly divided into two categories. The first group of kernel functions consider the full adjacency matrix of graphs, and hence measured the global similarity of two graphs. These include product graph kernels [27], random walk based kernels [28], and kernels based on the shortest paths between a pair of nodes [29]. The second group of kernel functions tries to capture the local similarity of two graphs by counting the shared subcomponents of graphs. These include the subtree [30], cyclic [31], and spectrum kernels [24]. This section reviews the relevant work on these kernel functions.

Product graph kernels use a feature space of all possible node label sequences for walks in graphs. Since the number of possible walks are infinite, there is no way to enumerate all the features in kernel computation [27]. Instead, a *product graph* is computed in order to make the kernel function computation feasible.

Rather than computing the shared paths exactly, which has prohibitive computational cost for large graphs, the work of Kashima et al. [28] is based on the use of shared random label sequences in the computation of graph kernels. Their marginalized graph kernel uses a Markov model to randomly generate walks of a labeled graph. The random walks are created using a transition probability matrix combined with a walk termination probability. These collections of random walks are then compared and the number of shared sequences is used to determine the overall similarity between two molecules.

Spectrum kernels aim to simplify the aforementioned kernels by working in a finite-dimensional feature space based on a set of subgraphs (or as special cases, trees, cycles, and paths). The kernel function is computed as the inner product between two feature vectors (e.g., counts of subgraph occurrences) as in [24]. Transformations of the inner product (e.g., minmax kernel [32] and Tanimoto kernel [26]), are also widely used. The subtree kernel [33] is a variation on the spectrum kernel that uses subtrees instead of paths.

The optimal assignment kernel, described by Frölich et al. [10], differs significantly from the marginalized graph kernel. This kernel function first computes the similarity between all vertices in one graph and all vertices in another. The similarity between the two graphs is then computed by finding the maximal weighted bipartite graph between the two sets of vertices, called the optimal assignment. The authors investigate an extension of this method whereby certain structure patterns defined *a priori* by expert knowledge, are collapsed into single vertices, and this reduced graph is used as input to the optimal assignment kernel.

9.3.4 Wavelets Functions for Graphs

Crovella and Kolaczyk [11] developed a multiscale method for network traffic data analysis. For this application, they are attempting to determine the scale at which certain traffic phenomena occur. They represent traffic networks as graphs labeled with some measurement (e.g., bytes carried per unit time). In their method, they use the *hop* distance between vertices in a graph, defined as the length of the shortest path between them, and apply a weighted average function to compute the difference between the average of measurements close to a vertex and measurements that are far, up to a certain distance. This process produces a new measurement for a specific vertex that captures and condenses information about the vertex neighborhood. Figure 9.5 shows a diagram of wavelet function weights overlayed on a chemical structure.

Maggioni et al. [12] demonstrate a general purpose biorthogonal wavelet for graph analysis. In their method, they use the dyadic powers of an diffusion operator to induce a multiresolution analysis. While their method applies to a large class of spaces, (e.g., manifolds and graphs), the applicability of their method to attributed chemical structures is not clear. The major technical difficulty is how to incorporate node labels in a multiresolution analysis.

9.4   ALIGNMENT KERNELS WITH PATTERN-BASED FEATURES

Traditional approaches to graph similarity rely on the comparison of compounds using a variety of molecular attributes known *a priori* to be involved in the activity

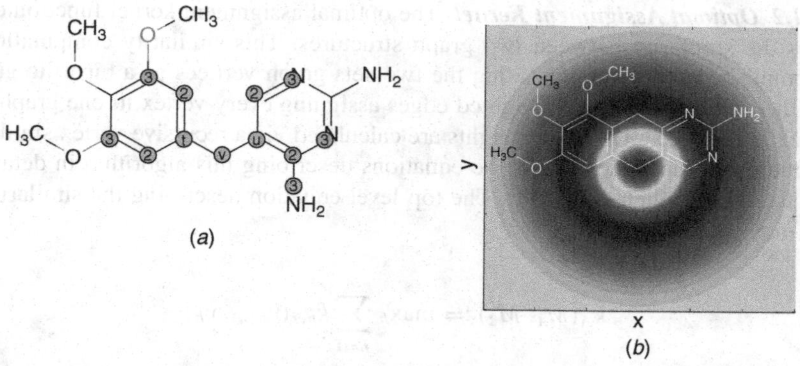

FIGURE 9.5   A chemical graph and hop distances. From [10], with permission.

of interest. Such methods are problem-specific, however, and provide little assistance when the relevant descriptors are not known in advance. Additionally, these methods lack the ability to provide explanatory information regarding what structural features contribute to the observed chemical activity. The method proposed here, referred to as OAPD for Optimal-Assignment with Pattern-Based Descriptors, alleviates both of these issues through the mining and analysis of structural patterns present in the data in order to identify highly discriminating patterns, which then augment a graph kernel function that computes molecular similarity.

9.4.1 Structure-Based Pattern Mining for Chemical Compound Classification

The following sections outline the algorithm that drives the experimental method. In short, it measures the similarity of graph structures whose vertices and edges have been labeled with various descriptors. These descriptors represent physical and chemical information (e.g., atom and bond types). They are also used to represent the membership of atoms in specific structure patterns that have been mined from the data. To compute the similarity of two graphs, the vertices of one graph are aligned with the vertices of the second graph, such that the total overall similarity is maximized with respect to all possible alignments. Vertex similarity is measured by comparing vertex descriptors, and is computed recursively so that when comparing two vertices, it also compares the neighbors of those vertices, and their neighbors, and so on.

9.4.1.1 Structure Pattern Mining The frequent subgraph mining problem can be phrased as such: Given a set of labeled graphs, the support of an arbitrary subgraph is the fraction of all graphs in the set that contain that subgraph. A subgraph is frequent if its support meets a certain minimum threshold. The goal is to enumerate all the frequent, connected subgraphs in a graph database. The extraction of important subgraph patterns can be controlled by selecting the proper frequency threshold, as well as other parameters (e.g., size and density) of subgraph patterns.

9.4.1.2 Optimal Assignment Kernel The optimal assignment kernel function computes the similarity between two graph structures. This similarity computation is accomplished by first representing the two sets graph vertices as a bipartite graph, and then finding the set of weighted edges assigning every vertex in one graph to a vertex in the other. The edge weights are calculated via a recursive vertex similarity function. This section presents the equations describing this algorithm in detail, as discussed by Frölich et al. [34]. The top-level equation describing the similarity of two molecular graphs is

$$k_A(M_1, M_2) := \max_\pi \sum_{h=1}^{m} k_{nei}(v_{\pi(h)}, v_h) \qquad (9.2)$$

where π denotes a permutation of a subset of graph vertices, and m is the number of vertices in the smaller graph. This information is needed to assign all vertices of the smaller graph to vertices in the large graph. The k_{nei} function, which calculates the similarity between two vertices using their local neighbors, is given as follows:

$$k_{nei}(v_1, v_2) := k_v(v_1, v_2) + R_0(v_1, v_2) + S_{nei}(v_1, v_2) \qquad (9.3)$$

$$S_{nei}(v_1, v_2) := \sum_{l=1}^{L} \gamma(l) R_l(v_1, v_2) \qquad (9.4)$$

The functions k_v and k_e compute the similarity between vertices (atoms) and edges (bonds), respectively. These functions could take a variety of forms, but in the OA kernel they are RBF functions between vectors of vertex–edge labels.

The $\gamma(l)$ term is a decay parameter that weights the similarity of neighbors according to their distance from the original vertex. The l parameter controls the topological distance within which to consider neighbors of vertices. The R_l equation, which recursively computes the similarity between two specific vertices, is given by the following equation:

$$R_l(v_1, v_2) = \frac{1}{|v_1||v_2|} \sum_{i,j} R_{l-1}(n_i(v_1), n_j(v_2)) \qquad (9.5)$$

where $|v|$ is the number of neighbors of vertex v, and $n_k(v)$ is the set of neighbors of v. The base case for this equation is R_0, defined by

$$R_0(v_1, v_2) := \frac{1}{|v_1|} \max_\pi \sum_{i=1}^{|v_2|} (k_v(a, b)|k_e(x, y)) \qquad (9.6)$$

$$a = n_{\pi(i)}(v_1), \quad b = n_i(v_2) \qquad (9.7)$$

$$x = v_1 \to n_{\pi(i)}(v_1), \quad y = v_2 \to n_i(v_2) \qquad (9.8)$$

The notation $v \rightarrow n_i(v)$ refers to the edge connecting vertex v with the ith neighboring vertex. The functions k_v and k_e are used to compare vertex and edge descriptors, by counting the total number of descriptor matches.

9.4.1.3 Reduced Graph Representation

One way in which to utilize the structure patterns that are mined from the graph data is to collapse the specific subgraphs into single vertices in the original graph. This technique is explored by Frölich et al. [10] with moderate results, although they use predefined structure patterns, so called pharmacophores, identified *a priori* with the help of expert knowledge. The method proposed here ushers these predefined patterns in favor of the structure patterns generated via frequent subgraph mining.

The use of a reduced graph representation has some advantages. First, by collapsing substructures, an entire set of vertices can be compared at once, reducing the graph complexity and marginally decreasing computation time. Second, by changing the substructure size, the resolution at which graph structures are compared can be adjusted. The disadvantage of a reduced graph representation is that substructures can only be compared directly to other substructures, and cannot align partial structure matches. As utilized in Frölich et al. [34], this is not as much of a burden since they have defined the best patterns *a priori* using expert knowledge. In the case of the method presented here, however, this is a significant downside, as there is no *a priori* knowledge to guide pattern generation and we wish to retain as much structural information as possible.

9.4.1.4 Pattern-Based Descriptors

The loss of partial substructure alignment following the use of a reduced graph representation motivated us to find another way of integrating this pattern-based information. Instead of collapsing graph substructures, vertices are simply annotated with additional descriptor labels indicating the vertex's membership in the structure patterns that were previously mined. These pattern-based descriptors are calculated for each vertex and are used by the optimal assignment kernel in the same way that other vertex descriptors are handled. In this way, substructure information can be captured in the graph vertices without needing to alter the original graph structure.

9.4.2 Experimental Study

Classification experiments were conducted on five different biological activity data sets, and measured SVM classifier prediction accuracy for several different feature generation methods. The data sets and classification methods are described in more detail in the following sections, along with the associated results. Figure 9.6 gives a graphical overview of the process.

All of the experiments were performed on a desktop computer with a 3-GHz Pentium 4 processor and 1 GB of RAM. Generating a set of frequent subgraphs is very quick, generally a few seconds. Optimal assignment requires significantly more computation time, but not intractable, at less than one-half of an hour for the largest data set.

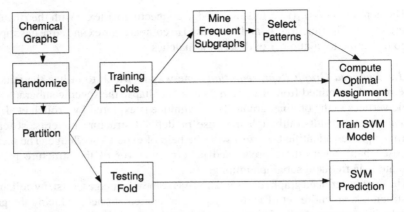

FIGURE 9.6 Experimental workflow for a cross-validation trial with frequent subgraph mining.

9.4.2.1 Data Sets Five data sets used in various problem areas were selected to evaluate classifier performance. The predictive toxicology challenge (PTC) data set, discussed by Helma et al. [35], contains a set of chemical compounds classified according to their toxicity in male rats (PTC–MR), female rats (PTC–FR), male mice (PTC-MM), and female mice (PTC–FM). The human intestinal absorption (HIA) dataset (Wessel et al. [36]) contains chemical compounds classified by intestinal absorption activity. Also included were two different virtual screening data sets (VS-1 and VS-2) used to predict various binding inhibitors from Fontaine et al. [37] and Jorissen and Gilson [38]. The final data set (MD) is from Patterson et al. [39], and was used to validate certain molecule descriptors. Various statistics for these data sets can be found in Table 9.1.

9.4.2.2 Methods The performance of the SVM classifier was evaluated by training with several different feature sets. The first set of features (FSM) consists only of frequent subgraphs. Those subgraphs are mined using the FFSM software [23] with

TABLE 9.1 Data Set Statistics for OAPD Experiments

Data Set	Number of Compunds	Number of Positives	Number of Negatives	Average Compund Size
HIA	86	47	39	22.45
MD	310	148	162	10.38
VS-1	435	279	156	59.81
VS-2	1071	125	946	39.33
PTC–MR	344	152	192	25.56
PTC–MM	336	129	207	25.05
PTC–FR	351	121	230	26.08
PTC–FM	349	143	206	25.25

minimum subgraph frequency of 50%. Each chemical compound is represented by a binary vector with length equal to the number of mined subgraphs. Each subgraph is mapped to a specific vector index, and if a chemical compound contains a subgraph then the bit at the corresponding index is set to one, otherwise it is set to zero.

The second feature set (optimal assignment, OA) consists of the similarity values computed by the optimal assignment kernel, as proposed by Frölich et al. [34]. Each compound is represented as a real-valued vector containing the computed similarity between it and all other molecules in the data set.

The third feature set optimal assignment reduced graph (OARG) is computed using the optimal assignment kernel as well, except that the frequent subgraph patterns are embedded as a reduced graph representation before computing the optimal assignment. The reduced graph representation is described by Frölich et al. as well, but they use *a priori* patterns instead of frequently mined ones.

Finally, the fourth feature set optimal assignment pattern discovery (OAPD) also consists of the subgraph patterns combined with the optimal assignment kernel, however, in this case a reduced graph is not derived, and instead annotate vertices in a graph with additional descriptors indicating its membership in specific subgraph patterns.

In the experiments, SVM classifier was used in order to generate activity predictions. The use of SVM has recently become quite popular for a variety of biological machine learning applications because of its efficiency and ability to operate on high-dimensional data sets. The SMO SVM classifier was used, implemented by Platt [40] and included in the Weka data-mining software package by Witten and Frenk [41]. The SVM parameters were fixed, with a linear kernel and $C = 1$. Classifier performance was averaged over a ten-fold cross-validation set.

Some feature selection was performed in order to identify the most discriminating frequent patterns. Using a simple statistical formula, known as the Pearson correlation coefficient (PCC), the correlation between a set of feature samples (in this case, the occurrences of a particular subgraph in each of the data samples) and the corresponding class labels was measured. Frequent patterns are ranked according to correlation strength, and the top patterns are selected.

9.4.2.3 Results

Table 9.2 contains results reporting the average and standard deviation of the prediction accuracy over the 10 cross-validation trials. The following observations can be made from this table:

First, notice that OAPD (and OARG) outperforms FSM methods in all of the tried data sets except one (FSM is better than OARG on the PTC–MR data set). This result indicate that use of frequent subgraphs alone without using the optimal alignment kernel, does not produce a good classifier. Although the conclusion is generally true, interestingly, for the PTC–MR data set, the FSM method outperforms both the OA and OARG methods, while the OAPD method outperforms FSM. This seems to suggest that important information is encoded in the frequent subgraphs, and is being lost in the OARG, but is still preserved in the OAPD method.

Second, notice that the OAPD (or OARG) method outperforms the original OA method in five of the tried eight data sets: The HIA, MD, PTC–FR, PTC–MM,

TABLE 9.2 **Average and Standard Deviation of 10-Fold Cross-Validation Accuracy for OAPD Experiments**

Data Set	Method			
	FSM	OA	OARG	OAPD
HIA	57.36 ± 19.11	63.33 ± 20.82	62.92 ± 22.56	65.28 ± 15.44
MD	68.39 ± 7.26	70.00 ± 6.28	69.35 ± 6.5	70.32 ± 5.65
VS-1	60.00 ± 5.23	64.14 ± 3.07	62.07 ± 4.06	63.91 ± 4.37
VS-2	90.29 ± 2.3	94.96 ± 1.88	93.18 ± 2.68	94.77 ± 2.17
PTC–MR	54.16 ± 5.82	61.35 ± 9.53	59.03 ± 6.46	59.29 ± 8.86
PTC–MM	63.28 ± 5.32	60.10 ± 9.21	64.68 ± 3.96	64.39 ± 3.6
PTC–FR	60.45 ± 3.87	62.16 ± 6.43	62.75 ± 7.69	63.05 ± 5.24
PTC–FM	58.42 ± 4.43	56.41 ± 6	54.07 ± 7.52	60.76 ± 7.32

PTC–MR. OAPD data sets have a very close performance to that of OA in the rest of the three data sets. The results indicate that the OAPD method provides good performance for diverse data sets that involve tasks (e.g., predicting chemical's toxicology, human intestinal absorption of chemicals, and virtual screening of drugs).

In addition to outperforming the previous methods, this method also reports the specific subgraph patterns that were mined from the training data and used to augment the optimal assignment kernel function. By identifying highly discriminative patterns, this method can offer additional insight into the structural features that contribute to a compound's chemical function. Table 9.3 contains the five highest ranked (using Pearson correlation coefficient) subgraph patterns for each data set, expressed as SMARTS strings that encode the specific pattern. Many of the patterns in all sets

TABLE 9.3 **SMARTS String of Highly Ranked Chemical Patterns from the OAPD Method**

HIA	MD	VS-1	VS-2
[NH^{3+}]C(C)C	C(=CC)(C)S	C(C=CC=C)C=C	C(=CCC)C
C(=C)(C)C	C(=CC=CC)(C)S	C(=CC)CNC	C=CCC
C(=CC)(C)C	C(=C)(C=CC=C)S	C(=C)CNC	[NH^{2+}](CC=C)CC
C(=CC)(C=C)C	C(=CCC)C=C	CC(=CC)N	[NH^{2+}](CCC)CC
C(=CC=C)(C=C)C	C(=CS)C=C	CNCC=C	[NH^{3+}]CC(=CC)C

PTC–MR	PTC–MM	PTC–FR	PTC–FM
[NH^{2+}]C(=C)C=C	[NH^{3+}]CC	[NH^{2+}]C(=CC)C=C	OCC=C
[NH^{2+}]C=CC	c1ccccc1	[NH^{2+}]C(=C)C=C	C(=CC)C(=C)C
[NH^{3+}]CC	C(=CC)C(=C)C	[NH^{3+}]CC	CCC=CC
CC=C	C(=CC=C)C	CC=C	C(=C)(C)C
C(CC)C	C(=C)C(=C)C	C(CC)C	c1ccccc1

denote various carbon chains (C(CC)C, C=CC, etc.), however, there seem to be some unique patterns as well. The MD data set contains carbon chain patterns with some sulfur atoms mixed in, while the VS-1 data set has carbon chains with nitrogen mixed in. The [NH^{2+}] and [NH^{3+}] patterns appear to be important in the VS-2 data set, as well as some of the PTC data sets.

9.4.3   Conclusions

Graph structures are a powerful and expressive representation for chemical compounds. This work presents a new method, termed OAPD, for computing the similarity of chemical compounds, based on the use of an optimal assignment graph kernel function augmented with pattern-based descriptors that have been mined from a set of molecular graphs. Experimental studies demonstrate that the OAPD method integrates the structural alignment capabilities of the existing optimal alignment kernel method with the substructure discovery capabilities of the frequent subgraph mining method and delivers better performance in most of the tried benchmarks. In the future, it may be possible to involve domain experts to evaluate the performance of this algorithm, including the prediction accuracy and the capability of identifying structure important features, in diverse chemical structure data sets.

9.5   ALIGNMENT KERNELS WITH APPROXIMATE PATTERN FEATURES

The work presented in this chapter aims to leverage existing frequent pattern mining algorithms and explore the application of kernel classifiers in building highly accurate graph classification algorithms. Toward that end, a novel technique is demonstrated called graph pattern diffusion kernel (GPD). In this method, all frequent patterns are first identified from a graph database. Then subgraphs are mapped to graphs in the graph database and nodes of graphs are projected to a high-dimensional space with a specially designed function. Finally, a novel graph alignment algorithm is used to compute the inner product of two graphs. This algorithm is tested using a number of chemical structure data sets. The experimental results demonstrate that this method is significantly better than competing methods (e.g., those based on paths, cycles, and other subgraphs).

9.5.1   Graph Pattern Diffusion Kernels for Accurate Graph Classification

Here we present the design of the pattern diffusion kernel. The section begins by first presenting a general framework. It is proved, through a reduction to the subgraph isomorphism problem, that the computational cost of the general framework can be prohibitive for large graphs. The pattern-based graph alignment kernel is then presented. Finally, a technique is shown called "pattern diffusion" that can significantly improve graph classification accuracy in practice.

9.5.1.1 Graph Similarity Measurement with Alignment An *alignment* of two graphs G and G' (assuming $|V[G]| \leq |V[G']|$) is a 1-1 mapping $\pi : V[G] \to V[G']$. Given an alignment π, define the similarity between two graphs, as measured by a kernel function k_A, below:

$$k_A(G, G') = \max_{\pi} \sum_{v} k_n(v, \pi(v)) + \sum_{u,v} k_e((u, v), (\pi(u), \pi(v))) \qquad (9.9)$$

The function k_n is a kernel function to measure the similarity of node labels and the function k_e is a kernel function to measure the similarity of edge labels. Equation (9.9) uses an additive model to compute the similarity between two graphs. The maximal similarity among all possible mappings is defined as the similarity between two graphs.

9.5.1.2 NP-Hardness of Graph Alignment Kernel Function It is no surprise that computing the graph alignment kernel is a nonpdynomial (NP)-hard problem. This has been proposed with a reduction from the graph alignment kernel to the subgraph isomorphism problem. Here, paragraphs, assuming there exists an efficient solver of the graph alignment kernel problem, it is shown that the same solver can be used to solve the subgraph isomorphism problem efficiently. Since the subgraph isomorphism problem is an NP-hard problem, with the reduction mentioned before, it is proved that the graph alignment kernel problem is therefore an NP-hard problem as well. *Note*: This section is a stand-alone component of this work, and readers who choose to skip this section should encounter no difficulty in reading the rest of the text.

Given two graphs G and G' (for simplicity, assume nodes and edges in G and G' are not labeled as usually studied in the subgraph isomorphism problem), use a node kernel function that returns a constant 0. Define an edge kernel function $k_e : V[G] \times V[G] \times V[G'] \times V[G'] \to \mathbb{R}$ as

$$k_e((u, v), (u', v')) = \begin{cases} 1 & \text{if } (u, v) \in E[G] \text{ and } (u', v') \in E[G'] \\ 0 & \text{otherwise} \end{cases}$$

With the constant node and the specialized edge function, the kernel function of two graphs is simplified to the following format:

$$k_A(G, G') = \max_{\pi} \sum_{u,v} k_e((u, v), (\pi(u), \pi(v))) \qquad (9.10)$$

The NP-hardness of the graph alignment kernel is established with the following theorem.

Theorem 9.5.1 *Given two (unlabeled) graphs G and G' and the edge kernel function k_e defined previously, G is subgraph isomorphic to G' if and only if $K_a(G, G') = |E[G]|$.*

Proof: If: Notice from the definition of k_e that the maximal value of $K_a(G, G')$ is $|E[G]|$. Given $K_a(G, G') = |E[G]|$, it is claimed that there exists an alignment function $\pi : V[G] \rightarrow V[G']$ such that for all $(u, v) \in E[G]$, $(\pi(u), \pi(v)) \in E[G']$. The existence of such a function π guarantees that graph G is a subgraph of G'.

Only if: Given G is a subgraph of G', there is an alignment function $\pi : V[G] \rightarrow V[G']$ such that for all $(u, v) \in E[G]$, $(\pi(u), \pi(v)) \in E[G']$. According to Eq. (9.10), $K_a(G, G') = |E[G]|$. $\qquad\square$

Theorem 9.5.1 shows that the graph alignment kernel problem is no easier than the subgraph isomorphism problem. Hence, it is at least NP-hard in complexity.

9.5.1.3 Graph Node Alignment Kernel To derive an efficient algorithm scalable to large graphs, the idea is that a function f is used to map nodes in a graph to a high (possibly infinite)-dimensional feature space that captures not only the node label information, but also the neighborhood topological information around the node. If such a function f is obtained, the graph kernel function may be simplified with the following formula:

$$k_M(G, G') = \max_{\pi} \sum_{v \in V[G]} k_n(f(v), f(\pi(v))) \qquad (9.11)$$

Where $\pi : V[G] \rightarrow V[G']$ denotes an alignment of graph G and G'. $f(v)$ is a set of "features" associated with a node.

With this modification, the optimization problem that searches for the best alignment can be solved in polynomial time. To derive a polynomial running time algorithm, a weighted complete bipartite graph is constructed by making every node pair $(u,v) \in V[G] \times V[G']$ incident on an edge. The weight of the edge (u,v) is $k_n(f(v), f(u))$. Figure 9.7, shows a weighted complete bipartite graph for $V[G] = \{v_1, v_2, v_3\}$ and $V[G'] = \{u_1, u_2, u_3\}$. Highlighted edges $(v1, u2)$, $(v2, u1)$, $(v3, u3)$ have larger weights than the rest of the edges (dashed).

With the bipartite graph, a search for the best alignment becomes a search for the maximum weighted bipartite subgraph from the complete bipartite graph. Many network flow-based algorithms (e.g., linear programming) can be used to obtain the maximum weighted bipartite subgraph. The Hungarian algorithm is used with complexity $O(|V[G]|^3)$. For details of the Hungarian algorithm see [42].

Applying the Hungarian algorithm to graph alignment was first explored by [34] for chemical compound classification. In contrast to their algorithm, which utilized domain knowledge of chemical compounds extensively and developed a complicated recursive function to compute the similarity between nodes, a new framework is developed here that maps such nodes to a high-dimensional space in order to measure the similarity between two nodes without assuming any domain knowledge. Even in cheminformatics, experiments show that this technique generates similar and sometimes better classification accuracies compared to the method reported in [34].

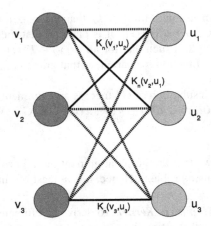

FIGURE 9.7 A maximum weighted bipartite graph for graph alignment.

Unfortunately, using the Hungarian algorithm for assignment, as used by [34] is not a true Mercer kernel. Since the kernel function proposed here uses this algorithm as well, it is also not a Mercer kernel. As seen in [34], however, this kernel still performs competitively.

9.5.1.4 Pattern Diffusion This section introduces a novel technique "pattern diffusion" to project nodes in a graph to a high-dimensional space that captures both node labeling and local topology information. This design has the following advantages as a kernel function:

The design is generic and does not assume any domain knowledge from a specific application. The diffusion process may be applied to graphs with dramatically different characteristics.

The diffusion process is straightforward to implement and can be computed efficiently.

Below, the pattern diffusion kernel is outlined in three steps.

In the first step, a seed is identified as a starting point for the diffusion. In this design, a "seed" could be a single node, or a set of connected nodes in the original graph. In the experimental study, frequent subgraphs are used for seeds since a seed can easily be compared from one graph to a seed in another graph. However, there is no requirement that frequent subgraphs must be used for the seed.

In the second step given a set of nodes S as seed, recursively define f_t in the following way.

The base f_0 is defined as

$$f_0(u) = \begin{cases} 1/|S| & \text{if } u \in S \\ 0 & \text{otherwise} \end{cases}$$

Given some time t, define f_{t+1} ($t \geq 0$) with f_t in the following way:

$$f_{t+1}(v) = f_t(v) \times (1 - \frac{\lambda}{d(v)}) + \sum_{u \in N(v)} f_t(u) \times \frac{\lambda}{d(u)} \qquad (9.12)$$

In this notation, $N(v)$ is the set of nodes that connects to v directly. The parameter $d(v)$ is the node degree of v, or $d(v) = |N(v)|$ and λ is a parameter that controls the diffusion rate.

Equation (9.12) describes a process where each node distributes a λ fraction of its value to its neighbors evenly and in the same way receives some value from its neighbors. Call it "diffusion" because the process simulates the way a value is spreading in a network. The intuition is that the distribution of such a value encodes information about the local topology of the network.

To constrain the diffusion process to a local region, one parameter, called diffusion time, is used and is denoted by τ, to control the diffusion process. Specifically, the diffusion process is limited to a local region of the original graph with nodes that are at most τ hops away from a node in the seed S. For this reason, the diffusion is referred to as "local diffusion".

Finally, for the seed S, define the mapping function f_S as the limit function of f_t as t approaches infinity, or

$$f_S = \lim_{t \to \infty} f_t \qquad (9.13)$$

9.5.1.5 Pattern Diffusion Kernel and Graph Classification
This section summarizes the discussion of kernel functions and shows how they are utilized to construct an efficient graph classification algorithm at both the training and testing phases.

Training Phase. In the training phase, divide graphs of the training data set $D = \{(G_i, T_i,)\}_{i=1}^n$ into groups according to their class labels. For example, in binary classification there are two groups of graphs: positive or negative. For multiclass classification, there are multiple groups of graphs where each group contains graphs with the same class label. The training phase is composed of four steps:

1. Obtain frequent subgraphs for seeds. Identify frequent subgraphs from each graph group and take union of the subgraph sets together as the seed set S.
2. For each seed $S \in S$ and for each graph G in the training data set, use f_S to label nodes in G. Thus the feature vector of a node v is a vector $L_V = \{f_{S_i}(v)\}_{i=1}^m$ with length $m = |S|$.
3. For two graphs G, G', construct the complete weighted bipartite graph as described in Section 9.5.1.3 and compute the kernel $K_a(G, G')$ using Eq. (9.11).
4. Train a predictive model using a kernel classifier.

Testing Phase. In the testing phase, the kernel function is computed for graphs in the testing and training data sets. The trained model is used to make predictions about graph in the testing set.

- For each seed $S \in \mathcal{S}$ and for each graph G in the testing data set, f_S is used to label nodes in G and create feature vectors as done in the training phase.
- Equation (9.11) computes the kernel function $K_a(G, G')$ for each graph G in the testing data set and for each graph G' in the training data set.
- Use kernel classifier and trained models to obtain prediction accuracy of the testing data set

9.5.2 Experimental Study

Classification experiments were conducted using 10 different biological activity data sets, and compared cross-validation accuracies for different kernel functions. The following sections describe the data sets and the classification methods in more detail along with the associated results.

All of the experiments were performed on a desktop computer with a 3 GHz Pertium 4 processor and 1 GB of RAM. Generating a set of frequent subgraphs is efficient, generally taking a few seconds. Computing alignment kernels somewhat takes more computation time, typically in the range of a few minutes.

In all kernel classification experiments, the LibSVM software [43] was used as the kernel classifier. The nu-SVC type classifier was used with nu = 0.5, the LibSVM default. To perform a fair comparison, model selection was not performed, the SVM parameters were not tuned to favor any particular method, and default parameters were used in all cases. The classifiers CBA and Xrule were downloaded as instructed in the related papers, and default parameters were used for both. The classification accuracy is computed by averaging over 10 trials of a 10-fold cross-validation experiment. Standard deviation is computed similarly.

9.5.2.1 *Data Sets*   Ten data sets were selected covering typical chemical benchmarks in drug design to evaluate our classification algorithm performance.

The first five data sets are from drug virtual screening experiments taken from [38]. In this data set, the target values are drugs' binding affinity to a particular protein. Five proteins also are used in the data set including: CDK2, COX2, FXa, PDE5, and A1A, where each symbol represents a specific protein. For each protein, the data provider carefully selected 50 chemical structures that clearly bind to the protein (active ones). The data provider also deliberately listed chemical structures that are very similar to the active ones (judged with domain knowledge), but clearly do not bind to the target protein. This list is known as the "decoy" list and 50 chemical structures were randomly sampled.

The next data set, from Wessel et al. [37] includes compounds classified by affinity for absorption through human intestinal lining. Moreover, the PTC [35] data sets were included, which contain a series of chemical compounds classified according to their toxicity in male and female rats and male and female mice.

TABLE 9.4   Data Set and Class Statistics for GPD Experiments

Data Set	No. G	No. P	No. N
CDK2 inhibitors	100	50	50
COX2 inhibitors	100	50	50
Fxa inhibitors	100	50	50
PDE5 inhibitors	100	50	50
A1A inhibitors	100	50	50
Intestinal absorption	310	148	162
Toxicity (female mice)	344	152	192
Toxicity (female rats)	336	129	207
Toxicity (male mice)	351	121	230
Toxicity (male rats)	349	143	206

The same protocol was used as in [23] to transform chemical structure data sets to graphs. Table 9.4 lists the total number of chemical compounds in each data set, as well as the number of positive and negative samples. In the table, no. G-number of samples (chemical compounds) in the data set, no. P-positive samples and no. N-negative samples

9.5.2.2 Feature Sets Frequent patterns were exclusively used from graph representations of chemicals in our study. Such frequent subgraphs were generated from a data set using two different graph mining approaches: that with exact matching [23] and that of approximate matching. In the approximate frequent subgraph mining, a pattern *matches* with a graph as long as there are up to $k > 0$ node label mismatches. For chemical structures, typical mismatch tolerance is small, that is k values are 1, 2, and so on. In the experiments, approximate graph mining with $k = 1$ was used.

Once frequent subgraphs are mined, three feature sets are generated: (1) general subgraphs (all of mined subgraphs), (2) tree subgraphs, and (3) path subgraphs. Cycles were examined as well, but were not included in this study, since typically less than two cyclic subgraphs were identified in a data set. These feature sets are used for constructing kernel functions as discussed below.

9.5.2.3 Classification Methods The performance of the following classifiers was evaluated:

CBA. The first is a classifier that uses frequent item set mining, known as CBA [14]. In CBA mined frequent subgraphs are treated as item sets.

Graph Convolution Kernels. This type of kernel include the mismatch kernel (MIS) and the min–max (MNX) kernel. The former is based on the normalized Hamming distance of two binary vectors, and the latter is computed as the ratio between two sums: The numerator is the sum of the minimum between each feature pair in two binary vectors, and the denominator is the same, except it sums the maximum. See [32] for details about the min–max kernel.

SVM Built-in Kernels. A linear kernel (Linear) and radial basis function (RBF) kernel were used.

GPD. The graph pattern diffusion kernel was implemented, as discussed in Section 9.5.1. The default parameter for the GPD kernel is a diffusion rate of $\lambda = 20\%$ and the diffusion time $\tau = 5$.

9.5.2.4 Experimental Results

Here we present the results of our graph classification experiments. One round of experiments was performed to evaluate the methods based on exact subgraph mining, and another round of experiments were with approximate subgraph mining. For both subgraph mining methods, patterns were selected that were general graphs, trees, and paths.

A simple feature selection method is applied in order to identify the most discriminating frequent patterns. Using a simple statistical formula, PCC, the correlation is measured between a set of feature samples (in our case, the occurrences of a particular subgraph in each of the data samples) and the corresponding class labels. Frequent patterns are ranked according to correlation strength, and the top 10% patterns are selected to construct the feature set.

Comparison between Classifiers. The results of the comparison of different graph kernel functions are shown in Table 9.5. For these results, frequent subgraph mining using exact matching was used. In the table that uses general subgraphs (the first 10 rows in Table 9.5), it is shown that for exact mining of general subgraphs, in 4 of the 10 data sets, the GPD method provides mean accuracy that is significantly better (at least two standard deviations above the next best method). In another, 4 data sets, GPD gives the best performance, but the difference is less significant and is still >1 standard deviation). In the last two data sets, other methods perform better, but not significantly better. The mismatch and min–max kernels all give roughly the same performance. Hence, only the results of the mismatch kernel are shown. The GPD's superiority is also confirmed in classifications where tree and path patterns are used.

Table 9.6 compares the performance of our GPD kernel to the classification based on association (CBA) method. In general it shows comparable performance to the other methods. In one data set, it does show a noticeable increase over the other methods. This is expected since CBA is designed specifically for discrete data such as the binary feature occurrences used here. Despite the strengths of CBA, the GDA method still gives the best performance for six of the seven data sets. These data sets were also tested using the recursive optimal-assignment kernel included in the JOELib2 computational chemistry library. It's results are comparable to those of the CBA method, and hence were not included here as separate results.

In addition, a classifier called XRules was tested. XRules is designed for classification of tree data [13]. Chemical graphs, while not strictly trees, often are close to trees. To run the XRules executable, a graph is transformed to a tree by randomly selecting a spanning tree of the original graph. Our experimental study shows the application of XRules on average delivers incompetent results

TABLE 9.5   Comparison of Different Graph Kernel Functions and Feature Sets in GPD Experiments, With Strict Subgraph Matching

Subgraph Type	Data Set	MIS[a]		GPD[a]		Linear[a]		RBF	
	CDK2	76.3	2.06	87.2*	2.04	76.3	2.06	77.9	1.6
	COX2	85.1*	0.99	83.2	0.79	85.1*	0.99	84.5	1.08
	FXa	87	0.94	87.6*	0.52	87	0.94	86.2	0.42
	PDE5	83.2*	0.63	82.8	1.4	83.2*	0.63	83	0.67
General	A1A	84.8	0.63	90.9*	0.74	85	0.94	88.7	1.06
	Int. abs.	49.53	4.82	56.86*	3.12	50.7	4.56	47.56	3.44
	Toxicity (FM)	51.46	3.4	54.81*	1.16	51.95	3.26	50.95	2.75
	Toxicity (FR)	52.99	4.33	56.35*	1.13	49.57	4.71	51.94	3.34
	Toxicity (MM)	49.64	3.43	60.71*	1.16	49.38	1.96	51.16	2.28
	Toxicity (MR)	50.44	3.06	56.83*	1.17	49.91	3.09	54.3	2.59
	CDK2	76.3	2.06	87.2*	2.04	76.3	2.06	77.9	1.6
	COX2	85.1*	0.99	83.2	0.79	85.1*	0.99	84.5	1.08
	FXa	87	0.94	87.6*	0.52	87	0.94	86.2	0.42
	PDE5	83.2*	0.63	82.8	1.4	83.2*	0.63	83	0.67
Trees	A1A	84.8	0.63	90.9*	0.74	85	0.94	88.7	1.06
	Int. abs.	49.53	4.82	56.86*	3.12	50.7	4.56	47.56	3.44
	Toxicity (FM)	51.46	3.4	54.81*	1.16	51.95	3.26	50.95	2.75
	Toxicity (FR)	52.99	4.33	56.35*	1.13	49.57	4.71	51.94	3.34
	Toxicity (MM)	49.64	3.43	60.71*	1.16	49.38	1.96	51.16	2.28
	Toxicity (MR)	50.44	3.06	56.83*	1.17	49.91	3.09	54.3	2.59
	CDK2	76.3	0.82	86.2*	2.82	76.4	0.97	77.1	0.74
	COX2	85*	0	83.7	0.48	85*	0	85*	0
	FXa	86.8	0.79	87.6*	0.52	86.8	0.79	86.6	0.84
	PDE5	82.6	0.84	83*	1.25	82.6	0.84	82.7	0.95
Paths	A1A	84.1	0.88	91.2*	1.14	84	0.67	85.7	0.67
	Int. abs.	49.07	7.16	54.07*	3.52	50.58	4.32	50	4.72
	Toxicity (FM)	50.14	3.41	54.79*	2.13	50.37	2.59	50.14	4.38
	Toxicity (FR)	47.83	6.85	55.93*	2.44	48.32	7.83	50.09	4.37
	Toxicity (MM)	46.85	3.57	58.81*	1.07	48.6	4.78	50.33	2.29
	Toxicity (MR)	50.26	3.13	54.71*	1.38	48.69	3.93	54.27	3.04

[a] The asterisk represents the best accuracy in the column.

among the group of classifiers (e.g., 50% accuracy on the CDK2 inhibitor data set), which may be due to the particular way a graph is transformed to a tree. Since tree patterns are computed for the rule based classifier CBA in our comparison, XRules was not explored further.

A method based on a recursive optimal assignment [10] was also tested using biologically relevant chemical descriptors labeling each node in a chemical graph. In order to perform a fair comparison with this method to the other methods, the chemical descriptors are ignored and the focus is instead on the structural alignment. In these experiments, the performance of this method is very similar to CBA. Hence, only the results of CBA are shown here.

TABLE 9.6   Comparison of GPD Kernel to CBA

Data Set	GPD[a]	CBA[a]
CDK2 inhibitors	88.6*	80.46
COX2 inhibitors	82.7*	77.86
Fxa inhibitors	89.3*	86.87
PDE5 inhibitors	81.9	87.14*
A1A inhibitors	91.4*	87.76
Intestinal absorption	63.14*	54.36
Toxicity (male rats)	56.66*	55.95

[a] The asterisk represents the best accuracy in the column.

Comparison between Descriptor Sets. Various types of subgraphs (e.g., trees, paths, and cycles) have been used in kernel functions between chemical compounds. In addition to exact mining of general subgraphs, approximate subgraph mining was also used to generate the features for our respective kernel methods. In both cases, the general subgraphs mined are filtered into sets of trees and sets of paths as well.

The results for all kernels using exact tree subgraphs are identical to those for exact general subgraphs. This is not surprising, given that most chemical fragments are structured as trees. The results using exact path subgraphs, however, do show some shifts in accuracy, but the difference is not significant. These results are not recorded here since they add no appreciable information to the evaluation of the various methods.

The results using approximate subgraph mining (shown in Table 9.7) are similar to those for exact subgraph mining (shown in Table 9.5). In contrast to the hypothesis that using approximate subgraph mining might improve the classification accuracy, the data show that there is no significant difference between the set of features. However, it is clear that GPD is still better than the competing kernel functions.

Effect of Varying GPD Diffusion Rate and Time. This section evaluates the sensitivity of the GPD methods to its two parameters: diffusion rate λ and diffusion time. Different diffusion rate λ values and diffusion time values were tested. Figure 9.8 shows that the GPD algorithm is not very sensitive to the two parameters at the range that was tested. Although only three data sets are shown in Figure 9.8, the observation is true for other data sets in the experiments.

9.5.3   Conclusions

With the rapid development of fast and sophisticated data collection methods, data has become complex, high-dimensional, and noisy. Graphs have proven to be powerful tools for modeling complex, high-dimensional, and noisy data; building highly accurate predictive models for graph data is a new challenge for the data-mining community. This work demonstrates the utility of a novel graph kernel function, graph

TABLE 9.7   Comparison of Different Graph Kernel Functions and Feature Sets in GPD Experiments, With Approximate Subgraph Matching

Subgraph Type	Data Set	MIS[a]		GPD[a]		Linear[a]		RBF[a]	
General	CDK2	76.3	2.06	85.7*	1.49	76.3	2.06	77.9	1.6
	COX2	85*	0	83	0.67	85*	0	85*	0
	FXa	86.4	0.52	87.5*	0.53	86.4	0.52	86.1	0.32
	PDE5	83.3*	0.67	83.3*	1.64	83.3*	0.67	82.9	0.74
	A1A	86.2	1.81	88.7*	0.82	86.2	1.81	88.7	0.48
	Int. abs.	51.28	4.3	60.81*	2.63	52.67	4.07	51.86	6.18
Trees	CDK2	76.3	2.06	85.7*	1.49	76.3	2.06	77.9	1.6
	COX2	85*	0	83	0.67	85*	0	85*	0
	FXa	86.4	0.52	87.5*	0.53	86.4	0.52	86.1	0.32
	PDE5	83.3*	0.67	83.3*	1.64	83.3*	0.67	82.9	0.74
	A1A	86.2	1.81	88.7*	0.82	86.2	1.81	88.7*	0.48
	Int. abs.	51.28	4.3	60.81*	2.63	52.67	4.07	51.86	6.18
Paths	CDK2	76.3	0.82	86.1*	2.13	76.4	0.97	77.1	0.74
	COX2	85*	0	83.4	0.7	85*	0	85*	0
	FXa	86	0	88*	0.82	86	0	86	0
	PDE5	83.1	0.57	83.8*	2.53	83.1	0.57	82.9	0.57
	A1A	83.6	0.7	88.6*	0.7	83.6	0.7	85.7	0.67
	Int. abs.	49.88	4.3	60.23*	4.34	51.05	3.82	49.65	3.76

[a] The asterisk represents the best accuracy in the column.

pattern diffusion kernel (GPD kernel). It is shown that the GPD kernel can capture the intrinsic similarity between two graphs and has the lowest testing error in many of the data sets evaluated. Although a very efficient computational framework was developed, computing a GPD kernel may be hard for large graphs. Future work will concentrate on improving the computational efficiency of the GPD kernel for very

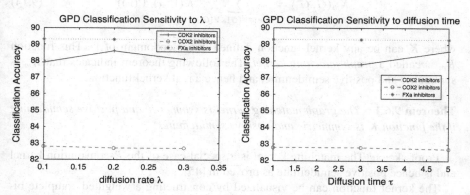

FIGURE 9.8 Effect of diffusion rate and time on GPD classification accuracy. From [8], with permission.

large graphs, as well as performing additional comparisons between this method and other two-dimensional (2D)-descriptor and QSAR-based methods.

9.6 MATCHING KERNELS WITH APPROXIMATE PATTERN-BASED FEATURES

This chapter expands on the GPD kernel presented in Chapter 8, by defining a similar kernel function that uses a matching-based set kernel instead of an alignment kernel. This method is termed a graph pattern matching (GPM) kernel. The advantage of this modification is that the GPM kernel, unlike GPD, is guaranteed to be positive semidefinite, and hence a true Mercer kernel. This algorithm was tested using 16 chemical structure data sets. The experimental results demonstrate that this method outperforms existing state-of-the-art methods with a large margin.

9.6.1 Graph Pattern Matching Kernel with Diffusion for Accurate Graph Classification

This section presents the design of a graph matching kernel with diffusion. The section begins by first presenting a general framework for graph matching. Then the pattern-based graph matching kernel is presented. Finally, a technique called "pattern diffusion" is discussed that significantly improves graph classification accuracy in practice.

9.6.1.1 Graph Matching Kernel To derive an efficient algorithm scalable to large graphs, a function $\Gamma : V \rightarrow \mathbb{R}^n$ is used to map nodes in a graph to an n-dimensional feature space that captures not only the node label information, but also the neighborhood topological information around the node. If there is such a function Γ, the following graph kernel may be defined

$$K_m(G, G') = \sum_{(u,v) \in V[G] \times V[G']} K(\Gamma(u), \Gamma(v)) \qquad (9.14)$$

where K can be any kernel function defined in the codomain of Γ. This function K_m is called a *graph matching kernel*. The following theorem indicates that K_m is symmetric and positive semidefinite, and hence a real kernel function.

Theorem 9.6.1 *The graph matching kernel is symmetric and positive semidefinite if the function K is symmetric and positive semidefinite.*

Proof sketch: The matching kernel is a special case of the R-convolution kernel and is hence positive semidefinite as proved in [45].

The kernel function can be visualized by constructing a weighted complete bipartite graph: connecting every node pair $(u,v) \in V[G] \times V[G']$ with an edge. The weight of the edge (u,v) is $K(\Gamma(v), \Gamma(v))$. Figure 9.6 shows a weighted complete bipartite graph for $V[G] = \{v_1, v_2, v_3\}$ and $V[G'] = \{u_1, u_2, u_3\}$. Highlighted edges $(v1, u2), (v2, u1), (v3, u3)$ have larger weights than the rest of the edges (dashed).

We can see from the figure that if two nodes are quite dissimilar, the weight of the related edge is small. Since dissimilar node pairs usually outnumber similar node pairs, if a linear kernel is used for nodes, the kernel function may be noisy, and hence lose the signal. In this design, the RBF kernel function is used, as specified below, to penalize dissimilar node pairs.

$$K(X, Y) = e^{\frac{-\|X-Y\|_2^2}{2}} \tag{9.15}$$

where $\|X\|_2^2$ is the squared L_2 norm of a vector X.

9.6.1.2 Graph Pattern Matching Kernel One way to design the function Γ is to take advantage of frequent patterns mined from a set of graphs. Intuitively, if a node belongs to a subgraph F, there is some information about the local topology of the node. Following the intuition, given a node v in a graph G and a frequent subgraph F, a function Γ_F is designed such that

$$\Gamma_F(v) = \begin{cases} 1 & \text{if } u \text{ belongs an embedding of } F \text{ in } G \\ 0 & \text{otherwise} \end{cases}$$

The function Γ_F is called a "pattern membership function" since this function tests whether a node occurs in a specific subgraph feature (membership to a subgraph).

Given a set of frequent subgraphs $\mathcal{F} = F_1, F_2, \ldots, F_n$, each membership function is treated as a dimension and the function $\Gamma_{\mathcal{F}}$ is defined as

$$\Gamma_{\mathcal{F}}(v) = (\Gamma_{F_i}(v))_i^n \tag{9.16}$$

In other words, given an n frequent subgraph, the function Γ maps a node v in G to an n-dimensional space, indexed by the n subgraphs, where values of the features indicate whether the node is part of the related subgraph in G.

Example 9.2   Figure 9.9, shown that two subgraph features, F_1 and F_2, where F_1 is embedded in Q at $\{q_1, q_2\}$ and F_2 occurs in Q at $\{q_1, q_3\}$. The occurrences are depicted using shadings with different color and orientations. For node q_1, a subgraph F_1 is considered as a feature, and $\Gamma_{F_1}(q_1) = 1$ since q_1 is part of an embedding of F_1 in Q. Also, $\Gamma_{F_1}(q_3) = 0$ since q_3 is not part of an embedding of F_1 in Q. Similarly, $\Gamma_{F_2}(q_1) = 1$ and $\Gamma_{F_2}(q_3) = 1$. Hence, $\Gamma_{F_1,F_2}(q_1) = (1, 1)$ and $\Gamma_{F_1,F_2}(q_3) = (0, 1)$. The values of the function Γ_{F_1,F_2} are also illustrated in the same figure using the annotated Q.

9.6.1.3 Graph Pattern Matching Kernel with Pattern Diffusion This section introduces a better technique than the pattern membership function to capture the local

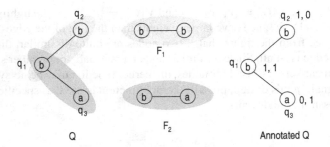

FIGURE 9.9 Example pattern membership functions for GPM kernel. From [9], with permission.

topology information of nodes. This technique is called "pattern diffusion". The design here has the following advantages:

It is generic and does not assume any domain knowledge from a specific application. The diffusion process may be applied to graphs with dramatically different characteristics.

The diffusion process is straightforward to implement and can be computed efficiently.

It is proof that the diffusion process is related to the probability distribution of a graph random walk. This explains why the simple process may be used to summarize local topological information.

Below, the pattern diffusion kernel is outlined in three steps.

In the first step, a seed is identified as a starting point for the diffusion. In this design, a "seed" could be a single node, or a set of connected nodes in the original graph. In the experimental study, frequent subgraphs are always used for seeds since a seed from one graph can be easily compared to a seed in another graph.

In the second step, given a set of nodes S as seed, a diffusion function f_t is recursively defined in the following way:

The base f_0 is defined as

$$f_0(u) = \begin{cases} 1/|S| & \text{if } u \in S \\ 0 & \text{otherwise} \end{cases}$$

Define f_{t+1} ($t \geq 0$) with f_t in the following way:

$$f_{t+1}(v) = f_t(v) \times (1 - \frac{\lambda}{d(v)}) + \sum_{u \in N(v)} f_t(u) \times \frac{\lambda}{d(u)} \tag{9.17}$$

In the notation, $N(v) = \{u | (u, v) \text{ is an edge}\}$ is the set of nodes that connects to v directly and $d(v) = |N(v)|$ is the node degree of v. The parameter λ controls the diffusion rate.

Equation (9.17) describes a process where each node distributes a λ fraction of its value to its neighbors evenly and in the same way receives some value from its neighbors. It is called "diffusion" because the process simulates the way a value is spreading in a network. The intuition is that the distribution of such a value encodes information about the local topology of the network.

To constrain the diffusion process to a local region, one parameter called diffusion time, denoted by τ, is used to control the diffusion process. Specifically, the diffusion process is limited to a local region of the original graph with nodes that are at most τ hops away from a node in the seed S. In this sense, the diffusion should be named "local diffusion".

Finally, in the last step for the seed S, define the mapping function Γ_S^d as the limit function of f_t as t approaches to infinity, or

$$\Gamma_S^d = \lim_{t \to \infty} f_t \qquad (9.18)$$

And given a set of frequent subgraph $\mathcal{F} = F_1, F_2, \ldots, F_n$ as seeds, define the pattern diffusion function $\Gamma_{\mathcal{F}}^d$ as

$$\Gamma_{\mathcal{F}}^d(v) = (\Gamma_{F_i}^d(v))_i^n \qquad (9.19)$$

9.6.1.4 Connections of Other Graph Kernels

Connection to Marginalized Kernels. Here the connection of pattern matching kernel function to the marginalized graph kernel [28] is shown, which uses a Markov model to randomly generate walks of a labeled graph.

Given a graph G with nodes set $V[G] = \{v_1, v_2, \ldots, v_n\}$, and a seed $S \subseteq V[G]$, for each diffusion function f_t, construct a vector $U_t = (f_t(v_1), f_t(v_2), \ldots, f_t(v_n))$. According to the definition of f_t, $U_{t+1} = M \times U_t$, where the matrix M is defined as

$$M(i, j) = \begin{cases} \frac{\lambda}{d(v_j)} & \text{if } i \neq j \text{ and } i \in N(j) \\ 1 - \frac{\lambda}{d(v_i)} & i = j \\ 0 & \text{otherwise} \end{cases}$$

In this representation, compute the stationary distribution ($f_S = \lim_{t \to \infty} f_t$) by computing $M^\infty \times U_0$.

Note that the matrix M corresponds to a probability matrix corresponding to a Markov chain since

- All entries are non-negative.
- Column sum is 1 for each column.

Therefore the vector $M^\infty \times U_0$ corresponds to the stationary distribution of the local random walk as specified by M. In other words, rather than using random walk to retrieve information about the local topology of a graph, the stationary distribution is used to retrieve information about the local topology.

The experimental study shows that this in fact is an efficient method of graph classification.

Connection to Optimal Assignment Kernel. The optimal assignment (OA) kernel [34] carries the same spirit of the graph pattern matching kernel in that OA uses pairwise node kernel function to construct a graph kernel function. The OA kernel has been utilized for cheminformatics applications and is found to deliver good results empirically.

There are two major differences between GPM and the OA kernel. (1) The OA kernel is not positive semidefinite, and hence is not a Mercer kernel in a strict sense. Non-Mercer kernel functions are used to train SVM models and the problem is that the convex optimizer utilized in SVM will not converge to a global optimal and hence the performance of the SVM training may not be reliable. (2) The OA utilizes a complicated recursive function to compute the similarity between nodes, which make the computation of the kernel function run slowly for large graphs [10].

9.6.1.5 Pattern Diffusion Kernel and Graph Classification This section summarizes the discussions presented so far and shows how the kernel function is utilized to construct an efficient graph classification algorithm in both the training and testing phases.

Training Phase. In the training phase, graphs of the training data set $D = \{(G_i, T_i,)\}_{i=1}^n$ are divided into groups according to their class labels. For example in binary classification there are two groups of graphs: positive or negative. For multiclass classification, graphs are partitioned according to their class label, where graphs having the same class labels are grouped together. The training phase is composed of four steps:

1. Obtain frequent subgraphs. Identify frequent subgraphs from each graph group and union the subgraph sets together as the seed set $\mathcal{F}$.
2. For each graph G in the training data set, use the node pattern diffusion function $\Gamma_{\mathcal{F}}^d$ to label nodes in G. Thus the feature vector of a node v is a vector $L_V = (\Gamma_{F_i}^d(v))_{i=1}^m$ with length $m = |\mathcal{F}|$.
3. For two graphs G, G', construct the complete weighted bipartite graph as described in Section 9.6.1.1 and compute the kernel $K_m(G, G')$ using Eqs. (9.14) and (9.15).
4. Train a predictive model using a kernel classifier.

Testing Phase. In the testing phase, the kernel function is computed for graphs in the testing and training data sets. The trained model is used to make predictions about graph in the testing set.

- For each graph G in the testing data set, use $\Gamma_{\mathcal{F}}^d$ to label nodes in G and create feature vectors as in the training phase.
- Use Eqs. (9.14) and (9.15) to compute the kernel function $K_m(G, G')$ for each graph G in the testing data set and for each graph G' in the training data set.
- Use kernel classifier and trained models to obtain prediction accuracy of the testing data set

9.6.2 Experimental Study

Classification experiments were conducted using six different graph kernel functions, including the pattern diffusion kernel, on 16 different data sets. There are 12 chemical–protein binding data sets, and the rest are chemical toxicity data sets. All of the experiments were performed on a desktop computer with a 3-GHz Pertium 4 processor and 1 GB of RAM. The following sections describe the data sets and the classification methods in more detail along with the associated results.

In all classification experiments, the LibSVM [44] was used as kernel classifier. The nu-SVC was used with default parameter $\nu = 0.5$. The classification accuracy (TP+TN/S, TP: true positive, TN: true negative, S: total number of testing samples) is computed by averaging over a 10-fold cross-validation experiment. Standard deviation is computed similarly. To have a fair comparison, default SVM parameters were used in all cases, and were not tuned to increase the accuracy of any method.

9.6.2.1 Data Sets Sixteen data sets were selected, covering prediction of chemical–protein binding activity and chemical toxicity. The first seven data sets are manually extracted from the BindindDB database [45]. The next five are established data sets taken from Jorissen and Gilson [38]. The last four are from the predictive toxicology challenge [35] (PTC). Detailed information for the data sets is available in Table 9.8 where no. G-number of samples (chemical compounds) in the data set, no. P-positive samples, and no. N-negative samples .

BindingDB Sets. The BindingDB database contains >450 proteins. For each protein, the database record chemicals that bind to the protein. Two types of activity measurements K_i and IC_{50} are provided. Both measurements measure

TABLE 9.8   Characteristics of Data Sets in GPM Experiments

Source	Data Set	No. G	No. P	No. N
	AChE	138	69	69
	ALF	93	47	46
	EGF–R	377	190	187
BindingDB	HIV–P	202	101	101
	HIV–RT	365	183	182
	HSP90	82	41	41
	MAPK	255	126	129
	CDK2	100	50	50
	COX2	100	50	50
Jorissen	FXa	100	50	50
	PDE5	100	50	50
	A1A	100	50	50
Predictive	PTC–FM	344	152	192
Toxicology	PTC–FR	336	129	207
Challenge	PTC–MM	351	121	230
	PTC-MR	349	143	206

inhibition–dissociation rates between a proteins and chemicals. From BindingDB, 7 proteins were manually selected with a wide range of known interacting chemicals (ranging from tens to several hundreds). These data sets are AChE, ALF, EGF-R, HIV-P, HIV-RT, HSP90, and MAPK.

Jorissen Sets. The Jorissen data sets also contains information about chemical–protein binding activity. In this case, the provider of the data set carefully selected positive and negative samples, and hence is more reliable than the data sets created from BindingDB. For more information about the creation of the data sets, see [38] in details. The data sets from this study are CDK2, COX2, FXa, PDE5, and A1A.

PTC Sets. The PTC data sets contain a series of chemical compounds classified according to their toxicity in male and female rats and male and female mice. While chemical–protein binding activity is an important type of chemical activity, it is not the only type. Toxicity is another important, though different, kind of chemical activity necessary to predict in drug design. These data sets (PTC–FR/FM/MR/MM) are well curated and highly reliable.

9.6.2.2 Kernel Functions

Six different kernel functions were selected for evaluation: marginalized [28], spectrum [24], tanimoto [26], subtree [33], optimal assignment [34], together with the graph pattern matching kernel.

Four kernel functions (marginalized, spectrum, tanimoto, and subtree) are computed using the open source Chemcpp v1.0.2 package [47]. The optimal assignment kernel was computed using the JOELib2 package, and is not strictly a kernel function, but still provides good prediction accuracy. The graph pattern matching kernel was computed using MATLAB code.

9.6.2.3 Experimental Results

Comparison between Kernel Functions. This section presents the results of our graph classification experiments with various kernel functions. Figure 9.10 shows the classification accuracy for different kernel functions and data sets, averaged over a 10-fold cross-validation experiment. The standard deviations (omitted) of the accuracies are generally very high, from 5–10%, so statistically significant differences between kernel functions are generally not observed.

The data shows that the GPM method is competitive for all 16 data sets. If the accuracy of each kernel function averaged over all data sets is examined, the GPM kernel performs the best overall. Again, the standard deviations are high so the differences between the top performing kernels are not statistically significant. Still, with 16 different data sets some trends are clear: GPM kernel delivers the highest classification accuracy in 8 out of the 16 data sets, with tanimoto kernel best in 4, marginalized best in 2, subtree in 2, optimal assignment in 1, and spectrum in none.

Although GPM does not work well on a few data sets (e.g., AChE, HIV–RT, MAPK, and PTC–FR/MR), overall it performs better when compared to any other

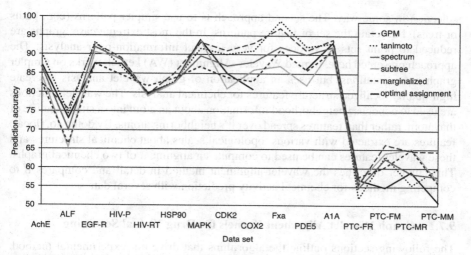

FIGURE 9.10   Average accuracy for kernel functions and data sets in GPM experiments. From [9], with permission.

kernels for a majority of data sets. It is better than every other kernel function in at least 10 of the 16 data sets.

In general the GPM, spectrum and tanimoto kernels perform the best, with an overall average accuracy of ~80%. The subtree, optimal assignment, and marginalized also perform very good, in the mid to high 70%. The min–max tanimoto kernel performed much worse than the other methods, and hence were not included in the figure. Note that the optimal assignment kernel is missing a prediction accuracy for the FXa data set, which was due to a terminal error in the JOELib2 software used to calculate this kernel on this data set.

9.6.3   Conclusions

Graphs have proven to be powerful tools for modeling complex and high-dimensional biological data; building highly accurate predictive models for chemical graph classification is a goal for cheminformatics and drug design. This work demonstrates the utility of a novel graph kernel function, graph pattern matching kernel (GPM kernel). It is shown that the GPM kernel can capture the intrinsic connection between a chemical and its class label and has the lowest testing error in a majority of the data sets we evaluated.

9.7   GRAPH WAVELETS FOR TOPOLOGY COMPARISON

Previous kernels such as the alignment kernel or other substructure-based kernels attempt to mitigate the high-dimensionality of graphs in different ways. The first possibility is to use complex patterns (e.g., general subgraphs), but restrict pattern selection in some way. The second approach is to use simpler patterns (e.g., paths or trees), but retain the set of feature patterns. In the most extreme case, graphs are reduced to point sets of vertices for very fast but information-poor analysis. The approach presented here, termed Wavelet–Alignment (WA) kernel, works on simpler graph representations, but uses an application of graph wavelet analysis to create high-quality localized structure features for chemical analysis. The wavelet functions are used to condense neighborhood information about an atom into a single feature of that atom, rather than features spread over it's neighboring atoms. By doing so, (local) features are extracted with various topological scales about chemical structures and these wavelet features can be used to compute an alignment of two chemical graphs. This chapter describes the wavelet-alignment method in detail and compares it to competing methods for chemical activity prediction with several data sets.

9.7.1 Graph Wavelet Alignment Kernels for Drug Virtual Screening

The following sections outline the algorithms that drive our experimental method. This method measures the similarity of graph structures whose nodes and edges have been labeled with various features. These features represent different kinds of chemical structure information including atoms and chemical bond types, among others. To compute the similarity of two graphs, the nodes of one graph are aligned with the nodes of the second graph, such that the total overall similarity is maximized with respect to all possible alignments. Vertex similarity is measured by comparing vertex descriptors, and is computed recursively so that when comparing two nodes, the immediate neighbors of those nodes are also compared, and the neighbors of those neighbors, and so on.

9.7.1.1 Graph Alignment Kernel An *alignment* of two graphs G and G' (assuming $|V[G]| \leq |V[G']|$) is a 1-1 mapping $\pi : V[G] \to V[G']$. Given an alignment π, define the similarity between two graphs, as measured by a kernel function k_A, below:

$$k_A(G, G') := \max_\pi \sum_{v \in V[G]} k_n(v, \pi(v)) + \sum_{u,v} k_e((u, v), (\pi(u), \pi(v))) \quad (9.20)$$

The function k_n is a kernel function to measure the similarity of nodes and the function k_e is a kernel function to measure the similarity of edges. Intuitively, Eq. (9.20) uses an additive model to compute the similarity between two graphs by computing the sum of the similarity of nodes and the similarity of edges. The maximal similarity among all possible alignments is defined as the similarity between two graphs.

9.7.1.2 Simplified Graph Alignment Kernel A direct computation of the graph alignment kernel is computationally intensive and is unlikely scalable to large graphs. With no surprise, the graph alignment kernel computation is no easier than the subgraph isomorphism problem, a known NP-hard problem. (Formally, showing a reduction from the graph alignment kernel to the subgraph isomorphism problem is needed. The details of such reduction are omitted due to their loose connection to

the main theme of the current paper, which is an advanced data-mining approach, as applied to cheminformatics applications.) To derive efficient algorithms scalable to large graphs, the graph kernel function is simplified with the following formula:

$$k_M(G, G') = \max_{\pi} \sum_{v \in V[G]} k_a(f(v), f(\pi(v))) \qquad (9.21)$$

Where $\pi : V[G] \to V[G']$ denotes an alignment of graph G and G'. The parameter $f(v)$ is a set of features associated with a node that not only include node features, but also include information about topology of the graph where v belongs.

Equation (9.21), computes a maximal weighted bipartite graph, which has an efficient solution known as the Hungarian algorithm. The complexity of the algorithm is $O(|V[G]|^3)$. See [34] for further details.

Provided below is an efficient method, based on graph wavelet analysis, to create features to capture the topological structure of a graph.

9.7.1.3 Graph Wavelet Analysis
Originally proposed to analyze time series signals, wavelet analysis transforms a series of signals to a set of summaries with different scale. Two of the key insights of wavelet analysis of signals are (1) using localized basis functions and (2) analysis with different scales. Wavelet analysis offers efficient tools to decompose and represent a function with arbitrary shape [47, 48]. Since invented, wavelet analysis has quickly gained popularity in a wide range of applications outside time series data, (e.g., image analysis and geography data analysis). In all these applications, the level of detail, or *scale*, is considered as an important factor in data comparison and compression. Figure 9.11 shows two examples of wavelet functions in a 3D space, the Haar and Mexican Hat.

> *Intuition.* With wavelet analysis, as applied to graph representations of chemical structure features about each atom and its local environment are collected at different scales. For example, information can be collected about the average charge of an atom and it's surrounding atoms, then assign the average value

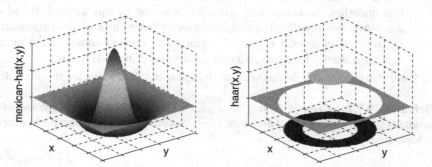

FIGURE 9.11 Two wavelet functions in three dimensions (3 Ds), Mexican hat and Haar. From [10], with permission.

as a feature to the atom. Information can also be collected about whether an atom belongs to a nearby functional group, whether the surrounding atoms of a particular atom belong to a nearby functional group, and the local topology of an atom to its nearby functional groups.

In summary, conceptually the following two types of insights are gained about the chemicals after applying wavelet analysis to graph represented chemical structure:

1. *Analysis With Varying Levels of Scale.* Intuitively, at the finest level, two chemical structures are compared by matching the atoms and chemical bonds in the two structures. At the next level, comparison of two regions is performed (e.g., chemical functional groups). At an even coarser level, small regions may be grouped into larger ones (e.g., pharmacophore), and two chemicals are compared by matching the large regions and the connections among large regions.

2. *Nonlocal Connection.* In a chemical structure, two atoms that are not directly connected by a chemical bond may still have some kind of interaction. Therefore when comparing two graphs, their vertices cannot depend only on the *local environment* immediately surrounding an atom, but rather must consider both the local and nonlocal environment.

Though conceptually appealing, current wavelet analysis is often limited to numerical data with regular structures (e.g., matrices and images). Graphs, however, are arbitrarily structured and may represent innumerable relationships and topologies between data elements. In order to define a reasonable graph wavelet function, the following two important concepts are introduced (1) h-hop neighborhood and (2) discrete wavelet functions.

The former (h-hop neighborhood) is essentially used to project graphs from a high-dimensional space with arbitrary topology into a Euclidean space suitable for operation with wavelets. The h-hop measure defines a distance metric between vertices that is based on the shortest path between them. The discrete wavelet function then operates on a graph projection in the h-hop Euclidean space to compactly represent the information about the local topology of a graph. It is the use of this compact wavelet representation in vertex comparison that underlies the complexity reduction achieved by this method. Based on the h-hop neighborhood, a discrete wavelet function is used to summarize information in a local region of a graph and create features based on the summarization. These two concepts are discussed in detail below.

h-hop Neighborhood. In this section, the following definitions are introduced.

Definition 9.7.1   *Given a node v in a graph G the h-**hope neighborhood** of v, denoted by $N_h(v)$, is the set of nodes that are (according to the shortest path) exactly h-hops away from v.*

For example if $h = 0$, then $N_0(v) = v$ and if $h = 1$, then $N_1(v) = \{u | (u, v) \in E[G]\}$.

Here, f_v denotes the feature vector associated with a node v in a graph G. The parameter $|f|$ is the feature vector length (number of features in the feature vector). The average feature measurement, denoted by $\overline{f}_j(v)$ for nodes in $N_j(v)$, is

$$\overline{f}_j(v) = \frac{1}{|N_j(v)|} \sum_{u \in N_j(v)} f_u \qquad (9.22)$$

Example 9.3   Figure 9.5(*a*) shows a chemical graph. Given a node v in the graph G, label the shortest distance of nodes to v in G. In this case, $N_0(v) = v$ and $N_1(v) = \{t, u\}$. If the feature vector contains a single feature of atomic number, $\overline{f}_1(v)$ is the average atomic number of atoms that are at most 1-hop away from v. In this case, since $N_1(v) = \{t, u\}$ and $\{t, u\}$ are both carbon with an atomic number equal to eight, then $\overline{f}_1(v)$ is equal to eight as well.

Discrete Wavelet Functions.   In order to adapt a wavelet function to a discrete structure (e.g., graphs), a wavelet function $\psi(x)$ must be applied to the h-hop neighborhood. Toward that end, a wavelet function $\psi(x)$ (e.g., the Haar or Mexican Hat) can be scaled to have support on the domain $[0, 1)$, with integral 0, and partition the function into $h + 1$ intervals. Then, compute the average, $\psi_{j,h}$, as the average of $\psi(x)$ over the jth interval, $0 \leq j \leq h$ as

$$\psi_{j,h} \equiv \frac{1}{h+1} \int_{j/(h+1)}^{(j+1)/(h+1)} \psi(x)dx \qquad (9.23)$$

With neighborhood and discrete wavelet functions, wavelet analysis can be applied to graphs. This analysis is called *wavelet measurements*, denoted by $\Gamma_h(v)$, for a node v in a graph G at scale up to $h > 0$.

$$\Gamma_h(v) = C_{h,v} * \sum_{j=0}^{h} \psi_{j,h} * \overline{f}_j(v) \qquad (9.24)$$

where $C_{h,v}$ is a normalization factor with $C(h, v) = (\sum_{j=0}^{h} \frac{\psi_{j,h}^2}{|N_k(v)|})^{-1/2}$

Define $\Gamma^h(v)$ as the sequence of wavelet measurements as applied to a node v with scale value up to h. That is $\Gamma^h(v) = \{\Gamma_1(v), \Gamma_2(v), \ldots, \Gamma_h(v)\}$. Call $\Gamma^h(v)$ the *wavelet measurement vector* of node v. Finally insert the wavelet measurement vector into the alignment kernel with the following formula:

$$k_\Gamma(G, G') = \max_\pi \sum_{v \in V[G]} k_a(\Gamma^h(v), \Gamma^h(\pi(v))) \qquad (9.25)$$

where $k_a(\Gamma^h(v), \Gamma^h(\pi(v)))$ is a kernel function defined on vectors. Two popular choices are linear kernel and radius-based function kernel.

Example 9.4   Figure 9.5(*b*) shows a chemical graph overlayed with a wavelet function centered on a specific vertex. It is clear how the wavelet is most intense at the central vertex, hop distance of zero, corresponding to a strongly positive region of the wavelet function. As the hop distance increases, the wavelet function becomes strongly negative, roughly at hop distances of one and two. At hop distance >2, the wavelet function returns to zero intensity, indicating negligible contribution from vertices at this distance.

9.7.2   Experimental Study

Classification experiments were conducted on five different biological activity data sets, and measured SVM classifier prediction accuracy for several different feature generation methods. The following sections describe the data sets and classification methods in more detail, along with the associated results.

We performed all experiments on a desktop computer with a 3-GHz Pertium 4 processor and 1 GB of RAM.

9.7.2.1 *Data Sets*   Five data sets were selected to represent typical chemical benchmarks in drug design to evaluate the classifier performance. The PTC data set, discussed by Helma et al. [35], contains a set of chemical compounds classified according to their toxicity in male rats (PTC–MR), female rats (PTC–FR), male mice (PTC–MM), and female mice (PTC–FM). The human intestinal absorption (HIA) data set (Wessel et al. [36]) contains chemical compounds classified by intestinal absorption activity. The remaining data set (MD) is from Patterson et al. [40], and was used to validate certain molecule descriptors. Various statistics for these data sets can be found in Table 9.9.

All of these data sets exist natively as binary classification problems, therefore in the case of the MD and HIA data sets, some preprocessing is required to transform them into regression and multiclass problems. For regression, this is a straightforward process of using the compound activity directly as the regression target. In the case of multiclass problems, the transformation is not as direct. A histogram of compound activity values was chosen to visualize which areas of the activity space are more dense, allowing natural and intuitive placement of class separation thresholds.

9.7.2.2 *Methods*   The performance of the SVM classifier trained with different methods was evaluated. The first two methods (WA–linear, WA–RBF) are both computed using the wavelet-alignment kernel, but use different functions for computing atom–atom similarity; both a linear and RBF function were tested here. Different hop distance thresholds were evaluated and fixed to $h = 3$ in all experiments.

The method OA consists of the similarity values computed by the optimal assignment kernel, as proposed by Frölich et al. [34]. There are several reasons that we consider OA as the current state-of-the-art graph-based chemical structure classification method. First, the OA method is developed specifically for chemical graph classification. Second the OA method contains a large library to compute different features for chemical structures. Third, the OA method has developed a sophisticated

TABLE 9.9   Data Set and Class Statistics for WA Experiments

Data Set	No. Graphs	Class	Labels	Count
		Regression	0–100	86
		Binary	0	39
			1	47
HIA	86	Multiclass	1	21
			2	18
			3	21
			4	26
		Regression	0–7000	310
		Binary	0	162
			1	148
MD	310	Multiclass	1	46
			2	32
			3	37
			4	35
PTC–MR	344	Binary	0	192
			1	152
PTC–MM	336	Binary	0	207
			1	129
PTC–FR	351	Binary	0	230
			1	121
PTC–FM	349	Binary	0	206
			1	143

kernel function to compute the similarity between two chemical structures. The experimental study shows that the wavelet analysis obtains performance profiles comparable to, and sometimes exceeding that of the existing state-of-the-art chemical classification approaches. In addition, a significant computation time reduction was achieved by using the wavelet analysis. The details of the experimental study are shown below.

In these experiments, the SVM classifier was used in order to generate activity predictions. The LibSVM classifier was used, as implemented by Chang et al. [43] and included in the Weka data-mining software package by Witten et al. [42]. The SVM parameters were fixed across all methods, and we use a linear kernel. For (binary) classification, nu-SVC was used for multiclass classification with nu = 0.5. The Haar wavelet function was used in the WA experiments. Classifier performance was averaged over a 10-fold cross-validation set.

Most of the algorithms were developed and tested under the MATLAB programming environment. The OA software was provided by [34] as part of their JOELib software, a computational chemistry library implemented in java [23]

9.7.2.3 Results Below are results of the experimental study of the wavelet-alignment kernel with two focuses: (1) classification accuracy and (2) computational efficiency.

TABLE 9.10   Prediction Results of Cross-Validation Trials for WA Experiments

Data Set	Labels	OA[a]	WA–RBF[a]	WA–linear[a]
HIA	Real	979.82(32.48)*	989.72(33.60)	989.31(24.62)
	Binary	51.86(3.73)	61.39(2.77)*	57.67(3.54)
	Multiclass	29.30(2.23)	39.06(0.63)*	29.76(5.73)
MD	Real	3436395(1280)	3436214(1209)*	3440415(1510)
	Binary	67.16(0.86)*	52.51(3.34)	65.41(0.42)
	Multiclass	39.54(1.65)*	33.35(3.83)	33.93(1.87)
PTC–FM	Binary	58.56(1.53)*	51.46(3.45)	55.81(1.31)
PTC–FR	Binary	58.57(2.11)	52.87(2.65)	59.31(1.95)*
PTC–MM	Binary	58.23(1.25)	52.36(0.93)	58.91(2.078)*
PTC–MR	Binary	51.51(1.20)	52.38(3.48)	52.09(2.61)*

[a] The asterisk represents the best accuracy in the column.

9.7.2.4 Classification Accuracy Table 9.10 reports the average and standard deviation of the prediction results over 10 trials. The best results are marked with an asterisk. For classification problems, results are in prediction accuracy, and for regression problems they are in mean-squared-error (MSE) per sample. From the table, observe that for the HIA data set, WA–RBF kernel significantly outperforms OA for both binary and multiclass classification. For the MD data set, OA does best for both classification sets, but WA–linear is best for regression. For the PTC binary data, the WA–linear method outperforms the others in three of the four sets.

9.7.2.5 Computational Efficiency In Table 9.11, the kernel computation time for both OA and WA methods was documented using six different data sets. The runtime advantage of the WA algorithm over OA is clear, showing improved computation efficiency by factors of >10-fold for the WA–linear kernel and over fivefold for the WA–RBF kernel.

Figure 9.12 shows the kernel computation time across a range of data set sizes, with chemical compounds sampled from the HIA data set. Using simple random sampling with replacement, data sets were created sized from 50 to 500. The OA method was not run on even larger data sets since the experimental results clearly demonstrate the efficiency of the WA kernel already.

What these run time results do not demonstrate is the *even greater* computational efficiency afforded by the WA algorithm when operating on general, non-chemical graph data. Chemical graphs have some restrictions on their general structure, specifically, the number of atom neighbors is bound by a small constant (4 or so). Since the OA computation time is much more dependent on the number of neighbors, WA is even more advantageous in these circumstances. Unfortunately, since the OA software is designed as part of the JOELib cheminformatics library specifically for use with chemical graphs, it will not accept generalized graphs as input, and hence this aspect of the algorithm could not be empirically demonstrated

TABLE 9.11   Running Time Results for WA Experiments

Data Set	Kernel	Time	Speedup
HIA	OA	75.87	
	WA–RBF	13.76	5.51
	WA–linear	4.91	15.45
MD	OA	350.58	
	WA–RBF	50.85	6.89
	WA–linear	26.82	13.07
PTC–FM	OA	633.13	
	WA–RBF	103.95	6.09
	WA–linear	44.87	14.11
PTC–FR	OA	665.95	
	WA–RBF	116.89	5.68
	WA–linear	54.64	12.17
PTC–MM	OA	550.41	
	WA–RBF	99.39	5.53
	WA–linear	47.51	11.57
PTC–MR	OA	586.12	
	WA–RBF	101.68	5.80
	WA–linear	45.93	12.73

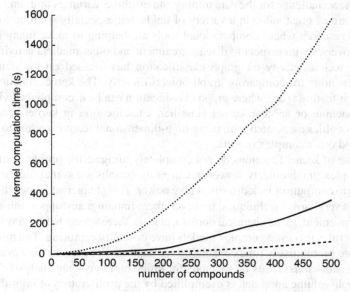

FIGURE 9.12 Comparison of computation times between methods for WA experiments. From [10], with permission.

9.7.3 Conclusions

Graph structures are a powerful and expressive representation for chemical compounds. This work presents a new method *wavelet-assignment*, for computing the similarity of chemical compounds, based on the use of an optimal assignment graph kernel function augmented with pattern and wavelet-based descriptors. The experimental study demonstrates that this wavelet-based method delivers an improved classification model, along with an order of magnitude speedup in kernel computation time. For high-volume, real-world data sets, this algorithm is able to handle a much greater number of graph objects, demonstrating it's potential for processing both chemical and non-chemical data in large amounts. In the present study, only a limited number of atom features are used. In the future, domain experts can be involved to evaluate the performance of these algorithms, including the prediction accuracy and the capability for identifying important features in diverse chemical structure data sets.

9.8 CONCLUSIONS

Graph structures are a powerful and expressive representation for many kinds of data. With the rapid development of fast and sophisticated data collection methods, data has become complex, high-dimensional, and noisy. Graphs have proven to be powerful tools for modeling such data. Building highly accurate predictive models for graph data is a new challenge for the data mining and machine learning communities. These methods are of great value in a variety of fields, but especially so in biological and chemical research where computational tools are helping to make many important new discoveries with respect to disease treatment and other medical activities.

Much recent activity on graph classification has focused on the definition of kernel functions for comparing graph objects directly. The kernel function defines an implicit feature space where graph classification can be accomplished via support vector machine or another kernel classifier. Classification in kernel space avoids many difficulties associated with using high-dimensional feature vectors to represent graphs and other complex objects.

The use of kernel functions do not completely mitigate the problems of working with complex graph objects, however. Currently established kernel functions are either slow to compute or lack discriminative power. This chapter addresses these issues through several novel techniques, however, there remain many opportunities for further improvement. In the chemical domain, at least, there appear to be many high-level structural rules that even complex models have difficulty capturing. The most precise models are prohibitively time consuming for databases of the size now available.

Future work *must* focus on methods for efficient, large-scale analysis. The value of this high-volume approach is exemplified by the proliferation of high-throughput screening technology, which has drastically accelerated the analysis of chemicals and biological molecules. The ability to accurately and quickly analyze databases in the millions of compounds using only computer models offers unprecedented opportunities for learning about biological systems.

Ultimately, the result of improved computer models is a better understanding and control of complex phenomena. Biological systems, though an important beneficiaries of such models, are only a single area of potential application. Graphs are fundamental to our general understanding of many concepts. Therefore, only by fully understanding graphs can these concepts themselves be fully modeled and understood.

REFERENCES

1. N. Tolliday, P. A. Clemons, P. Ferraiolo, A. N. Koehler, T. A. Lewis, X. Li, S. L. Schreiber, D. S. Gerhard, and S. Eliasof (2006), Small molecules, big players: the national cancer institute's initiative for chemical genetics. *Cancer Res.*, 66:8935–8935.

2. C. P. Austin, L. S. Brady, T. R. Insel, and F. S. Collins (2004), Nih molecular libraries initiative. *Science*, 306(5699):1138–1139.

3. Y. Xue, H. Li, C. Y. Ung, C. W. Yap, and Y. Z. Chen (2006), Classification of a diverse set of tetrahymena pyriformis toxicity chemical compounds from molecular descriptors by statistical learning methods. *Chem. Res. Toxicol.*, 19 (8).

4. R. Put, Q. S. Xu, D. L. Massart, and Y. V. Heyden (2004), Multivariate adaptive regression splines (mars) in chromatographic quantitative structure-retention relationship studies. *J Chromatogr A.*, 1055(1–2).

5. V. Svetnik, A. Liaw, C. Tong, J. C. Culberson, R. P. Sheridan, and B. P. Feuston (2003), Random forest: A classification and regression tool for compound classification and qsar modeling. *J. Chem. Information Computer Sci.*, 43,

6. D. Haussler (1999), Convolution kernels on discrete structures. *Technical Report UCSC-CRL099-10, Computer Science Department, UC Santa Cruz.*

7. A. Smalter, J. Huan, and G. Lushington (2008), Structure-based pattern mining for chemical compound classification. *Proceedings of the 6th Asia Pacific Bioinformatics Conference,* Kyato, Japan.

8. A. Smalter, J. Huan, and G. Lushington (2008), Gpd: A graph pattern diffusion kernel for accurate graph classification. *Proceedings of the 8th International Workshop on Data Mining in Bioinformatics,* Las Vegas, NE.

9. A. Smalter, J. Huan, and G. Lushington (2008), Gpm: A graph pattern matching kernel with diffusion for accurate graph classification. *Proceedings of the 8th IEEE International Conference on BioInformatics and BioEngineering,* Athens, Greece.

10. A. Smalter, J. Huan, and G. Lushington (2009), Graph wavelet alignment kernels for drug virtual screening. *J. Bioinformatics Computational Bio.*, 7:473–497.

11. M. Crovella and E. Kolaczyk (2003), Graph wavelets for spatial traffic analysis. *Infocom,* 3:1848–1857.

12. M. Maggioni, J. Bremer, Jr, R. Coifman, and A. Szlam (2005), Biorthogonal diffusion wavelets for multiscale representations on manifolds and graphs. *Proc. SPIE Wavelet XI,* Vol. 5914.

13. M. J. Zaki and C. C. Aggarwal (2006), Xrules: An effective structural classifier for xml data. *Machine Learning J. Special Issue Stat. Relational Learning Multi-Relational Data Mining,* 62(1–2):137–170.

14. B. Liu, W. Hsu, and Y. Ma (1998), Integrating classification and association rule mining. *Proceedings of the Fourth International Conference on Knowledge Discovery and Data Mining, NY.*

15. J. R. Quinlan (1993), *C4.5 : Programs for Machine Learning*. Morgan Kaufmann.

16. V. Vapnik (1998), *Statistical Learning Theory*. John Wiley & Sons, Inc. NY.

17. A. Inokuchi, T. Washio, and H. Motoda (2000), An apriori-based algorithm for mining frequent substructures from graph data. *PKDD'00*, Lyon, France, 13–23.

18. M. Kuramochi and G. Karypis (2001), Frequent subgraph discovery. *Proc. International Conference on Data Mining'01*, San Diego, CA, pp. 313–320.

19. X. Yan and J. Han (2002), gspan: Graph-based substructure pattern mining. *Proc. International Conference on Data Mining'02*, Masbashe City, Japan, 721–724.

20. W. Wang, J. Huan, and J. Prins (2003), Efficient mining of frequent subgraphs in the presence of isomorphism. In *Proceeding of ICDM,* Melbourne, FL.

21. J. Huan, W. Wang, J. Prins, and J. Yang (2004), SPIN: Mining maximal frequent subgraphs from graph databases, Seattle, WA, 581–586.

22. S. Nijssen and J. N. Kok (2004), A quickstart in frequent structure mining can make a difference. *Proceedings of the 10th ACM SIGKDD International Conference on Knowledge Discovery and Data Mining*, Seattle, WA, 647–652.

23. J. Huan, W. Wang, and J. Prins (2003), Efficient mining of frequent subgraph in the presence of isomorphism. *Proceedings of the 3rd IEEE International Conference on Data Mining (ICDM)*, Melbourne, FL, pp. 549–552.

24. M. Deshpande, M. Kuramochi, and G. Karypis (2005), Frequent sub-structure-based approaches for classifying chemical compounds. *IEEE Trans. on Knowledge Data Eng.*, 1768:1036–1050.

25. T. Kudo, E. Maeda, and Y. Matsumoto (2004), An application of boosting to graph classification. *NIPS*, Vancaurce, Canada.

26. L. Ralaivola, S. J. Swamidass, H. Saigo, and P. Baldi (2005), Graph kernels for chemical informatics. *Neural Networks*, 18:1093–1110.

27. T. Gärtner, P. Flach, and S. Wrobel (2003), On graph kernels: Hardness results and efficient alternatives. *Sixteenth Annual Conference on Computational Learning Theory and Seventh Kernel Workshop,* Washington, DC.

28. H. Kashima, K. Tsuda, and A. Inokuchi (2003), Marginalized kernels between labeled graphs. *Proceedig of the Twentieth International Conference on Machine Learning (ICML)*, Washington, DC.

29. K. M. Borgwardt and H. P. Kriegel (2005), Shortest-path kernels on graphs. *Proceeding of the International Conference on Data Mining*, Houston, TX, 27–31, NY.

30. J. Ramon and T. Gärtner (2003), Expressivity versus efficiency of graph kernels. In *Technical Report, First International Workshop on Mining Graphs, Trees and Sequences,* Carat. Dubrounik, Groatia.

31. T. Horvath, T. Gartner, and S. Wrobel (2004), Cyclic pattern kernels for predictive graph mining. *SIGKDD*, Seattle, WA.

32. N. Wale, I. Watson, and G. Karypis (2007), Comparison of descriptor spaces for chemical compound retrieval and classification. *Knowledge Infor. Systems*, 14(3):347–375.

33. P. Mahe and J. P. Vert (2006), Graph kernels based on tree patterns for molecules. Technical Report HAL:ccsd-00095488, Ecoles des Mines de Paris.

34. H. Fröhlich, J. Wegner, F. Sieker, and A. Zell, (2006), Kernel functions for attriubted molecular graphs - a new similarity-based approach to adme prediction in classification. *QSAR Combinatorial Sci.*, 25(4):317–326.

35. C. Helma, R. King, and S. Kramer (2001), The predictive toxicology challenge 2000–2001. *Bioinformatics*, 17(1):107–108.

36. M. Wessel, P. Jurs, J. Tolan, and S. Muskal (1998), Prediction of human intestinal absorption of drug compounds from molecular structure. *J. Chem. Inf. Comput. Sci.*, 38(4):726–735.

37. F. Fontaine, M. Pastor, I. Zamora, and F. Sanz (2005), Anchor-grind: Filling the gap between standard 3d qsar and the grid-independent descriptors. *J. Med. Chem.*, 48:2687–2694.

38. R. Jorissen and M. Gilson (2005), Virtual screening of molecular databases using a support vector machine. *J. Chem. Inf. Model.*, 45(3):549–561.

39. D. Patterson, R. Cramer, A. Ferguson, R. Clark, and L. Weinberger (1996), Neighbourhood behaviour: A useful concept for validation of "molecular diversity" descriptors. *J. Med. Chem.*, 39:3049–3059.

40. J. Platt (1998), *Fast Training of Support Vector Machines using Sequential Minimal Optimization*. MIT Press, Cambridge, MA.

41. I. Witten and E. Frank (2005), *Data Mining: Practical machine learning tools and techniques*, 2nd ed. Morgan Kaufmann, San Francisco, CA.

42. R. Ahuja, T. Magnanti, and J. Orlin (1995), Network flows, *SIAM Rev.*, 37 (1).

43. C. Chang and C. Lin (2001), Libsvm: a library for support vector machines, Available at http://www.csie.ntu.edu.tw/ cjlin/libsvm.

44. S. Lyu (2005), Mercer kernels for object recognition with local features. *IEEE Computer Vision and Pattern Recognition*, San Diego, CA, 223–229.

45. T. Liu, Y. Lin, X. Wen, R. N. Jorrisen, and M. K. Gilson (2007), Bindingdb: a web-accessible database of experimentally determined protein-ligand binding affinities. *Nucleic Acids Res.*, 35:D198–D201.

46. J. L. Perret, P. Mahe, and J. P. Vert (2007), Chemcpp: an open source c^{++} toolbox for kernel functions on chemical compounds, Available at http://chemcpp.sourceforge.net.

47. A. Deligiannakis and N. Roussopoulos (2003), Extended wavelets for multiple measures. *Proceedings of the 2003 ACM SIGMOD International Conference on Management of Data* San Diego, CA.

48. M. Garofalakis and A. Kumar (2005), Wavelet synopses for general error metrics. *ACM Tran. Database Systems (TODS)*, 30(4):888–928.

10

IN SILICO DRUG DESIGN USING A COMPUTATIONAL INTELLIGENCE TECHNIQUE

SOUMI SENGUPTA AND SANGHAMITRA BANDYOPADHYAY

10.1 INTRODUCTION

Discovery of novel lead molecules has always been a long, time consuming, and expensive process in traditional drug discovery. It involves searching a chemical space of $> 10^{18}$ compounds [1] to find a suitable small molecule that can act as a drug and is safe to be administered. Finding a suitable molecule with the desired chemical property from such a large search space is a very complex problem. With the advent of new technologies and the abundance of three-dimensional (3D) structures of proteins, the scientific fraternity can exploit this structural information in order to design novel ligands possessing high-binding affinity to selective target proteins. This approach of finding novel ligand molecules using the structure information of the receptor is usually referred to as structure-based drug design.

Several Lead molecules have been discovered using the structure-based drug design approach. A few of them are approved drugs and many others are under clinical trials. Prostaglandin D synthase inhibitors [2] and X-linked inhibitor of apoptosis protein inhibitors [3] are most recent examples of drug design using fragment-based Lead design. The success of this approach inspired the scientists to apply computational technologies to aid the drug discovery process. The main objectives of the computational methods was to reduce the time and expense of the drug discovery process. One of the earliest such approaches for computer-aided drug design or rational drug design is DOCK [4]. This approach is a virtual screening method. It searches

Computational Intelligence and Pattern Analysis in Biological Informatics, Edited by Ujjwal Maulik,
Sanghamitra Bandyopadhyay, and Jason T. L. Wang
Copyright © 2010 John Wiley & Sons, Inc.

the database of 3D ligands to find the most suitable small molecule for a given target protein. To find the goodness of a ligand, it docks the ligand to the given receptor and gauges the stability of the complex. There is another approach to address the problem. Instead of searching among known 3D molecules to find a suitable molecule, algorithms can be developed to design molecules with desired chemical features.

The problem of Lead optimization, be it by searching known 3D molecules or by conceiving novel molecular scaffolds, is a search and optimization problem. In such a scenario, application of genetic algorithms (GAs) [5, 6] seems natural and appropriate. These GAs are a family of search and optimization techniques inspired by the principles of evolution.

A few earlier applications of GAs for efficient ligand design are [7–9]. Budin et al., [10] developed a GA based approach for building peptides. However, a seed has to be provided to the program for building the final ligand. Globus et al., proposed another GA based approach to evolve small molecules represented as graphs, with atoms as nodes and bonds between the atoms as edges [11]. Goh and Foster [8] proposed a GA based ligand design framework that uses a tree structure encoding for representing the ligands. The trees representing the ligands contain a functional group, selected from a given library, at each leaf. But, it had an important limitation. This approach used a fixed tree length for encoding the ligands. Ligands can never be of the same size for every target, rather the ligand size would vary with the active site geometry of different targets. To overcome this, Bandyopadhyay et al., proposed a method based on variable length genetic algorithm (VGA) [7]. This approach was more realistic as it used a variable length tree for encoding ligand as chromosomes. Consideration of the variable tree length allowed ligand size to vary with different active site geometries [7]. But again this approach also builds two-dimensional (2D) ligands. Therefore, solutions provided by the approach may not be as good when conceived in 3Ds. This chapter endeavors to improve this work by mining the active site from a given protein structure, building 3D ligands, considering different energy components for optimization, a much larger suite of functional groups for constructing the ligand, both inter- and intramolecular interactions for optimization and domain specific crossover and mutation operators. Experiments have also been conducted to study the contribution of the intramolecular and the intermolecular energy components in virtual screening. The effectiveness of the algorithm is established through a comparative analysis of the results of proposed methods to VGA and two other existing approaches for ligand design, namely, NEWLEAD [12] and LigBuider [13].

10.2 PROPOSED METHODOLOGY

This chapter discusses a genetic algorithm-based approach to *de novo* ligand design and emphasizes the importance of the contribution of intramolecular and intermolecular interaction energy for optimizing the ligands. The program takes the protein data bank (PDB) structure files of the target proteins as input. From these input files, the active site of the target protein is mined. According to the geometry and chemistry of the target active site, the core ligand molecules are built while initialization. These molecules are evolved using specially tailored domain specific genetic operators according to the value of the optimization parameter. Intramolecular and intermolecular interaction energy are the optimization criteria computed by the fitness function. Intramolecular energy is a sum of bond stretching, angle bending, angle rotation, van der Waals, and electrostatic energy components. The intermolecular interaction energy is a sum of van der Waals and electrostatic energy components. We have obtained the fitness value as a weighted sum of the intramolecular and intermolecular energies to investigate the importance of their contribution for the Lead optimization problem. Further, to validate our results we have docked the ligands built using the proposed algorithm, VGA, NEWLEAD, and LigBuilder with their target proteins employing an already established software InsightII [MSI/Accelrys, San Diego, CA] and have compared them to their similar molecules present in Cambridge structural database (CSD).

10.2.1 Active Site Processing

The steps involved in active site identification for ligand building are accounted for in Section 10.2.1.1–10.2.1.3.

10.2.1.1 Active Site Identification Preliminary information about the geometry and chemical composition of either the target active site or the natural ligand of the target is required to address the Lead molecule design problem. The program that we have developed requires the geometry and chemistry of the active site to build its corresponding ligands. The geometry of the target active site determines the size of the ligand and the chemical composition actuate the desired chemical property of the ligand. To mark the active site in the given protein, its coordinates obtained from the PDB are fit into a grid with a spacer of 0.5 Å. Grids containing protein coordinates are labeled as "full". If the input file is a ligand–protein complex, then grids occupied by the ligand coordinates are labeled as "empty" and this group of grids is treated as the active site. If an isolated protein molecule is input, then empty grids containing nothing are labeled "empty" and the largest assembly of such "empty" grids is considered as the active site.

10.2.1.2 Active Site Surface Marking After identifying the active site, the dimensions and chemical property of the active site is determined. Therefore, as the next step the surface of the active site is marked and the amino acids on its surface are also marked. To find the active site surface each "empty" grid comprising the active site is filled with a water molecule of radius 1.4 Å. After placing the water molecule in each grid, the distance between the water molecule and the nearest protein coordinate is calculated. If the distance is 0.5 Å or less, then that particular grid containing the coordinate of the protein molecule is labeled as "surface" and the atom on that coordinate is noted. The atoms on the surface of the active site are responsible for the biological functionality of the protein. So, these atoms are necessary to be considered while building a ligand that is supposed to bind to it. These atoms are responsible for the protein–ligand interaction. The center of the active site is detected by calculating the median of the set of grid points considered as the active site. The ligand building starts from this point.

10.2.1.3 Building Preference Matrix The atoms on the surface of the active site are marked to design ligands that can bind efficiently to the target protein. A preference matrix is constructed to make a sequential list of every fragment being in the vicinity of a particular atom in the active site. The preference matrix contains atoms of the receptor protein comprising the active site in its rows while columns contain the estimation of the different fragments, as mentioned in Figure 10.1, of being in the vicinity of the given atom in the specific row.

To estimate the probability of a fragment being in the neighborhood of a particular active site atom, first the nonbonding interactions (NBI) between all the fragments and each of the atoms constituting the active site are calculated. These interactions are calculated as

$$\text{NBI}_{i, f'} = \sum_{i=1}^{|f'|} \left[\frac{C_n}{r_{ij}^6} - \frac{C_m}{r_{ij}^{12}} + \frac{(q_i \times q_j)}{(4 \times \pi \times \epsilon_0 \times \epsilon \times r_{ij}^2)} \right]. \tag{10.1}$$

Equation (10.1) considers van der Waals and electrostatic interactions. Here, C_n and C_m are constants, r_{ij} is the distance between the ith atom of the fragment f' and jth interacting atom on the receptor active site, and q_i, q_j are charges on i and j, respectively.

Then the probability of each fragment f', $f' = 0, 1, 2, \ldots, 40$, to be considered in the neighborhood of a given atom j on the receptor active site, is calculated as

$$\text{prob}_{j, f'} = \frac{NBI_{j, f'}}{\sum_{f'=0}^{40}[\text{NBI}_{j, f'}]} \tag{10.2}$$

Here, $\text{prob}_{j, f'}$ is the probability of the fragment f' being in proximity of the atom j, in the active site of the receptor. The numerator is the NBI energy between atom j on the receptor active site and a fragment f'. The denominator is the sum of the NBI energies between each fragment and the atom j of the receptor active site.

10.2.2   Genetic Algorithm-Based Ligand Design

A GA based *de novo* ligand design algorithm is described here. This algorithm uses the fragment-based approach for designing ligands. The fragment library that it uses for ligand building is shown in Figure 10.1. Chromosome representation, population initialization, fitness computation, and genetic operators of the proposed algorithm for ligand design are explained in Sections 10.2.2.1–10.2.2.4.

10.2.2.1 Chromosome Representation and Population Initialization The present work uses 41 fragments, as shown in Fig. 10.1, for constructing the ligands. Table 10.1 gives the valencies corresponding to each fragment. For example, fragment number 9 is a nitrogen atom and and it has a valency of 3 (i.e., it can form three more bonds to join itself to other fragments). The ligand size may vary according to the different target active sites. Therefore, to allow construction of ligands with varying length, a chromosome is encoded as a variable length tree like structure. Each gene of a chromosome or each node of the tree representing a ligand is a structure containing 3

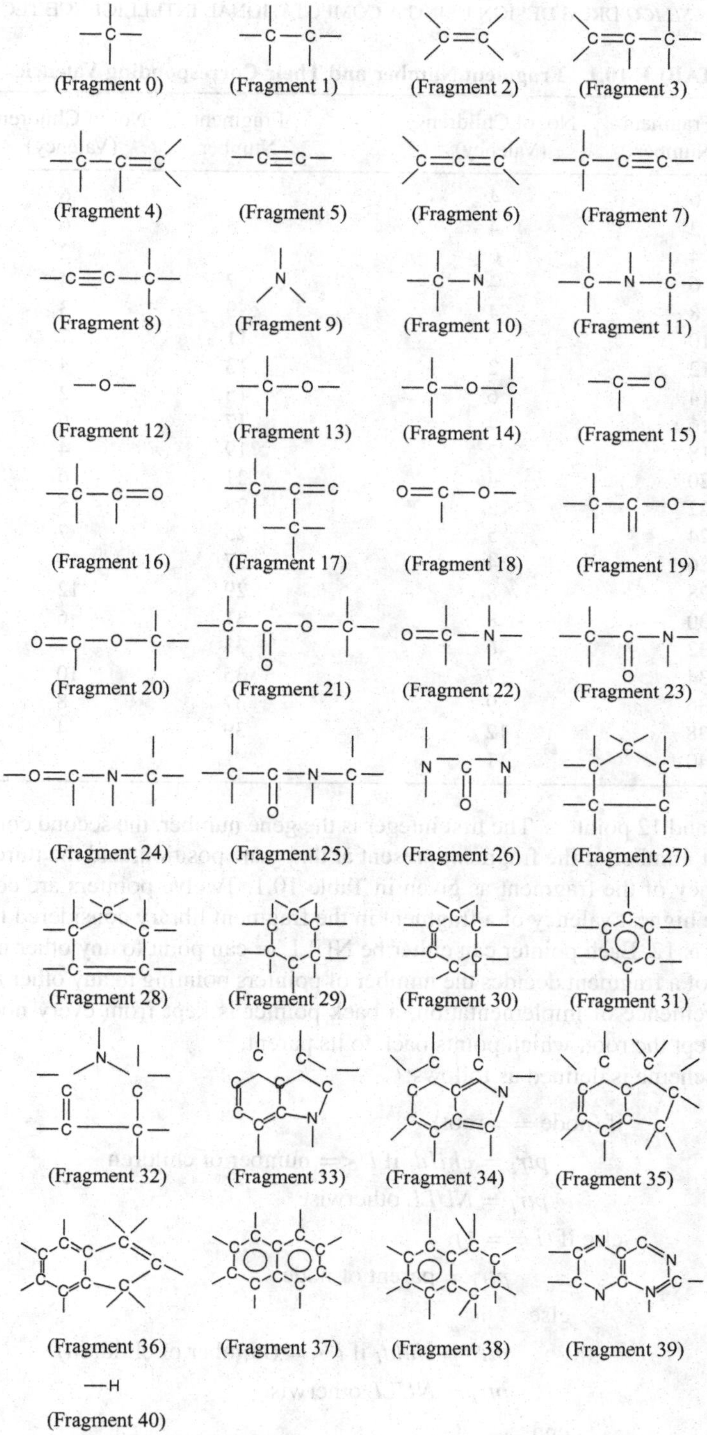

(Fragment 0)

(Fragment 1)

(Fragment 2)

(Fragment 3)

(Fragment 4)

(Fragment 5)

(Fragment 6)

(Fragment 7)

(Fragment 8)

(Fragment 9)

(Fragment 10)

(Fragment 11)

(Fragment 12)

(Fragment 13)

(Fragment 14)

(Fragment 15)

(Fragment 16)

(Fragment 17)

(Fragment 18)

(Fragment 19)

(Fragment 20)

(Fragment 21)

(Fragment 22)

(Fragment 23)

(Fragment 24)

(Fragment 25)

(Fragment 26)

(Fragment 27)

(Fragment 28)

(Fragment 29)

(Fragment 30)

(Fragment 31)

(Fragment 32)

(Fragment 33)

(Fragment 34)

(Fragment 35)

(Fragment 36)

(Fragment 37)

(Fragment 38)

(Fragment 39)

—H

(Fragment 40)

FIGURE 10.1 Forty-one fragments (groups) were used to build the ligands using the proposed method.

TABLE 10.1   Fragment Number and Their Corresponding Valencies

Fragment Number	No. of Children (Valency)	Fragment Number	No. of Children (Valency)
0	4	1	6
2	4	3	6
4	6	5	2
6	4	7	4
8	4	9	3
10	5	11	7
12	2	13	4
14	6	15	2
16	4	17	6
18	2	19	4
20	4	21	6
22	3	23	5
24	5	25	7
26	4	27	10
28	8	29	12
30	8	31	6
32	6	33	7
34	7	35	10
36	9	37	8
38	12	39	4
40	1		

integers and 12 pointers. The first integer is the gene number, the second contains the fragment number of the fragment present at that gene position, and the third denotes the valency of the fragment as given in Table 10.1. Twelve pointers are considered since the highest valency of a fragment in the fragment library considered for ligand building is 12. Each pointer can either be NULL or can point to any other node. The valency of a fragment decides the number of pointers pointing to any other node. For the convenience of implementation, a back pointer is kept from every node of the tree, except the root, which points back to its parent.

The scheme is defined as follows:

if (node $==$ root)
$\quad ptr_i = child_i$ if $i <=$ number of children
$\quad ptr_i = NULL$ otherwise
else if ($i == 1$)
$\quad ptr_i =$ parent of node
else
$\quad ptr_i = child_i$ if $i <=$ (number of children)
$\quad ptr_i = NULL$ otherwise
end

end

To initialize a chromosome i, the first gene position of the chromosome is filled by a fragment selected randomly from the fragment library, as mentioned in Figure 10.1. From the second gene position onward, each fragment is placed at every gene position and the fragment due to which the internal energy of the ligand is least is used for ligand extension. The ligand extension occurs as long as the ligand does not grow out of the active site. This incremental construction is done only for initializing the population with core ligands that are further evolved using the GA.

10.2.2.2 Fitness Evaluation   The fitness value of a ligand gauges the goodness of the solution. The goodness of a probable ligand is calculated as a function of its chemical composition and proximity to the target active site. The fitness function computes the intramolecular ligand energy and the intermolecular nonbonding interaction energy of the ligand and protein. Low intramolecular energy ensures a stable ligand and low inter molecular interaction energy warrants a stable ligand–protein complex implying better binding affinity. In this work, we have taken a weighted sum of the intramolecular and intermolecular interaction energy to enunciate their contributions in selectivity of ligands.

The van der Waals (vdw) energy is calculated using the following Lennard-Jones 6–12 potential function [14]

$$E_{vdw}(x, y) = \left(\frac{C_n}{r_{xy}^6} \right) - \left(\frac{C_m}{r_{xy}^{12}} \right) \tag{10.3}$$

Here, $E_{vdw}(x, y)$, C_n, C_m, and r_{xy} are the van der Waals interaction energy, constants and the distance between the interacting atoms x and y, respectively.

The electrostatic interaction energy $E_{el}(x, y)$ between two atoms x and y is calculated by [14]

$$E_{el}(x, y) = \frac{(q_x \times q_y)}{(4 \times \pi \times \epsilon_0 \times \epsilon \times r_{xy}^2)} \tag{10.4}$$

Here, q_x and q_y are formal charges of the interacting atoms, ϵ_0 is a constant, and r_{xy} is the distance between the interacting groups. Solvent water molecules are not considered for the calculations, so distance-dependent dielectric constant (ϵ) is used to mimic the solvent effect during calculation [15].

Equation (10.5) is used for calculating the bond-stretching energy $E_l(x, y)$ [14]

$$E_l(x, y) = \frac{k_l \times (l_{xy} - l_{xy,0})^2}{2} \tag{10.5}$$

Here, l_{xy} and $l_{xy,0}$ are the calculated bond length and reference bond length between the two atoms x and y, respectively. The bond-stretching constant is k_l.

The angle bending energy E_θ is calculated using the following equation [14]:

$$E_\theta = \frac{k_\theta \times (\theta - \theta_0)^2}{2} \tag{10.6}$$

Here, θ and θ_0 are the calculated angle and reference angle, respectively and k_θ is the angle-bending constant.

The torsional energy E_ϕ is calculated using the following expression [14]:

$$E_\phi = k_\phi \times (1 - \cos n \times (\phi - \phi_0)) \tag{10.7}$$

Here, ϕ and ϕ_0 are the calculated and reference torsion angles, respectively, k_ϕ is the torsion contribution constant, and n is the periodicity linked with the type of central bond of the torsion.

Therefore the intramolecular energy can be calculated by combining all the above mentioned energies as follows:

$$E_{\text{intra}} = \sum_{l'=1}^{\text{lig}} \sum_{l=1}^{l'-1} \left[E_{\text{vwd}}(l, l') + E_{el}(l, l') \right] + \sum_{\text{bonds}} E_l + \sum_{\text{angles}} E_\theta + \sum_{\text{torsion}} E_\phi \tag{10.8}$$

The intermolecular energy is

$$E_{\text{inter}} = \sum_{i=1}^{\text{lig}} \sum_{j=1}^{\text{receptor}} \left[E_{\text{vwd}}(i, j) + E_{el}(i, j) \right] \tag{10.9}$$

Here, lig and receptor are the number of groups in the ligand and the receptor, respectively. Sum of the intramolecular and intermolecular energy gives the total energy that determines the stability of the ligand, as well as the ligand–protein complex. But, as mentioned above, to enunciate the contributes of the E_{intra} and E_{inter} in ligand selection pressure weighted sum of both the energy components are considered. Therefore the total energy is calculated as

$$E_{\text{total}} = w \times E_{\text{intra}} + (1 - w) \times E_{\text{inter}} \tag{10.10}$$

Here, w, that varies between 0 and 1, controls the contributions of the two energy components toward the composite energy, E_{total}. Different values of w are used in the experiments in order to evaluate the relative importance of the two factors and to design an effective fitness function.

As mentioned before, lower energy corresponds to more stable ligands. Therefore the fitness value of a chromosome is set to be inversely proportional to the total energy value. In other words, the fitness value, F, of a chromosome is defined as

$$F = \frac{1}{E_{\text{total}}} \tag{10.11}$$

such that individuals with higher fitness correspond to ligands having lower energy values, and hence greater stability.

For refining the results, a few domain specific constraints are applied. Nonbonding interaction energy are is calculated for the functional group of the ligand lying at a distance not >5 Å and not <0.65 Å from the protein receptor molecule to avoid steric hindrance. Three dimensional conformation and orientation of a ligand is very important to make bonds with its target. For example, a polar hydroxyl group should lie close to an amine group or acidic amino acids to make stable hydrogen bonds. Similarly, hydrophobic interactions will occur only when hydrophobic atoms of the ligand will face the hydrophobic amino acids on the active site of the target protein. Ligands violating these constraints are heavily penalized by adding a large positive integer to the total energy so that they will be automatically eliminated in the evolutionary process.

10.2.2.3 Genetic Operators The genetic operators used are selection, crossover, and mutation. Roulette wheel selection technique is employed. According to this selection strategy, more fit individuals are more probable to reproduce (i.e., a chromosome is more likely to be selected as a parent for reproduction if it has better fitness).

A crossover probability of cprob is adaptively set for application of the domain specific crossover operator, on a pair of parent chromosomes. For performing the crossover, the crossover points in both the parents are generated. A crossover point is a randomly generated gene number in a parent. The subtrees following these gene numbers on the crossover points are exchanged to obtain two new chromosomes. After the exchange, the pointers and the gene numbers are rearranged appropriately by following a breadth first traversal. According to the cprob, if the crossover is not to performed between a pair of parents, then they are simply copied to the next population. The adaptive crossover probability is calculated similarly to [16]. If f_{max} is the maximum fitness value of the current population, $\overline{f}$ is the average fitness value of the population and f' is the larger of the fitness values of the solutions to be crossed. Then the probability of crossover, cprob, can be calculated as

$$\text{cprob} = k_1 \times \frac{(f_{max} - f')}{(f_{max} - \overline{f})} \quad \text{if} \quad f' > \overline{f}, \quad \text{cprob} = k_3 \quad \text{if} \quad f' \leq \overline{f} \quad (10.12)$$

Here, similar to [16], the values of k_1 and k_3 are both considered as 1.0. Note that, when $f_{max} = \overline{f}$, then $f' = f_{max}$ and cprob attains the same value as k_3. The impetus for this adaptation is to achieve a trade-off between exploration and exploitation in a different manner. When two chromosomes with poor fitness are to be crossed, the cprob increases, but it decreases if the two solutions under consideration for crossover are good solutions. This adaptation increases the likelihood of the bad solution to be evolved and decreases the likelihood of disrupting a good solution by crossover.

Mutation is also performed with an adaptive mutation probability of mprob as described in [16]. A gene position is to be mutated or not is decided using the mutation probability mprob. If a gene position is found to be suitable for mutation then the preference matrix, described earlier, is consulted to replace the gene position with the most likely substitute. For finding the appropriate substitute, the nearest neighbor on the gene on the active site is located. Then, a roulette wheel selection scheme is employed to select an appropriate fragment from the preference matrix to replace the fragment in the selected gene position. The mprob is calculated using the following expression

$$\text{mprob} = k_2 \times \frac{(f_{\max} - f)}{(f_{\max} - \overline{f})} \quad \text{if} \quad f > \overline{f},$$
$$\text{mprob} = k_4 \quad \text{if} \quad f \leq \overline{f} \tag{10.13}$$

Here, values of k_2 and k_4 are set equal to 0.5. Adaptive mutation is an aid to GA for overcoming a local optimum.

Adaptive crossover and mutation probabilities are helpful in avoiding premature convergence of GA at local optima. When $(f_{\max} - \overline{f})$ decreases indicating an optima, both cprob and mprob increases preventing the convergence of the GA. But due to this phenomenon, disruption of the near-optimal solutions can occur in order to prevent the convergence of the GA at even the global optimum. But as cprob and mprob attain lower values for more fit solutions and attain higher values for less fit solutions, individuals with high fitness values help in the convergence of the GA while the individuals with low fitness values prevent the GA from getting stuck at a local optimum. For solutions with the maximum fitness value, cprob and mprob are both zero.

10.2.2.4 Elitism The termination criterion for the algorithm is a specified number of generations. Elitism is incorporated in each generation. The best solution observed till a generation is stored in the next population, as well as in a location outside the population, is referred to as the elite population. Note that the size of the elite population is equal to the number of generations executed.

10.2.3 Postprocessing of the Ligand

The proposed algorithm is executed with the value of w as 0, 0.25, 0.50, 0.75, and 1. Elite and final populations are screened to identify the three top scoring individuals for each run of the proposed algorithm with w as 0, 0.25, 0.50, 0.75, and 1. A total of 15 high-scoring ligands were screened from the solution pool obtained using the proposed algorithm with various weights of inter- and intramolecular energy and are further analyzed for their goodness. For this analysis, the "Docking" module of Insight II [MSI/Accelrys, San Diego, CA] is used. Three ligands corresponding to the weight producing best results are chosen and are further compared with the output of VGA [7], NEWLEAD [12], and LigBuilder [13]. The optimized 3D structure of the 2D ligands designed by VGA are obtained by using a "Build" module of Insight II [MSI/Accelrys, San Diego, CA]. This module has a built in optimization routine to find the most stable conformation of the input ligand. Similar to comparing the activity of the ligands designed using the proposed algorithm, VGA, NEWLEAD, and LigBuilder, they are docked using the "Docking" module of Insight II [MSI/Accelrys,

San Diego, CA]. To study if it was possible to synthesize the designed ligands, CSD, a library of >450,000 small molecules, is searched using ConQuest [17] to find molecules similar to the designed ligands. These are considered for further docking and comparative analyses. The idea behind the comparison of the real molecules, retrieved from CSD, to the designed molecules, is that if any derivative of the designed molecule has already been synthesized, then perhaps the designed molecules can also be synthesized. Therefore, the corresponding real molecule can also assist in finding out the activity of the designed molecules. Moreover, if the similar real molecule is found to posses high-binding affinity to the given target, then both the real molecule and the designed molecules could be investigation worthy.

10.3   EXPERIMENTAL RESULTS AND DISCUSSION

C programming language has been used to develop the proposed algorithm on the UNIX platform. The performance of GA depends on the choice of the control parameters. Hence, the mutation and crossover probability are adaptively set as suggested in [16]. The number of generations and the population size are set to 1000 and 100, respectively.

The drug targets considered for the study are HIV-1 Protease and Thrombin. The posttranscriptional processing of viral gag and gag-pol proteins for the production of functional viral proteins are assisted by HIV-l Protease. The structural proteins of virion core (i.e., p17, p24, p7, and p6) are transcribed and translated from the gag gene. Gag-pol is responsible for the release of viral replicative enzymes (protease, reverse transcriptase, and integrase), necessary for its retroviral life cycle. Thrombin is a serine protease prominently participating in blood coagulation. It hydrolyzes fibrinogen to fibrin for activating platelets to form the clot. Thrombin can be used as a tool to control coagulation cascade and ameliorate specific diseases [18]. A wide variety of binding modes and geometries of thrombin has been revealed by many scientists. According to [19] thrombin contains three principal interaction sites, namely, S1, D, and P. The S1 site contains an aspartic acid residue. Both D and P sites contain hydrophobic pockets. All three sites are responsible for the specificity of thrombin. The PDB entries 1AAQ and 1DWD [19, 20], the structure of HIV-1 Protease and Thrombin, respectively, are used as input files to the program. Both NAPAP and Ritonavir are the known synthetic inhibitors of Thrombin and HIV-1 Protease, respectively. Therefore, the ligands designed using the proposed algorithm, VGA, NEWLEAD, and LigBuilder are compared with these molecules to estimate their goodness.

10.3.1   Comparative Analyses of the Contribution of Intramolecular and Intermolecular Energy for Ligand Designing

The three top scoring individuals obtained after each run of the proposed algorithm using the value of w as 0, 0.25, 0.50, 0.75, and 1 corresponding to each of the target proteins are docked to their respective receptors. Their corresponding energy values

TABLE 10.2   Interaction Energies for the Ligands Designed Using the Proposed Method With the Weight as 0, 0.25, 0.50, 0.75, and 1 for HIV-1 Protease and Thrombin[a]

Protein	Ligand	Interaction Energy (kcal mole⁻¹)				
		w = 0	w = 0.25	w = 0.5	w = 0.75	w = 1
HIV-1	*ligand₁*	−2.52	−3.88	−9.35	−3.69	1.02
Protease	*ligand₂*	−2.67	−3.56	−8.54	−3.66	1.96
	ligand₃	0.19	−2.11	−6.23	−3.24	2.5
Thrombin	*ligand₁*	−5.45	−2.98	−10.33	−1.24	2.55
	ligand₂	−4.11	−2.24	−9.42	0.56	3.01
	ligand₂	−4.86	−1.29	−9.11	0.98	3.51

[a] In kcal mole⁻¹.

are given in Table 10.2. The results shows that the ligand target complexes possess less energy when the ligands are designed with $w = 0.5$. This observation indicates that the ligands designed using the equal contribution of intramolecular and intermolecular energy are better in comparison to the ligands designed with unequal contribution of the intermolecular and intramolecular energy. The reason behind such an observation could be that the ligands that are being designed need to have a stable conformation for itself and should be able to bond well to its target. It can also be observed from Table 10.2 that the ligands designed considering only intermolecular energy ($w = 0$) are better than the ligands designed using only intramolecular energy ($w = 1$). The reason for this is that while designing ligands for a given target, the interaction of the target to the protein must be considered so as to get an approximate estimate of the binding affinity of the designed molecule to its given target. In fact, the work in [7] used only this component of the energy. Though the intermolecular interaction energy is more important to be evaluated than *de novo* ligand design, the efficacy of the algorithm increases when intramolecular energy is incorporated. Therefore, we conclude that the fitness function for evolving small drug-like molecules should give equal importance to both intramolecular and intermolecular interaction. Further analysis of the results for the comparative study with other existing approaches are obtained using $w = 0.5$.

10.3.2   Comparative Analyses of Interaction Energy and Hydrogen-Bond Interaction

The ligands designed by the proposed algorithm (VGA, NEWLEAD, and LigBuilder) for HIV-1 Protease and Thrombin are docked with their corresponding receptor proteins using the "Docking" module of Insight II [MSI/Accelrys, San Diego, CA]. The corresponding interaction energies are provided in Table 10.3. The significantly lower energy values of the molecules designed using the proposed algorithm indicate that these produce more stable receptor ligand complexes. The ligands designed for HIV-1 Protease by each of the *de novo* design scheme and their docked complexes with the protein are shown in Figure 10.2. The ligands designed by the proposed algorithm

TABLE 10.3   Interaction Energies for the Ligands Designed Using the Proposed Method, VGA, NEWLEAD, and LigBuilder for HIV-1 Protease and Thrombin[a]

| Protein | Ligand | Interaction Energy (kcal mole^{-1}) | | | |
		Proposed method	VGA	NEWLEAD	LigBuilder
HIV-1	$ligand_1$	−9.35	2.53	−7.98	−8.67
Protease	$ligand_2$	−8.54	5.76	−6.14	−7.11
	$ligand_3$	−6.23	0.23	−4.32	−6.02
	Average interaction energy	−8.04	2.84	−6.14	−7.26
Thrombin	$ligand_1$	−10.33	−2.53	−5.80	−8.97
	$ligand_2$	−9.42	−2.23	−5.64	−8.56
	$ligand_2$	−9.11	−1.52	−4.28	−7.79
	Average interaction energy	−9.62	−2.09	−5.24	−8.44

[a] In kcal mol^{-1}.

are generally smaller and comprise less aromatic groups (see Figure 10.2), causing less stearic hindrance and better interaction with the target protein, in comparison to the ligands designed by the other methods.

Hydrogen bonds in a protein–ligand complex are very essential since the binding affinity between the protein and the ligand is dependent on them. Therefore, the interacting residues of the protein–ligand complex are observed to identify the hydrogen bonds.

Tables 10.4–10.6 give the hydrogen-bond details for the protein–ligand interaction. From these tables, it is evident that ligands designed by the proposed algorithm are in general forming more hydrogen bonds with their target proteins, implying a more stable docked complex.

The rationale behind the formation of more and good hydrogen bonds between the target and the ligand designed by the proposed algorithm could be better genetic operators, bigger fragment libraries, and building 3D ligands. The proposed algorithm builds 3D ligands, therefore it can be expected that the ligands designed by it will always dominate results of VGA since 3D adaptation will allow better exploration of the search space. Consideration of preference matrix for mutation makes the process knowledge based and thus the algorithm is able to evolve a more fit individual in comparison to NEWLEAD and LigBuilder. The fragment library of the proposed algorithm is a balanced combination of the chemical fragments and atoms making the algorithm more flexible while designing small molecules. It is not compelled to grow ligands using only fragments, unlike LigBuilder, or only atoms, unlike [21,22]. It can grow ligands using both fragments and atoms as per requirement. References [21,22] have a comparatively large time complexity due to usage of atoms for building ligands. Therefore, the type of fragment library modeled for this algorithm increases the precision of the algorithm and reduces the time complexity.

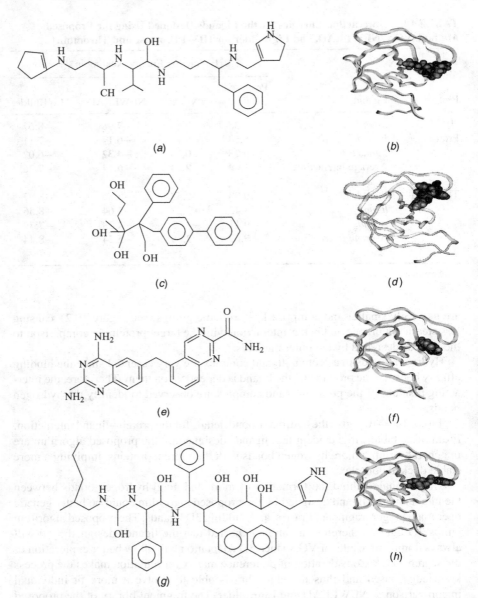

FIGURE 10.2   Structure of a ligand and the docked protein–ligand complex obtained by (*a* and *b*) the proposed method, (*c* and *d*) VGA, (*e* and *f*) NEWLEAD, and (*g* and *h*) LigBuilder for HIV-1 Protease (visualized using Insight II [MSI/Accelrys, San Diego, CA], where the protein is represented in ribbons and the ligands are represented in CPK).

TABLE 10.4 H-Bond Interactions of *Ligand*₁ Designed by the Proposed Method, VGA, NEWLEAD, and LigBuilder With HIV-1 Protease and Thrombin

Approach	Protein	H-Bond Donor	H-Bond Acceptor	H-Bond Distance
Proposed method	HIV-1	Protein:48:HN	Ligand:2:OH	2.38
	Protease	Ligand:2:HH	Protein:48:N	2.36
		Ligand:2:HH	Protein:48:O	2.48
	Thrombin	Ligand:3:O	Protein:96:O	1.43
		Ligand:7:NH	Protein:98:HH	2.07
VGA	HIV-1	Protein:87:HH	Ligand:3:OH	2.13
	Protease	Ligand:3:HH	Protein:87:NH	2.30
	Thrombin	Ligand:2:HH	Protein:102:NH	2.02
NEWLEAD	HIV-1	Protein:29:OH	Ligand:5:HH	1.13
	Protease	Ligand:5:HH	Protein:29:NH	2.05
	Thrombin	Ligand:3:HH	Protein:94:OH	1.67
		Ligand:4:HH	Protein:94:O	2.11
LigBuilder	HIV-1	Protein:48:N	Ligand:7:HH	2.08
	Protease	Ligand:5:HH	Protein:49:NH	2.28
	Thrombin	Protein:97:HN	Ligand:2:HH	2.87
		Ligand:2:HH	Protein:97:N	2.76

TABLE 10.5 H-Bond Interactions of *Ligand*₂ Designed by the Proposed Method, VGA, NEWLEAD, and LigBuilder With HIV-1 Protease and Thrombin

Approach	Protein	H-Bond Donor	H-Bond Acceptor	H-Bond Distance
Proposed method	HIV-1	Ligand:2:HH	Protein:87:NH	2.14
	Protease	Ligand:4:HH	Protein:27:O	0.25
		Ligand:7:HH	Protein:48:O	2.48
	Thrombin	Ligand:1:NH	Protein:94:HH	1.82
		Ligand:10:OH	Protein:96:HH	1.87
VGA	HIV-1	Protein:87:HH	Ligand:4:OH	2.13
	Protease	Ligand:4:HH	Protein:87:NH	1.46
	Thrombin	Ligand:2:OH	Protein:102:HH	2.94
NEWLEAD	HIV-1	Protein:48:NH	Ligand:5:HH	1.13
	Protease	Ligand:5:HH	Protein:48:NH	1.75
	Thrombin	Ligand:1:HH	Protein:98:O	2.05
		Ligand:3:HH	Protein:94:N	2.87
LigBuilder	HIV-1	Protein:48:NH	Ligand:7:HH	2.46
	Protease	Protein:48:NH	Ligand:6:OH	2.35
	Thrombin	Protein:98:NH	Ligand:5:OH	2.43
		Ligand:5:OH	Protein:98:NH	2.35

TABLE 10.6 H-Bond Interactions of *Ligand₃* Designed by the Proposed Method, VGA, NEWLEAD, and LigBuilder With HIV-1 Protease and Thrombin

Approach	Protein	H-Bond Donor	H-Bond Acceptor	H-Bond Distance
Proposed method	HIV-1 Protease	Protein:27:HN	Ligand:2:HH	1.08
		Ligand:2:HH	Protein:27:N	0.96
	Thrombin	Ligand:2:HH	Protein:94:O	1.87
		Ligand:3:HH	Protein:94:O	2.27
VGA	HIV-1 Protease	Protein:89:HH	Ligand:5:OH	2.05
		Ligand:6:HH	Protein:89:NH	2.16
	Thrombin	Ligand:4:HH	Protein:93:OH	2.84
NEWLEAD	HIV-1 Protease	Protein:30:HH	Ligand:4:NH	1.62
		Ligand:4:HH	Protein:30:NH	1.78
	Thrombin	Ligand:7:OH	Protein:96:HH	2.11
LigBuilder	HIV-1 Protease	Protein:27:HH	Ligand:3:NH	2.12
		Ligand:3:HH	Protein:27:NH	2.28
	Thrombin	Ligand:4:HH	Protein:83:O	2.32

To investigate the synthesizability of the ligands designed by the proposed method, VGA, NEWLEAD, and LigBuilder, analogous real molecules, are retrieved from CSD using the search module "ConQuest" [17]. When CSD is searched using the proposed ligands as query, several similar molecules are reported by ConQuest. Among these, the molecules that form a stable docked complex with their receptors are reported. The CSD Ref Codes, along with the interaction energy with their corresponding target proteins, HIV-1 Protease, and Thrombin are reported in Table 10.7. As seen earlier, the interaction energies are found to be smaller for the real CSD molecules that are similar to the ligands designed by the proposed algorithm in

TABLE 10.7 Comparison of the Interaction Energies for the Molecules Obtained from CSD for HIV-1 Protease and Thrombin

Ligand Building Scheme	Protein	CSD Ref Code	Energy kcal mol^{-1}
Proposed method	HIV-1 Protease	SEWZOJ	−24.76
	Thrombin	VELTIP	−19.04
VGA	HIV-1 Protease	VEHMUQ	−17.76
	Thrombin	EADPUU	−12.34
NEWLEAD	HIV-1 Protease	AMPTRA	−18.10
	Thrombin	EHIYAV	−10.43
LigBuilder	HIV-1 Protease	QUIASP	−22.86
	Thrombin	INITAA10	−16.90

TABLE 10.8   RMSD Values, (Å) between NAPAP and Ligands Designed Using the Computational Approaches for Thrombin

The Proposed Method	VGA	NEWLEAD	LigBuilder
0.76	8.54	3.62	1.04

comparison to the molecules designed by VGA, NEWLEAD, and LigBuilder. The results point out that the molecules designed by the proposed algorithm form more stable docked complexes than the other three approaches.

10.3.3   Comparative Study Using Root-Mean-Square Deviation Analysis

In order to compare the RMSD values between the known protein inhibitor and the ligands designed by the proposed method (VGA, NEWLEAD, and LigBuilder), the protein Thrombin is considered. Pymol [23] is used for aligning the two molecules appropriately and computing the RMSD values. The comparative results are reported in Table 10.8. As seen, the ligands designed using the proposed method and LigBuilder have small RMSD values, indicating their high similarity to the know inhibitor for Thrombin, NAPAP. The poor performance of VGA is expected since it builds the ligand in 2D space. Figures 10.3 (a) (b) show the ligands designed by LigBuilder and the proposed method, respectively, superimposed over NAPAP. For HIV-1 Protease, the known inhibitor is Ritonavir. A result for LigBuilder is unavailable for this protein. The ligand designed using the proposed method superimposed on Ritonavir is shown in Figure 10.3 (c). As seen, the proposed molecule is highly similar to the known inhibitor, with an RMSD value, computed using PyMol, of 1.97 Å.

10.4   CONCLUSION

Traditional drug discovery is a well-established process that involves large amounts of time and money. Though there is no substitute for the methodology, the advancement of science and technology have definitely found various ways to assist the procedure to reduce its time consumption and expense. Rational drug design tries to do the same thing (i.e., it helps reducing time and cost of the process by reducing the search space for wet experiments). This chapter describes a rational drug design technique for *de novo* ligand design. The program illustrated in this chapter takes the structure files of the target proteins in PDB file format and mines the active site from it. A preference matrix is built using the chemical property of the active site that is further used to evolve the ligands. It uses a library of 41 fragments for building ligands. The program uses genetic algorithm to search the chemical space and find an appropriate ligand for the given target. It uses a variable length tree-like structure for chromosome representation and domain-specific genetic operators. Though the chromosome representation involves memory overhead, it is manageable as the ligands designed

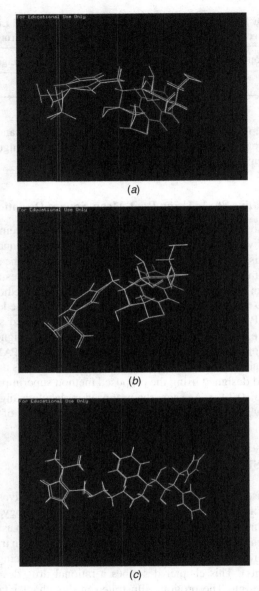

FIGURE 10.3 (*a*) Ligand built using grow module of LigBuilder (White) superimposed with NAPAP (Grey). (*b*) Ligand built using the proposed method (White) superimposed with NAPAP (Grey). (*c*) Ligand built using the proposed method (White) superimposed with Ritonavir (Grey).

are usually small. The fitness function of the algorithm computes bond stretching, dihedral angle, angle bending, electrostatic, and van der Waals energy components.

The results can be further improved if the algorithm amalgamates hydrophobic interaction and desolvation energies with the present fitness function for evaluating the goodness of the solutions. Usage of Lipinski rule of five, QSAR properties, and ADMET properties for ligand building can also improve results. Inclusion of these properties will assist in deciding the safety and efficacy of the ligands designed. The memory overhead also needs to be reduced using some other chromosome representation. The ligands designed using the proposed methodology are flexible, but while designing ligands, receptor proteins are considered rigid. To improve the algorithm, receptor flexibility needs to be incorporated.

REFERENCES

1. W. P. Walters, M. T. Stahl, and M. A. Murcko (1998), Virtual screening - an overview. *Drug Disc. Today*, 3:160–178.

2. M. Hohwy, L. Spadola, B. Lundquist, P. Hawtin, J. Dahmén, I. Groth-Clausen, E. Nilsson, S. Persdotter, K. v. Wachenfeldt, R. H. A. Folmer, and K. Edman (2008), Novel prostaglandin d synthase inhibitors generated by fragment-based drug design. *J. Med. Chem.*, 51(7):2178–2186.

3. J-W. Huang, Z. Zhang, B. Wu, J. F. Cellitti, X. Zhang, R. Dahl, C-W. Shiau, K. Welsh, A. Emdadi, J. L. Stebbins, J. C. Reed, and M. Pellecchia (2008), Fragment-based design of small molecule x-linked inhibitor of apoptosis protein inhibitors. *J. Med. Chem.*, 51(22):7111–7118.

4. I. D. Kuntz, E. C. Blaney, S. J. Oatley, R. Langridge, and T. E. Ferrin (1982), A Geometric Approach to Macromolecule-Ligand Interactions. *J. Mol. Biol.*, 161:269–288.

5. D. E. Goldberg (1989), *Genetic Algorithms in Search, Optimization and Machine Learning*. Addison-Wesley, NY.

6. J. H. Holland (1975), *Adaptation in Natural and Artificial Systems*. The University of Michigan Press, AnnArbor, MI.

7. S. Bandyopadhyay, A. Bagchi, and U. Maulik (2005), Active Site Driven Ligand Design: An Evolutionary Approach. *J. Bioinformatics Compu. Biol.*, 3:1053–1070.

8. G. Goh and J. A. Foster (2000), Evolving molecules for drug design using genetic algorithm via Molecular Tree. Proceedings of the Genetic and Evolutionary Computation Conference (GECCO '00), Morgan Kaufmann, Las Vegas, Nevada, USA, pp. 27–33.

9. S. C. Pegg, J. J. Haresco, and I. D. Kuntz (2001), A Genetic Algorithm for Structure-based De Novo Design. *J. Comput. Aided. Mol. Des.*, 15:911–933.

10. N. Budin, N. Majeux, C. Tenette Souaille, and A. Caflisch (2001), Structure-based Ligand Design by a Build-up Approach and Genetic Algorithm Search in Conformational Space. *J. Comput. Chem.*, 22:1956–1970.

11. A. Globus, J. Lawton, and T. Wipke (1999), Automatic Molecular Design Using Evolutionary Techniques. *Sixth Foresight Conference on Molecular Nanotechnology, 1998, Nanotechnology*, 10:290–299.

12. V. Tschinke and N. C. Cohen (2006), The NEWLEAD program: a new method for the design of candidate structures from pharmacophoric hypothesis. *J. Med. Chem.*, 45A:1834–1837.

13. R. Wang, T. Gao, and L. Lai (2000), Ligbuilder: A multi-purpose program for structure-based drug design. *J. Mol. Model.*, 6:498–516.

14. A. R. Leach (2001), *Molecular Modelling Principles and Applications*. Prentice Hall, NY.

15. J. M. Yang and C. Y. Kao (2000), Flexible Ligand Docking Using a Robust Evolutionary Algorithm. *J. Comput. Chem.*, 21:988–998.

16. M. Srinivas and L. M. Patnaik (1994), Adaptive Probabilities of Crossover and Mutation in Genetic Algorithms. *IEEE Transactions on Syatem, Man And Cybernatics*, 24:656–667.

17. I. J. Bruno, J. C. Cole, P. R. Edgington, M. Kessler, C. F. Macrae, P. McCabe, J. Pearson, and R. Taylor (2002), New software for searching the cambridge structural database and visualizing crystal structures. *Acta Crystallogra. Sect. B*, 58:389–397.

18. B. Blomback, M. Blomback, B. Hessel, and S. Iwanaga (1967), Structures of N-Terminal Fragments of Fibrinogen and Specificity of Thrombin. *Nature (London)*, 215:1445–1448.

19. D. W. Banner and P. Hadvary (1991), Crystallographic analysis at 3.0-a resolution of the binding to human thrombin of four active site-directed inhibitors. *J. Biol. Chem.*, 266:20085–20093.

20. G. B. Dreyer, D. M. Lambert, T. D. Meek, T. J. Carr, T. A. Tomaszek, Jr. A. V. Fernandez, H. Bartus, E. Cacciavillani, and A. M. Hassell (1992), Hydroxyethylene isostere inhibitors of human immunodeficiency virus-1 protease: structure-activity analysis using enzyme kinetics, x-ray crystallography, and infected T-cell assays. *Biochemistry*, 31:6646–6659.

21. R. S. Bohacek and C. McMartin (1994), Multiple highly diverse structures complementary to enzyme binding sites: Results of extensive application of a de novo design method incorporating combinatorial growth. *J. Am. Chem. Soc.*, 116:5560–5571.

22. Y. Nishibata and A. Itai (1993), Confirmation of usefulness of a structure construction program based on three-dimensional receptor structure for rational lead generation. *J. Med. Chem.*, 36:2921–2928.

23. W. L. DeLano (2002), The pymol molecular graphics system. Technical report, San Carlos, CA.

PART IV

MICROARRAY DATA ANALYSIS

11

INTEGRATED DIFFERENTIAL FUZZY CLUSTERING FOR ANALYSIS OF MICROARRAY DATA

Indrajit Saha and Ujjwal Maulik

11.1 INTRODUCTION

In recent years, DNA microarrays has been developed as a popular technique for gathering a substantial amount of gene expression data that is necessary to examine complex regulatory behavior of a cell [1]. Microarray gene expression data, consisting of $\mathcal{G}$ genes and $\mathcal{T}$ time points, is typically organized in a two-dimensional (**2D**) matrix $E = [e_{ij}]$ of size $\mathcal{G} \times \mathcal{T}$. Each element e_{ij} gives the expression level of the ith gene at the jth time point. Clustering [2–4], an important microarray analysis tool, is used to identify the sets of genes with similar expression profiles. Clustering methods partition the input space into K regions, depending on some similarity–dissimilarity metric, where the value of K may or may not be known *a priori*. The main objective of any clustering technique is to produce a $K \times n$ partition matrix $U(X)$ of the given data set X, consisting of n patterns, $X = \{x_1, x_2, \ldots, x_n\}$. The partition matrix may be represented as $U = [u_{k,j}]$, $k = 1, 2, \ldots, K$ and $j = 1, 2, \ldots, n$, where $u_{k,j}$ is the membership of pattern x_j to the kth cluster.

In 1995, Storn and Price proposed a new floating point encoded evolutionary algorithm for global optimization [5] and named it differential evolution [6,7], owing to a special kind of differential operator, which they invoked to create new offspring from parent vectors instead of classical mutation. The DE algorithm is a stochastic optimization [8] method minimizing an objective function that can model the

---

Computational Intelligence and Pattern Analysis in Biological Informatics, Edited by Ujjwal Maulik, Sanghamitra Bandyopadhyay, and Jason T. L. Wang

problem's objectives while incorporating constraints. The DE has been used in different fields of engineering and science including unsupervized image classification [9].

This chapter develops a differential evolution-based fuzzy clustering algorithm (DEFC). The superiority of the developed method over genetic algorithm-based fuzzy clustering (GAFC) [10], simulated annealing-based fuzzy clustering (SAFC) [11], and Fuzzy C-Means (FCM) [12], has been demonstrated on four publicly available benchmark microarray data sets, namely, yeast sporulation, yeast cell cycle, arabidopsis thaliana, and human fibroblasts serum. To improve the clustering result further, an SVM is trained with a fraction of the datapoints selected from different clusters based on their proximity to the respective centers. The clustering assignments of the remaining points are thereafter determined using the trained classifier. Finally, a biological significance test has been conducted on yeast sporulation microarray data to establish that the developed integrated technique produces functionally enriched clusters.

11.2 CLUSTERING ALGORITHMS AND VALIDITY MEASURE

This section describes some well-known clustering methods and cluster validity measures.

11.2.1 Clustering Algorithms

11.2.1.1 Fuzzy C-Means Fuzzy C-Means [12] is a widely used technique that uses the principles of fuzzy sets to evolve a partition matrix $U(X)$ while minimizing the measure

$$J_m = \sum_{j=1}^{n} \sum_{k=1}^{K} u_{k,j}^m D^2(z_k, x_j) \quad 1 \leq m \leq \infty \tag{11.1}$$

where n is the number of datapoints, K represents the number of clusters, u is the fuzzy membership matrix (partition matrix), and m denotes the fuzzy exponent. Here, x_j is the jth datapoint and z_k is the center of kth cluster, and $D(z_k, x_j)$ denotes the distance of datapoint x_j from the center of the kth cluster.

The FCM algorithm starts with random initial K cluster centers, and then at every iteration it finds the fuzzy membership of each datapoint to every cluster using Eq. (11.2)

$$u_{k,i} = \frac{\left(\frac{1}{D(z_k, x_i)}\right)^{\frac{1}{m-1}}}{\sum_{j=1}^{K} \left(\frac{1}{D(z_j, x_i)}\right)^{\frac{1}{m-1}}} \quad \text{for} \quad 1 \leq k \leq K \quad 1 \leq i \leq n \tag{11.2}$$

for $1 \leq k \leq K$; $1 \leq i \leq n$, where $D(z_k, x_i)$ and $D(z_j, x_i)$ are the distances between x_i and z_k, and x_i and z_j, respectively. The value of m, the fuzzy exponent, is taken as 2. Note that while computing $u_{k,i}$ using Eq. (11.2), if $D(z_j, x_i)$ is equal to 0 for some

CLUSTERING ALGORITHMS AND VALIDITY MEASURE

j, then $u_{k,i}$ is set to zero for all $k = 1, \ldots, K$, $k \neq j$, while $u_{k,i}$ is set equal to 1. Based on the membership values, the cluster centers are recomputed using Eq. (11.3)

$$z_k = \frac{\sum_{i=1}^{n} u_{k,i}^m x_i}{\sum_{i=1}^{n} u_{k,i}^m} \quad 1 \leq k \leq K \tag{11.3}$$

The algorithm terminates when there is no further change in the cluster centers. Finally, each datapoint is assigned to the cluster to which it has maximum membership. The main disadvantages of the Fuzzy C-Means clustering algorithms are (1) it depends on the initial choice of the center and (2) it often gets trapped into some local optimum.

11.2.1.2 Genetic Algorithm based Fuzzy Clustering

Here we briefly discuss the use of genetic algorithms (GAs) [13] for fuzzy clustering. In GA based fuzzy clustering, the chromosomes are made up of real numbers that represent the coordinates of the centers of the partitions [14]. If chromosome i encodes the centers of K clusters in N-dimensional space, then its length l is $N \times K$. For initializing a chromosome, the K centers are randomly selected points from the data set while ensuring that they are distinct. The fitness of a chromosome indicates the degree of goodness of the solution it represents. In this chapter, J_m is used for this purpose. Therefore, the objective is to minimize J_m for achieving proper clustering. Given a chromosome, the centers encoded in it are first extracted. Let the chromosome encode K centers, and let these be denoted as $z_1, z_2, \ldots, z_K$. The membership values $u_{k,i}$, $k = 1, 2, \ldots, K$ and $i = 1, 2, \ldots, n$ are computed as in Eq. (11.2). The corresponding J_m is computed as in Eq. (11.1). The centers encoded in a chromosome are updated using Eq. (11.3). Conventional proportional selection implemented by the roulette wheel strategy is applied on the population of strings. The standard single-point crossover is applied stochastically with probability μ_c. The cluster centers are considered to be indivisible, (i.e., the crossover points can only lie in between two clusters centers). In [14], each gene position of a chromosome is subjected to mutation with a fixed probability μ_m, resulting in the overall perturbation of the chromosome. A number $\pm$ in the range [0, 1] is generated with uniform distribution. If the value at a gene position is v, after mutation it becomes $(1 \pm 2 \times \delta) \times v$, when $v \neq 0$, and $\pm 2 \times \delta$, when $v = 0$. The $+$ or $-$ signs occurs with equal probability. Note that because of mutation more than one cluster center may be perturbed in a chromosome. The algorithm terminates after a fixed number of generations. The elitist model of GAs has been used, where the best chromosome seen so far are stored in a location within the population. The best chromosome of the last generation provides the solution to the clustering problem.

11.2.1.3 Simulated Annealing-Based Fuzzy Clustering

Simulated annealing (SA) [15] is an optimization tool that has successful applications in a wide range of combinatorial optimization problems. This fact motivated researchers to use a SA to optimize the clustering problem, where it provides near optimal solutions of an objective or fitness function in the complex, large, and multimodal landscapes. In SA based fuzzy clustering [11], a string or configuration encodes K cluster centers. The fuzzy membership of all the points that are encoded in the configuration is computed

p = Random initial configuration.

(Here each configuration encodes K cluster centres)

T = T_{max}.

$E(p)$ = Energy of p is computed using Eq. (11.1).

while(T $\geq T_{min}$)

for i = 1 to k

   s = Perturb (p).

   $E(s)$ = Energy of s is computed using Eq. (11.1).

   if ($E(s)$ - $E(p)$ < 0)

   Set $p = s$ and $E(p) = E(s)$

   else

   if (rand(0,1) < $\frac{exp(-(E(s)-E(p)))}{T}$)

   Set $p = s$ and $E(p) = E(s)$

   end if

   end if

end for

T= T×r. /* 0 < r < 1 */

end while

FIGURE 11.1   The SAFC algorithm.

by using Eq. (11.2). configuration. Subsequently, the string is updated using the new centers [Eq. (11.3)]. Thereafter, the energy function, J_m, is computed as per Eq. (11.1). The current string is perturbed using the mutation operation, as discussed for GAFC. This way, perturbation of a string yields a new string. It's energy is also computed in a similar fashion. If the energy of the new string ($E(s)$) is less than that of the current string ($E(p)$), the new string is accepted. Otherwise, the new string is accepted based on a probability $\frac{exp(-(E(s)-E(p)))}{T}$, where T is the current temperature of the SA process. Figure 11.1 demonstrates the SAFC algorithm.

11.2.2   Cluster Validity Indices

11.2.2.1 $\mathcal{I}$ index   A cluster validity index $\mathcal{I}$, proposed in [16] is defined as follows:

$$\mathcal{I}(K) = \left(\frac{1}{K} \times \frac{E_1}{E_K} \times D_K \right)^p \tag{11.4}$$

where K is the number of clusters. Here,

$$E_K = \sum_{i=1}^{K} \sum_{k=1}^{n} u_{i,k} \parallel z_i - x_k \parallel \tag{11.5}$$

and

$$D_K = \max_{i \neq j} \| z_i - z_j \| \tag{11.6}$$

The index $\mathcal{I}$ is a composition of three factors, namely, $1/K$; E_1/E_K, and D_K. The first factor will try to reduce index $\mathcal{I}$ as K is increased. The second factor consists of the ratio of E_1, which is constant for a given data set, to E_K, which decreases with an increase in K. To compute E_1, the value of K in Eq. (11.5) is taken as 1 (i.e., all the datapoints are considered to be in the same cluster). Hence, because of this term, index $\mathcal{I}$ increases as E_K decreases. This, in turn, indicates that formation of more clusters, which are compact in nature, would be encouraged. Finally, the third factor, D_K, which measures the maximum separation between two clusters over all possible pairs of clusters, will increase with the value of K. However, note that this value is upper bounded by the maximum separation between two datapoints in the data set. Thus, the three factors are found to compete with and balance each other critically. The power p is used to control the contrast between the different cluster configurations. In this chapter, $p = 2$.

11.2.2.2 Silhouette Index

The silhouette index [17] is a cluster validity index that is used to judge the quality of any clustering solution C. Suppose a represents the average distance of a datapoint from the other datapoints of the cluster to which the datapoint is assigned, and b represents the minimum of the average distances of the datapoint from the datapoints of the other clusters. Now, the silhouette width s of the datapoint is defined as

$$s = \frac{b - a}{\max\{a, b\}} \tag{11.7}$$

Silhouette index $s(C)$ is the average silhouette width of all the datapoints and reflects the compactness and separation of clusters. The value of the silhouette index varies from -1 to 1, and higher values indicate a better clustering result.

11.3   DIFFERENTIAL EVOLUTION BASED FUZZY CLUSTERING

11.3.1   Vector Representation and Population Initialization

Each vector is a sequence of real numbers representing the K cluster centers. For an N-dimensional space, the length of a vector is $l = N \times K$, where the first N positions represent the first cluster center. The next N positions represent those of the second cluster center, and so on. The K cluster centers encoded in each vector are initialized to K randomly chosen points from the data set. This process is repeated for each of the P vectors in the population, where P is the size of the population.

11.3.2 Fitness Computation

The fitness of each vector (J_m) is computed using Eq. (11.1). Subsequently, the centers encoded in a vector are updated using Eq. (11.3).

11.3.3 Mutation

The ith individual vector of the population at time-step (generation) t has l components, that is,

$$G_{i,l}(t) = [G_{i,1}(t), G_{i,2}(t), \ldots, G_{i,l}(t)] \tag{11.8}$$

For each target vector $G_{i,l}(t)$ that belongs to the current population, DE samples three other individuals, like $G_{x,l}(t)$, $G_{y,l}(t)$, and $G_{z,l}(t)$ (as describe earlier) from the same generation. Then, the (componentwise) difference is calculated, scale by a scalar F (usually $\in [0, 1]$), and creates a mutant offspring $\vartheta_{i,l}(t + 1)$.

$$\vartheta_{i,l}(t + 1) = G_{x,l}(t) + F\left(G_{y,l}(t) - G_{z,l}(t)\right) \tag{11.9}$$

11.3.4 Crossover

In order to increase the diversity of the perturbed parameter vectors, crossover is introduced. To this end, the trial vector:

$$U_{i,l}(t + 1) = [U_{i,1}(t + 1), U_{i,2}(t + 1), \ldots, U_{i,l}(t + 1)] \tag{11.10}$$

is formed, where

$$U_{ji,l}(t + 1) = \begin{cases} \vartheta_{ji,l}(t + 1) \\ \quad if\ rand_j(0, 1) \leq CR\ or\ j = rand(i) \\ G_{ji,l}(t) \\ \quad if\ rand_j(0, 1) > CR\ and\ j \neq rand(i) \end{cases} \tag{11.11}$$

In Eq. (11.11), $rand_l(0, 1)$ is the lth evaluation of a uniform random number generator with outcome $\in [0, 1]$, CR is the crossover constant $\in [0, 1]$ that has to be determined by the user. $rand(i)$ is a randomly chosen index $\in 1, 2, \ldots, l$ that ensures that $U_{i,l}(t + 1)$ gets at least one parameter from $\vartheta_{i,l}(t + 1)$.

11.3.5 Selection

To decide whether or not it should become a member of generation $G + 1$, the trial vector $U_{i,l}(t + 1)$ is compared to the target vector $G_{i,l}(t)$ using the greedy criterion. If vector $U_{i,l}(t + 1)$ yields a smaller cost function value than $G_{i,l}(t)$, then $U_{i,l}(t + 1)$ is set to $G_{i,l}(t)$; otherwise, the old value $G_{i,l}(t)$ is retained.

11.3.6   Termination Criterion

The processes of mutation, crossover, and selection are executed for a fixed number of iterations. The best vector seen up to the last generation provides the solution to the clustering problem.

11.4   EXPERIMENTAL RESULTS

11.4.1   Gene Expression Data Sets

11.4.1.1 Yeast Sporulation This data set [18] consists of 6118 genes measured across seven time points (0, 0.5, 2, 5, 7, 9, and 11.5 h) during the sporulation process of budding yeast. The data are then log-transformed. The sporulation data set is publicly available at the website http://cmgm.stanford.edu/pbrown/sporulation. Among the 6118 genes, the genes whose expression levels did not change significantly during the harvesting have been ignored from further analysis. This is determined with a threshold level of 1.6 for the root mean squares of the log2-transformed ratios. The resulting set consists of 474 genes.

11.4.1.2 Yeast Cell Cycle The yeast cell cycle data set was extracted from a data set that shows the fluctuation of expression levels of ~6000 genes over two cell cycles (17 time points). Out of these 6000 genes, 384 genes have been selected to be cell-cycle regulated [19]. This data set is publicly available at http://faculty.washington.edu/kayee/cluster.

11.4.1.3 Arabidopsis Thaliana This data set consists of expression levels of 138 genes of Arabidopsis Thaliana. It contains expression levels of the genes over eight time points, namely, 15, 30, 60, 90 min, 3, 6, 9, and 24 h [20]. It is available at http://homes.esat.kuleuven.be/»thijs/Work/Clustering.html.

11.4.1.4 Human Fibroblasts Serum This data set [21] contains the expression levels of 8613 human genes. This data set has 13 dimensions corresponding to 12 time points (0, 0.25, 0.5, 1, 2, 4, 6, 8, 12, 16, 20, and 24 h) and one unsynchronized sample. A subset of 517 genes whose expression levels changed substantially across the time points have been chosen. The data is then log2-transformed. This data set is available at http://www.sciencemag.org/feature/data/984559.shl.

All the data sets are normalized so that each row has mean 0 and variance 1.

11.4.2   Performance Metrics

For evaluating the performance of the clustering algorithms, J_m [12], $\mathcal{I}$ [16], and the silhouette index $s(C)$ [17] are used for four real-life gene expression data sets, respectively. Also, two cluster visualization tools, namely, Eisen plot and cluster profile plot, have been utilized.

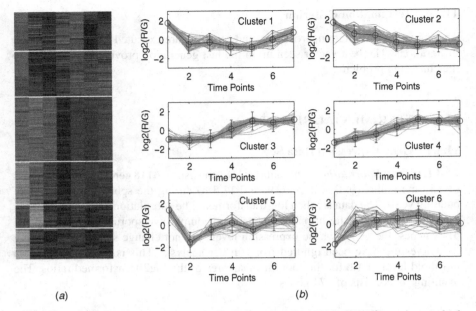

FIGURE 11.2   Yeast sporulation data clustered using the DEFC–SVM clustering method. (*a*) Eisen plot and (*b*) cluster profile plots.

11.4.2.1 Eisen Plot In Eisen plot [22] [e.g., Fig. 11.2(*a*)], the expression value of a gene at a specific time point is represented by coloring the corresponding cell of the data matrix with a color similar to the original color of its spot on the microarray. The shades of red represent higher expression levels, the shades of green represent lower expression levels, and the colors toward black represent absence of differential expression. In our representation, the genes are ordered before plotting so that the genes that belong to the same cluster are placed one after another. The cluster boundaries are identified by white colored blank rows.

11.4.2.2 Cluster Profile Plot The cluster profile plot [e.g., Fig. 11.2(*b*)] shows the normalized gene expression values (light green) for each cluster of the genes of that cluster with respect to the time points. Also, the average expression values of the genes of a cluster over different time points are plotted as a black line together with the standard deviation within the cluster at each time point.

11.4.3   Input Parameters

The population size and number of generation used for DEFC, GAFC, SAFC algorithms are 20 and 100, respectively. The crossover probability (CR) and mutation factors (F) used for DEFC is taken to be 0.7 and 0.8, respectively. The crossover and

TABLE 11.1 Average J_m, $\mathcal{I}$, and $s(C)$ Index Values of > 50 Runs of Different Algorithms for the Four Gene Expression Data Sets

Data Sets	Algorithms	J_m	$\mathcal{I}$	$s(C)$
	DEFC	203.0207	1.2353	0.5591
Yeast Sporulation	GAFC	204.7375	1.0024	0.5421
	SAFC	207.0706	0.9324	0.5372
	FCM	211.5058	0.8447	0.5163
	DEFC	1010.3717	1.0251	0.4184
Yeast Cell Cycle	GAFC	1016.6305	0.9428	0.4006
	SAFC	1014.0771	0.9573	0.4084
	FCM	1020.5317	0.8562	0.3875
	DEFC	205.5307	0.3118	0.3813
Arabidopsis Thaliana	GAFC	209.7050	0.2703	0.3641
	SAFC	207.6405	0.2975	0.3702
	FCM	214.1337	0.2106	0.3351
	DEFC	864.0755	0.9307	0.3628
Human Fibroblasts Serum	GAFC	867.8371	0.9051	0.3443
	SAFC	870.9063	0.8623	0.3307
	FCM	877.5301	0.7885	0.3152

mutation probabilities used for GAFC are taken to be 0.8 and 0.3, respectively. The parameters of the SA based fuzzy clustering algorithm are as follows: $T_{max} = 100$, $T_{min} = 0.01$, $r = 0.9$, and $k = 100$. The FCM algorithm is executed till it converges to the final solution. Note that the input parameters used here are fixed either following the literature or experimentally. For example, the value of fuzzy exponent (m), the scheduling of simulated annealing follows the literature, whereas the crossover, mutation probability, population size, and number of generation is fixed experimentally. The number of clusters for the sporulation, cell cycle, arabidopsis, and serum data sets are taken as 6, 5, 4, and 6, respectively. This conforms to the findings in the literature [18–21].

11.4.4 Results

Table 11.1 reports the average values of J_m, $\mathcal{I}$, and $s(C)$ indices provided by DEFC, GAFC, SAFC, and FCM clustering of >50 runs of the algorithms for the four real-life data sets considered here. The values reported in the tables show that for all the data sets, DEFC provides the best J_m, $\mathcal{I}$, and $s(C)$ index score. For example, for the yeast sporulation data set, the average value of $s(C)$ produces by the DEFC algorithm is 0.5591. The $s(C)$ value produced by GAFC, SAFC and FCM are 0.5421, 0.5372, and 0.5163, respectively. Figures 11.3 and 11.4 demonstrate the boxplot as well as the convergence plot of different algorithms. However, the performance of the proposed DEFC is best for all the data sets.

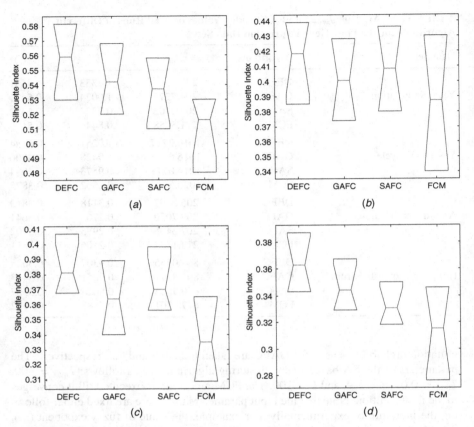

FIGURE 11.3 Boxplot of $s(C)$ for different clustering algorithms on (a) yeast sporulation, (b) yeast cell cycle, (c) Arabidopsis Thaliana, and (d) human fibroblasts serum.

11.5 INTEGRATED FUZZY CLUSTERING WITH SUPPORT VECTOR MACHINES

11.5.1 Support Vector Machines

Support vector machines (SVM) is a learning algorithm originally developed by Vapnik (1995). The SVM classifier is inspired by statistical learning theory and they perform structural risk minimization on a nested set structure of separating hyperplanes [22]. Viewing the input data as two sets of vectors in d-dimensional space, an SVM constructs a separating hyperplane in that space, one that maximizes the margin between the two classes of points. To compute the margin, two parallel hyperplanes are constructed on each side of the separating one, which are "pushed up against" the two classes of points. Intuitively, a good separation is achieved by the hyperplane that has the largest distance to the neighboring datapoints of both

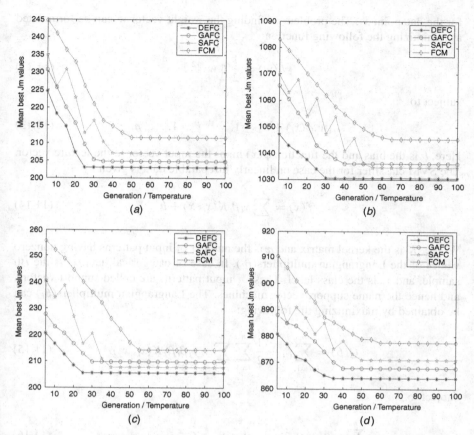

FIGURE 11.4   Convergence plot of different clustering algorithms on (*a*) yeast sporulation, (*b*) yeast cell cycle, (*c*) Arabidopsis Thaliana, and (*d*) human fibroblasts serum.

classes. The larger margins or distances between these parallel hyperplanes indicate a better generalization error of the classifier. Fundamentally, the SVM classifier is designed for two-class problems. It can be extended to handle multiclass problems by designing a number of one-against-all or one-against-one two-class SVMs. For example, a K-class problem is handled with K two-class SVMs.

For linearly nonseparable problems, SVM transforms the input data into a very high-dimensional feature space, and then employs a linear hyperplane for classification. Introduction of a feature space creates a computationally intractable problem. The SVM handle this by defining appropriate kernels so that the problem can be solved in the input space itself. The problem of maximizing the margin can be reduced to the solution of a convex quadratic optimization problem, which has a unique global minimum.

We consider a binary classification training data problem. Suppose a data set consists of n feature vectors $< x_i, y_i >$, where $y_i \in \{+1, -1\}$ denotes the class label for the datapoint x_i. The problem of finding the weight vector w can be formulated as minimizing the following function:

$$L(w) = \frac{1}{2} \parallel w \parallel^2 \tag{11.12}$$

subject to

$$y_i[w.\phi(x_i) + b] \geq 1, \qquad i = 1, \ldots, n \tag{11.13}$$

Here, b is the bias and the function $\phi(x)$ maps the input vector to the feature vector. The SVM classifier for the case on linearly inseparable data is given by

$$f(x) = \sum_{i=1}^{n} y_i \beta_i K(x_i, x) + b \tag{11.14}$$

Where, K is the kernel matrix and n is the number of input patterns having nonzero values of the Langrangian multipliers(β_i). In case of categorical data, x_i is the ith sample, and y_i is the class label. These n input patterns are called support vectors, and hence the name support vector machines. The Langrangian multipliers(β_i) can be obtained by maximizing the following:

$$Q(\beta) = \sum_{i=1}^{n} \beta_i - \frac{1}{2} \sum_{i=1}^{n} \sum_{j=1}^{n} y_i y_j \beta_i \beta_j K(x_i, x_j) \tag{11.15}$$

subject to

$$\sum_{i=1}^{n} y_i \beta_i = 0 \quad \text{and} \quad 0 \leq \beta_i \leq C \quad i = 1, \ldots, n \tag{11.16}$$

Where, C is the cost parameter, which controls the number of nonseparable points. Increasing C will increase the number of support vectors, thus allowing fewer errors, but making the boundary separating the two classes more complex. On the other hand, a low value of C allows more nonseparable points, and therefore, has a simpler boundary. Only a small fraction of the β_i coefficients are nonzero. The corresponding pairs of x_i entries are known as support vectors and they fully define the decision function. Geometrically, the support vectors are the points lying near the separating hyperplane, where $K(x_i, x_j) = \phi(x_i).\phi(x_j)$ is called the *kernel function*. The kernel function may be linear or nonlinear, like polynomial, sigmoidal, radial basis functions (RBF), and soon. The RBF kernels are of the following form:

$$K(x_i, x_j) = e^{-w|x_i - x_j|^2} \tag{11.17}$$

where x_i denotes the ith datapoint and w is the weight. In this chapter, the above mentioned RBF kernel is used. Also, the extended version of the two-class SVM

Step1: Execute fuzzy clustering to obtain a best solution vector consisting of cluster centers.

Step2: Select 50% of datapoints from each cluster which are nearest to the respective cluster centres. The class labels of the points are set to the respective cluster number.

Step3: Train a SVM classifier with the points selected in step 2.

Step4: Generatethe classlabelsfortheremaining points using thetrainedSVM classifier.

FIGURE 11.5   Algorithm of integrated fuzzy clusteing with SVM.

that deals with the multiclass classification problem by designing a number of one-against-all two-class SVMs, is used here.

11.5.2   Improving Fuzzy Clustering with SVM

This section describes the developed scheme for combining the fuzzy clustering algorithm (DEFC, GAFC, SAFC, or FCM) described in Sections 11.2 and 11.3 with the SVM classifier. This is motivated due to the fact that the presence of training points, supervised classification usually performs better than the unsupervised classification or clustering. In this chapter, we have exploited this advantage while selecting some training points using the differential evolution-based fuzzy clustering technique and the concept of proximity of the points from the respective cluster centers. The basic steps are described in Figure 11.5.

11.5.3   Results

Table 11.2 show the results in terms of $s(C)$ obtained by the integrated clustering algorithm for the four gene expression data sets, respectively. It can be seen from this table that irrespective of the clustering method used in the developed algorithm, the performance gets improved after the application of SVM. For example, in the case

TABLE 11.2   Average Values of $s(C)$ for the Integrated Fuzzy Clustering Algorithm Over 50 runs

Data Sets	Sporulation	Cell Cycle	Thaliana	Serum
DEFC–SVM	0.5797	0.4217	0.4037	0.3803
GAFC–SVM	0.5517	0.4113	0.3802	0.3592
SAFC–SVM	0.5404	0.4206	0.3931	0.3504
FCM–SVM	0.5233	0.3907	0.3408	0.3274

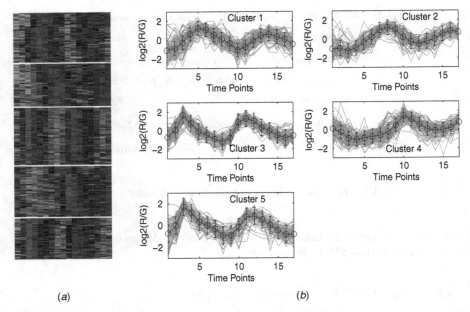

FIGURE 11.6   Yeast cell cycle data clustered using the DEFC–SVM clustering method. (*a*) Eisen plot and (*b*) cluster profile plots.

of yeast sporulation, the $s(C)$ values produced by DEAFC is 0.5591 while this gets improved to 0.5797 when SVM is used. A similar result is found for another data set also. The results demonstrate the utility of adopting the approach presented in this paper, irrespective of the clustering method used.

To demonstrate visually the result of DEFC–SVM clustering, Figures 11.2, 11.6–11.8 show the Eisen plot and cluster profile plots provided by DEFC–SVM on the two data sets, respectively. For example, the six clusters of the yeast sporulation data are very prominent, as shown in the Eisen plot [Fig. 11.2(*a*)]. It is evident from this figure that the expression profiles of the genes of a cluster are similar to each other and produce similar color patterns. The cluster profile plots [Fig. 11.2(*b*)] also demonstrate how the expression profiles for the different groups of genes differ from each other, while the profiles within a group are reasonably similar. A similar result is obtained for the other data set.

11.5.4   Biological Significance

The biological relevance of a cluster can be verified based on the statistically significant gene ontology (GO) annotation database (http://db.yeastgenome.org/cgi-bin/GO/goTermFinder). This is used to test the functional enrichment of a group of genes in terms of three structured, controlled vocabularies (ontologies), namely, associated biological processes, molecular functions, and biological components. The

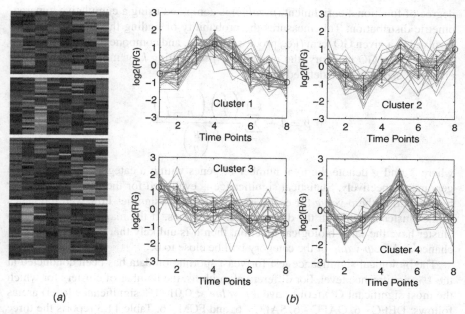

FIGURE 11.7 Arabidopsis Thaliana data clustered using the DEFC–SVM clustering method. (*a*) Eisen plot and (*b*) Cluster profile plots.

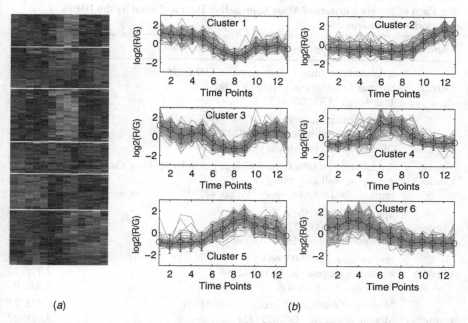

FIGURE 11.8 Human fibroblasts serum data clustered using the DEFC–SVM clustering method. (*a*) Eisen plot and (*b*) Cluster profile plots.

degree of functional enrichment (*p-value*) is computed using a cumulative hypergeometric distribution. This measures the probability of finding the number of genes involved in a given GO term (i.e., process, function, and component) within a cluster. From a given GO category, the probability p of getting k or more genes within a cluster of size n, can be defined as [23]:

$$p = 1 - \sum_{i=0}^{k-1} \frac{\binom{f}{i}\binom{g-f}{n-i}}{\binom{g}{n}} \tag{11.18}$$

where f and g denote the total number of genes within a category and within the genome, respectively. Statistical significance is evaluated for the genes in a cluster by computing the *p-value* for each GO category. This signifies how well the genes in the cluster match with the different GO categories. If the majority of genes in a cluster have the same biological function, then it is unlikely that this takes place by chance and the *p-value* of the category will be close to 0.

The biological significance test for yeast sporulation data has been conducted at the 1% significance level. For different algorithms, the number of clusters for which the most significant GO terms have a *p-value* < 0.01 (1% significance level) are as follows: DEFC - 6, GAFC - 6, SAFC - 6, and FCM - 6. Table 11.3 reports the three

TABLE 11.3 The Three Most Significant GO Terms and the Corresponding *p-Values* for Each of the Six Clusters of Yeast Sporulation Data as Found by the IDEFC Clustering Technique

Clusters	Significant GO term	*p-values*
Cluster1	Structural constituent of ribosome - GO:0003735 Structural molecule activity - GO:0005198 Translation - GO:0006412	1.13E-40 1.22E-35 1.73E-20
Cluster2	Glucose catabolic process - GO:0006007 Fungal-type cell wall - GO:0009277 Glucose metabolic process - GO:0006006	3.13E-06 5.02E-06 6.28E-05
Cluster3	Sporulation resulting in formation of a cellular spore - GO:0030435 Ascospore wall assembly - GO:0030476 Intracellular immature spore - GO:0042763	9.04E-22 9.52E-20 4.24E-8
Cluster4	Spindle - GO:0005819 M phase - GO:0000279 Microtubule cytoskeleton - GO:0015630	2.44E-06 3.31E-05 9.72E-05
Cluster5	Preribosome - GO:0030684 Ribosome biogenesis - GO:0042254 rRNA metabolic process - GO:0016072	2.64E-20 2.79E-14 2.03E-9
Cluster6	M phase of meiotic cell cycle - GO:0051327 Meiotic cell cycle - GO:0051321 Condensed nuclear chromosome - GO:0000794	3.53E-21 4.62E-22 4.17E-13

most significant GO terms (along with the corresponding *p-values*) shared by the genes of each of the six clusters identified by the DEFC technique (Fig. 11.2). As is evident from the table, all the clusters produced by DEFC clustering scheme are significantly enriched with some GO categories, since all the *p-values* are < 0.01 (1% significance level). This establishes that the developed DEFC clustering scheme is able to produce biologically relevant and functionally enriched clusters.

11.6 CONCLUSION

In this chapter, a differential evolution-based fuzzy clustering technique has been described for the analysis of microarry gene expression data sets. The problem of fuzzy clustering has been modeled as one of optimization of a cluster validity measure. Results on different gene expression date sets indicate that DEFC consistently performs better than GAFC, SAFC, and FCM clustering techniques. To improve the performance of clustering further, a SVM classifier is trained with a fraction of gene expression datapoints selected from each cluster based on the proximity to the respective cluster centers. Subsequently, the remaining gene expression datapoints are reassigned using the trained SVM classifier. Experimental results indicate that this approach is likely to yield better results irrespective of the actual clustering technique adopted.

As a scope of further research, the use of kernel functions other than RBF may be studied. A sensitivity analysis of the developed technique with respect to different setting of the parameters, including the fraction of the points to be used for training the SVM, needs to be carried out. Moreover, the DE based algorithm can be extended in the multiobject framework and the results need to be compared with other related techniques [12, 20].

REFERENCES

1. S. Bandyopadhyay, U. Maulik, and J. T. Wang (2007), *Analysis of Biological Data: A Soft Computing Approach.* World Scientific, NY.
2. B. S. Everitt (1993), *Cluster Analysis*, 3rd ed., Halsted Press, NY.
3. J. A. Hartigan (1975), *Clustering Algorithms*, Wiley, NY.
4. A. K. Jain and R. C. Dubes (1988), *Algorithms for Clustering Data*, Prentice-Hall, Englewood Cliffs, NJ.
5. R. Storn and K. Price (1995), Differential evolution—A simple and efficient adaptive scheme for global optimization over continuous spaces, *Tech. Rep. TR-95-012, International Computer Science Institute, Berkley.*
6. K. Price, R. Storn, and J. Lampinen (2005), *Differential Evolution—A Practical Approach to Global Optimization*, Springer, Berlin.
7. R. Storn and K. Price (1997), Differential evolution—A simple and efficient heuristic strategy for global optimization over continuous spaces, *J. Global Opt.*, 11:341–359.
8. A. Zilinska and A. Zhigljavsky (2008), *Stochastic global optimization*, Springer, NY.

9. M. Omran, A. Engelbrecht, and A. Salman (2005), Differential evolution methods for unsupervised image classification, *Proc. IEEE Int. Conf. Evol. Comput.*, 2:966–973.

10. M. K. Pakhira, S. Bandyopadhyay, and U. Maulik (2005), A study of some fuzzy cluster validity indices, genetic clustering and application to pixel classification, *Fuzzy Sets Systems*, 155:191–214.

11. S. Bandyopadhyay (2005), Simulated annealing using a reversible jump markov chain monte carlo algorithm for fuzzy clustering, *IEEE Trans. Knowledge Data Eng.*, 17(4):479–490.

12. J. C. Bezdek (1981), *Pattern Recognition with Fuzzy Objective Function Algorithms*, Plenum, New York.

13. D. E. Goldberg (1989), *Genetic Algorithms in Search, Optimization and Machine Learning*, Addison-Wesley, NY.

14. U. Maulik and S. Bandyopadhyay (2000), Genetic algorithm based clustering technique, *Pattern Recognition*, 33:1455–1465.

15. S. Kirkpatrik, C. D. Gelatt, and M. P. Vecchi (1983), Optimization by simulated annealing, *Science*, 220:671–680.

16. U. Maulik and S. Bandyopadhyay (2002), Performance evaluation of some clustering algorithms and validity indices, *IEEE Trans. Pattern Anal. Machine Intelligence*, 24(12):1650–1654.

17. P. J. Rousseeuw (1987), Silhouettes: a graphical aid to the interpretation and validation of cluster analysis, *J. Compt. App. Math*, 20:53–65.

18. S. Chu, J. DeRisi, M. Eisen, J. Mulholland, D. Botstein, P. O. Brown, and I. Herskowitz (1998), The transcriptional program of sporulation in budding yeast, *Science*, 282:699–705.

19. R. J. Cho et al. (1998), A genome-wide transcriptional analysis of mitotic cell cycle, *Mol. Cell.*, 2:65–73.

20. P. Reymonda, H. Webera, M. Damonda, and E. E. Farmera (2000), Differential gene expression in response to mechanical wounding and insect feeding in arabidopsis, *Plant Cell.*, 12:707–720.

21. V. R. Iyer, M. B. Eisen, D. T. Ross, G. Schuler, T. Moore, J. Lee, J. M. Trent, L. M. Staudt, J. J. Hudson, M. S. Boguski, D. Lashkari, D. Shalon, D. Botstein, and P. O. Brown (1999), The transcriptional program in the response of the human fibroblasts to serum, *Science*, 283:83–87.

22. M. B. Eisen, P. T. Spellman, P. O. Brown, and D. Botstein (1998), Cluster analysis and display og genome-wide expression patterns. *Proc. Nato. Acad. Scie.* USA, pp. 14863–14868.

23. S. Tavazoie, J. Hughes, M. Campbell, R. Cho, and G. Church (1999), Systematic determination of genetic network architecture, *Nature Genet.*, 22:281–285.

24. V. Vapnik (1998), *Statistical Learning Theory*, John Wiley & Sons, Inc., NY.

12

IDENTIFYING POTENTIAL GENE MARKERS USING SVM CLASSIFIER ENSEMBLE

ANIRBAN MUKHOPADHYAY, UJJWAL MAULIK, AND
SANGHAMITRA BANDYOPADHYAY

12.1 INTRODUCTION

An important task in modern data mining is to utilize advanced data analysis and integration tools in gene expression pattern discovery and classification. These tools include a number of machine learning techniques, which may help in identifying relevant features for diagnostic and system biology studies. Furthermore, discovery of novel automated techniques for intelligent information retrieval and knowledge representation are crucial for biological data analysis. When a living cell undergoes a biological process, not all of its genes are expressed at the same time. Function of a cell is critically related to the gene expression at a given time and their relative abundance. For understanding biological processes, it is usual to measure gene expression levels in different developmental phases, body tissues, clinical conditions, and organisms. This information of differential gene expression can be utilized in characterizing gene function, determining experimental treatment effects, and understanding other molecular biological processes. Traditional approaches to genomic research was based on examining and collecting data for a single gene locally. The progress in the field of microarray technology has made possible to the study of the expression levels of a large number of genes across different time points or tumor samples [1–5]. Microarray technology has its application in a wide variety of fields, including medical diagnosis and cancer classification. Supervised classification is usually used

Computational Intelligence and Pattern Analysis in Biological Informatics, Edited by Ujjwal Maulik,
Sanghamitra Bandyopadhyay, and Jason T. L. Wang
Copyright © 2010 John Wiley & Sons, Inc.

to classify the tissue samples into two classes, namely, normal (benign) and cancerous (malignant) or into their subclasses, considering the genes as classification features [6–9]. For successful diagnosis and treatment of cancer, it is important to have a precise and reliable classification of tumors. Classical methods for classifying human malignancies rely on various morphological, clinical, and molecular variables. In spite of recent progress, there are still uncertainties in diagnosis. Also, it is likely that the existing classes are heterogeneous and comprise diseases that are molecularly distinct and follow different clinical courses. Deoxyribonucleic acid (DNA) microarrays may be used to characterize the molecular variations among tumors by monitoring gene expression profiles on a genomic scale. This leads to a finer and more reliable classification of tumors, which in turn helps to identify marker genes that distinguish among these classes. Eventually this improves the ability to understand and predict cancer survival. There are several classification approaches studied by bioinformatics researchers, among which support vector machine (SVM) classifier [10, 11] has been widely used for this purpose [12–18]. The SVMs are powerful classification systems based on regularization techniques and provide excellent performance in many practical classification problems.

In this chapter, we have employed a SVM classifier to analyze a microarray matrix. The SVM classifiers use different kernel functions of which, four kernel functions, namely, *linear, polynomial, sigmoidal,* and *radial basis function (RBF)* are used. As different kernel functions can produce different classification results even when they are trained by the same set of samples, in this study we have used a majority voting ensemble technique to combine the classification results of the different kernel functions. Subsequently, this classification result is utilized to identify relevant gene markers based on SNR statistics followed by a feature selection method based on multiobjective genetic algorithm [19–21].

The performance of the proposed technique has been demonstrated on three publicly available benchmark cancer data sets, namely, leukemia, colon cancer, and lymphoma data. The experimental results establish the utility of the proposed ensemble classification technique. Moreover, relevant gene markers are identified from the four data sets that are responsible for different types of cancer.

12.2 MICROARRAY GENE EXPRESSION DATA

A microarray is typically a glass (or some other material) slide, on to which DNA molecules are attached at fixed locations (spots) [22]. There may be tens of thousands of spots on an array, each containing a huge number of identical DNA molecules (or fragments of identical molecules), of lengths from 20 to hundreds of nucleotides. Each of these molecules ideally should identify one gene or one exon in the genome. The chip is made of chemically coated glass, nylon, membrane, or silicon. Each grid cell of a microarray chip corresponds to a DNA sequence. For a cyclic DNA (cDNA) microarray experiment, the first step is to extract ribonucleic acid (RNA) from a tissue sample and amplification of RNA. Thereafter two messenger RNA (mRNA) samples are reverse transcribed into cDNA (targets) labeled using different fluorescent dyes (red-fluorescent dye Cy5 and green-fluorescent dye Cy3). Due to the complementary nature of the base pairs, the cDNA binds to the specific oligonucleotides on the array. In the subsequent stage, the dye is excited by a laser so that the amount of cDNA can be quantified by measuring the fluorescence intensities. The log ratio of two intensities of each dye is used as the gene expression profile.

$$\text{gene expression level} = \log_2 \frac{\text{Intensity(Cy5)}}{\text{Intensity(Cy3)}} \tag{12.1}$$

The spots are either printed on the microarrays by a robot, or synthesized by photolithography (as in computer chip productions), or by ink-jet printing. Many important questions can potentially be answered by analyzing and interpreting microarray data [23].

A microarray gene expression data consisting of s tissue samples and g genes are usually expressed as a real valued $s \times g$ matrix $M = [m_{ij}]$, $i = 1, 2, \ldots, s$ and $j = 1, 2, \ldots, g$. Here, each element m_{ij} represents the expression level of the jth gene in the ith sample.

$$M = \begin{bmatrix} m_{11} & m_{12} & \cdots & m_{1g} \\ m_{21} & m_{22} & \cdots & m_{2g} \\ \vdots & \vdots & \ddots & \vdots \\ m_{s1} & m_{s2} & \cdots & m_{sg} \end{bmatrix}$$

The raw gene expression data consists of noise, some variations arising from biological experiments and missing values. Hence, the raw data is preprocessed before it is used for any analysis. Two widely used preprocessing techniques are missing value estimation and standardization. Standardization is a statistical tool for transforming data into a format that can be used for meaningful analysis [4]. Normalization is a useful standardization process by which each row of the matrix M is standardized to have mean 0 and variance 1. The following preprocessing techniques are used here. First, some filtering is applied on the raw data to filter out those genes whose expression levels do not change significantly over different time points. Next, the expression values are log transformed and each row is normalized to have mean 0 and variance 1.

12.3 SUPPORT VECTOR MACHINE CLASSIFIER

Support vector machine classifiers are inspired by statistical learning theory and they perform structural risk minimization on a nested set structure of separating hyperplanes [10,11]. Viewing the input data as two sets of vectors in a d-dimensional space, an SVM constructs a separating hyperplane in that space, which maximizes the margin between the two classes of points. To compute the margin, two parallel hyperplanes are constructed on each side of the separating one, which are "pushed up against" the two classes of points (Fig. 12.1). Intuitively, a good separation is achieved by the hyperplane that has the largest distance to the neighboring datapoints of both classes. A larger margin or distance between these parallel hyperplanes indicates

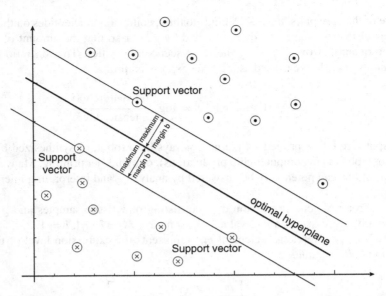

FIGURE 12.1 Example of maximally separating hyperplanes and support vectors for a linearly separable classes

a better generalization error of the classifier. Fundamentally, the SVM classifier is designed for two-class problems. It can be extended to handle multiclass problems by designing a number of one-against-all or one-against-one two-class SVMs.

Suppose a data set consisting of n feature vectors $< x_i, y_i >$, where $y_i \in \{+1, -1\}$, denotes the class label for the datapoint x_i. The problem of finding the weight vector w can be formulated as minimizing the following function:

$$L(w) = \frac{1}{2}||w||^2 \tag{12.2}$$

subject to

$$y_i[w.\phi(x_i) + b] \geq 1, \quad i = 1, \ldots, n \tag{12.3}$$

Here, b is the bias and the function $\phi(x)$ maps the input vector to the feature vector. The dual formulation is given by maximizing the following:

$$Q(\alpha) = \sum_{i=1}^{n} \alpha_i - \frac{1}{2} \sum_{i=1}^{n} \sum_{j=1}^{n} y_i y_j \alpha_i \alpha_j \mathcal{K}(x_i, x_j) \tag{12.4}$$

subject to

$$\sum_{i=1}^{n} y_i \alpha_i = 0 \quad \text{and} \quad 0 \leq \alpha_i \leq C, \quad i = 1, \ldots, n \tag{12.5}$$

Only a small fraction of the α_i coefficients are nonzero. The corresponding pairs of x_i entries are known as support vectors and they fully define the decision function. Geometrically, the support vectors are the points lying near the separating hyperplane. $\mathcal{K}(x_i, x_j) = \phi(x_i).\phi(x_j)$ is called the *kernel function*.

Kernel functions are used for mapping the input space to a higher dimensional feature space so that the classes become linearly separable. Use of four popularly used kernel functions has been studied in this chapter. These are

Linear: $K(x_i, x_j) = x_i^T x_j,$

Polynomial: $K(x_i, x_j) = (\gamma x_i^T x_j + r)^d,$

Sigmoidal: $K(x_i, x_j) = \tanh(\kappa(x_i^T x_j) + \theta), \kappa > 0, \theta < 0,$

RBF: $K(x_i, x_j) = e^{-\gamma|x_i - x_j|^2}, \gamma > 0.$

12.4   PROPOSED TECHNIQUE

The proposed method consists of two main phases. In the first phase, SVM classifier and ensembling is used for classification purposes. In the subsequent phase, the classification result is used to identify the gene markers.

12.4.1   Phase-I: SVM Classification and Ensemble

From the input preprocessed data set, 50% of the samples are chosen randomly as the training samples. These samples are used to train the four SVM classifiers with four kernel functions mentioned above, respectively. The remaining 50% of the samples are then classified by the four trained classifiers. This process is repeated 50 times resulting in 200 classification solutions. Finally, these solutions are combined through *majority voting ensemble* to produce a single classification of the samples. The whole process is repeated for 50 data sets created through bootstrapping of samples and genes and the best classification of samples (in terms of classification accuracy) is chosen finally for further processing.

12.4.2   Phase-II: Identification of Gene Markers

Phase two consists of two stages. First, most potential genes are selected based on signal-to-noise ratio (SNR) statistic. Thereafter, a multiobjective genetic algorithm-based feature selection method is employed in order to further reduce the number of selected gene markers.

Stage-I. The final classification result obtained in the previous phase is used to identify the relevant gene markers as follows: Each data set has two classes, one corresponds to normal samples and the other corresponds to malignant samples. For each gene, a statistic called SNR [8] is computed. The SNR is defined as

$$\text{SNR} = \frac{\mu_1 - \mu_2}{\sigma_1 + \sigma_2} \tag{12.6}$$

where μ_i and σ_i, $i \in \{1, 2\}$, denote the mean and standard deviation of class i for the corresponding gene. Note that a larger absolute value of SNR for a gene indicates that the gene's expression level is high in one class and low in another. Hence this bias is very useful in distinguishing the genes that are expressed differently in the two classes of samples.

After computing the SNR statistic for each gene, the genes are sorted in descending order of their SNR values. From the sorted list, the genes whose SNR values are grater than the average SNR value are selected. These genes are mostly responsible for distinguishing the two sample classes.

Stage-II. The set of genes obtained is further reduced by a feature selection technique based on multiobjective genetic algorithm. In this technique, each *chromosome* is represented as a binary string of length equal to the number of genes selected through the SNR method. The chromosomes encode the information of whether a gene is selected or not. For a chromosome, bit '1' indicates that the corresponding gene is selected, and bit '0' indicates that the corresponding gene is not selected. Here, we have used the nondominated sorting genetic algorithm-II (NSGA-II) [24], a popular multiobjective GA, as the underlying optimization tool. The two objective functions are the *classification accuracy* and the *number of selected genes*. The classification accuracy is computed by training a SVM classifier by half of the samples selected randomly, while predicting the class labels of the remaining samples by the trained SVM classifier. The same ensemble technique for combining the four different kernel solutions is used. Note that SVM training and testing is done for the subset of genes encoded in the chromosome. The goal is to maximize the first objective while minimizing the second one simultaneously. The crowded binary tournament selection method as used in [24] followed by conventional *uniform crossover* and *bit-flip mutation* operators are used to produce child population from a parent population. From the final nondominated front, the solution with the maximum classification accuracy is selected and the corresponding gene subset is selected as the final set of gene markers.

The different parameters of NSGA-II are selected as follows: number of generations = 100, population size = 50, crossover probability = 0.8, mutation probability = 0.1. All the parameters are set experimentally. Figure 12.2 summarizes the different steps of the two phases.

12.5 DATA SETS AND PREPROCESSING

Three publicly available benchmark cancer data sets, namely, leukemia, colon cancer, and lymphoma data sets have been used for experiments. The data sets and their preprocessing are described in this section.

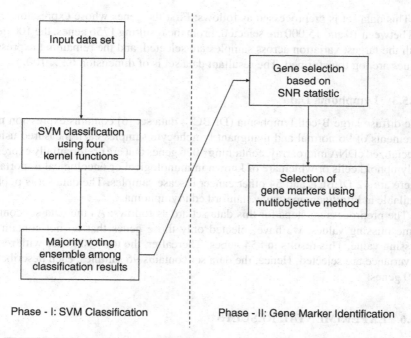

FIGURE 12.2 Summary of different steps of two phases of the proposed method

12.5.1   Leukemia Data

The leukemia data set [8] consists of 72 tissue samples. The samples consist of two types of leukemia, 25 of AML and 47 of ALL. The samples are taken from 63 bone marrow samples and 9 peripheral blood samples. There are 7129 genes in the data set. The data set is publicly available at http://www.genome.wi.mit.edu/MPR.

The data set is subjected to a number of preprocessing steps to find out the genes with most variability. The initial gene selection steps followed here are also completely unsupervised. However, more sophisticated methods for gene selection could have been applied. First, we have selected the genes whose expression levels fall between 100 and 15,000. From the resulting 1015 genes, the 100 genes with the largest variation across samples are selected, and the remaining expression values are log-transformed. The resultant data set is of dimension 72×100.

12.5.2   Colon Cancer Data

The colon cancer data set [7] consists of 62 samples of colon epithelial cells from colon cancer patients. The samples consists of tumor biopsies collected from tumors (40 samples), and normal biopsies collected from healthy parts of the colons (22 samples) of the same patient. The number of genes in the data set is 2000. The data set is publicly available at http://microarray.princeton.edu/oncology.

This data set is preprocessed as follows: First the genes whose expression levels fall between 10 and 15,000 are selected. From the resulting 1756 genes, the 100 genes with the largest variation across samples are selected, and the remaining expression values are log transformed. The resultant data set is of dimension 62×100.

12.5.3 Lymphoma Data

The diffuse large B-cell lymphoma (DLBCL) data set [6] contains expression measurements of 96 normal and malignant lymphocyte samples each measured using a specialized cDNA microarray, containing 4026 genes that are preferentially expressed in lymphoid cells or which are of known immunological or oncological importance. There are 42 DLBCL and 54 other cancer disease samples. The data set is publicly available at http://genome-www.stanford.edu/lymphoma.

The preprocessing steps for this data set are as follows: As the data set contains some missing values, we have selected only those genes that do not contain any missing value. This results in 854 genes. Thereafter, the top 100 genes with respect to variance are selected. Hence, the data set contains 96 samples, each described by 100 genes.

12.6   EXPERIMENTAL RESULTS

This section first demonstrates the utility of the proposed ensemble classifier method on the three publicly available microarray data sets used for experiments. Thereafter, we have discussed the gene markers identified in the second phase of the proposed technique.

12.6.1   Classification Results

Table 12.1 reports the percentage classification accuracy obtained by individual kernel functions, as well as by the majority voting ensemble method. It is evident from the table that the ensemble classification provides better classification accuracy compared to that provided by each of the kernel functions. This demonstrates the utility of the proposed ensemble classification technique.

TABLE 12.1   Percentage Classification Accuracy Obtained by Different Kernel Functions and Their Ensemble for All the Data Sets

SVM kernel	Leukemia	Colon	Lymphoma
Linear	76.2	75.0	71.4
Polynomial	80.9	87.5	86.3
Sigmoidal	85.7	90.3	82.6
RBF	90.4	89.4	84.6
Ensemble	95.2	92.5	89.5

TABLE 12.2   Number of Gene Markers Selected for Different Data Sets and Performance of Ensemble Classifier on the Set of all 100 Genes and on the Set of Marker Genes in Terms of Classification Accuracy

Data Set	No. Gene Markers	Ensemble Classifier on all 100 Genes	Ensemble Classifier on Marker Genes
Leukemia	11	95.2	100
Colon cancer	8	92.5	97.3
Lymphoma	9	89.5	93.8

12.6.2   Identification of Gene Markers

Table 12.2 reports the number of gene markers obtained as above for the three data sets. The numbers of gene markers for the three data sets are 11, 8, and 9, respectively. This table also reports the classification accuracy obtained by the proposed ensemble classification technique on the complete preprocessed data sets (with 100 genes) and on the reduced data set consisting of the marker genes only. It is evident from this table that the performance of the proposed technique gets improved when applied to the data set with the identified marker genes only. This indicates the ability of the gene markers to distinguish the two types of samples in all the data sets.

12.6.2.1 Gene Markers for Leukemia Data   In Figure 12.3, the heatmap of the gene versus sample matrix, where the rows correspond to the top 30 genes in terms of SNR statistic scores, and the columns correspond to the ALL and AML samples, is shown. The cells of the heatmap represent the expression levels of the genes in terms of colors. The shades of dark gray represent higher expression level, the shades of light gray represent low expression level, and the colors toward black represent absence of differential expression values. The eleven gene markers identified as discussed are placed at the top 11 rows of the heatmap. It is evident from the figure that these eleven gene markers discriminate the AML samples from the ALL ones. The characteristics of the gene markers are as follows: The genes M92287_at, HG1612-HT1612_at, X51521_at, Z15115_at, U22376_cds2_s_at, X67951_at are upregulated in the ALL samples and downregulated in the AML samples. On the other hand, the genes M63138_at, X62320_at, HG2788-HT2896_at, U46751,_at and L08246_at are downregulated in the ALL samples and upregulated in the AML samples. In Table 12.3, we have reported the eleven gene markers along with their description and associated gene ontological (GO) terms. It is evident from this table that all the eleven genes share most of the GO terms that indicating that these genes have similar molecular functions (mainly related to cell, cell part, and organelle).

12.6.2.2 Gene Markers for Colon Cancer Data   Figure 12.4 shows the heatmap of the gene versus sample matrix for the top 30 gene markers of colon cancer data. The eight gene markers identified as discussed are placed at the top eight rows

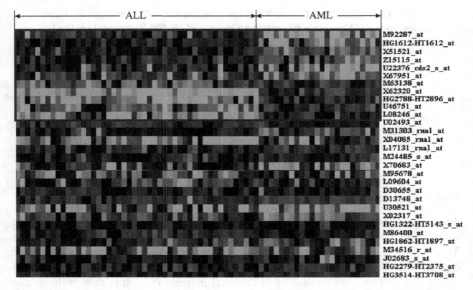

FIGURE 12.3 Heatmap of the expression levels of top 30 gene markers distinguishing the AML and ALL samples of leukemia data in terms of SNR statistic. Dark/light gray represent up/down regulation relative to black. The selected eleven markers are put in the first eleven rows.

TABLE 12.3 The Description and Associated Gene Ontological (GO) Terms for the Eleven Gene Markers Identified in Leukemia Data

AFFY_ID	Gene Description	Gene Function (GO Terms)
M92287_at	cyclin d3	cell, macromolecular complex, organelle, cell part
HG1612-HT1612_at	marcks-like 1	cell, cell part
X51521_at	villin 2 (ezrin)	cell, organelle, organelle part, cell part
Z15115_at	topoisomerase (dna) ii beta 180kda	cell, membrane-enclosed lumen, organelle, organelle part, cell part
U22376_cds2_s_at	v-myb myeloblastosis viral oncogene homolog (avian)	cell, membrane-enclosed lumen, macromolecular complex, organelle, organelle part, cell part
X67951_at	peroxiredoxin 1	cell, organelle, cell part
M63138_at	cathepsin d (lysosomal aspartyl peptidase)	extracellular region, cell, organelle, cell part
X62320_at	granulin	extracellular region, cell, organelle, extracellular region part, cell part
HG2788-HT2896_at	s100 calcium-binding protein a6 (calcyclin)	cell, envelope, organelle, organelle part, cell part
U46751_at	sequestosome 1	cell, organelle, cell part
L08246_at	myeloid cell leukemia sequence 1 (bcl2-related)	cell, envelope, organelle, organelle part, cell part

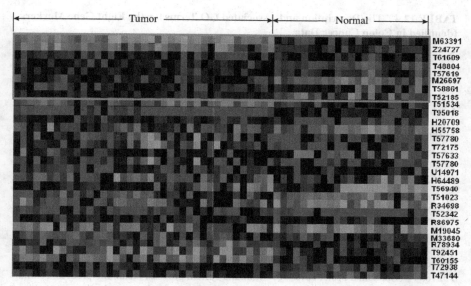

FIGURE 12.4 Heatmap of the expression levels top 30 gene markers distinguishing the tumor and normal samples of colon cancer data in terms of SNR statistic. Dark/light gray represent up–down regulation relative to black. The selected eight markers are put in the first eight rows.

of the heatmap. It is evident from visual inspection that these eight gene markers partitions the tumor samples from the normal ones. The characteristics of the gene markers are as follows: The genes M63391 and Z24727 are downregulated in the tumor samples and upregulated in the normal samples. On the contrary, the genes T61609, T48804, T57619, M26697, T58861, and T52185 are upregulated in the tumor samples and downregulated in the normal samples. In Table 12.4, the eight gene markers are described along with the associated GO terms. It is evident from this table that all eight genes are mainly take part in metabolic process, cellular process, gene expression, and share most of the GO terms. This indicates that these genes have similar molecular functions.

12.6.2.3 Gene Markers for Lymphoma Data In Figure 12.5, the heatmap for the top 30 gene markers for lymphoma data is shown. The topmost nine gene markers selected using the proposed method are placed at the top nine rows of the heatmap. Visual inspection reveals that these nine gene markers efficiently distinguish the DLBCL samples from the non-DLBCL ones. The characteristics of the gene markers are as follows: The genes 19335, 19338, 20344, 18344, 19368, 20392, and 16770 are upregulated in the non-DLBCL samples and downregulated in the DLBCL samples. On the other hand, the genes 13684 and 16044 are downregulated in the non-DLBCL samples and upregulated in the DLBCL samples. In Table 12.5, we have reported the nine gene markers along with their description and associated GO terms. It is evident from this table that all nine genes share most of the GO terms (mainly related to different kinds of binding functions), indicating that these genes have similar molecular functions.

TABLE 12.4   The Description and Associated GO Terms for the Eight Gene Markers Identified in Colon Cancer Data

Gene_ID	Gene Description	Gene Function (GO Terms)
M63391	desmin	cellular process, multicellular organismal process, biological regulation
Z24727	tropomyosin 1 (alpha)	cellular process, multicellular organismal process, localization biological regulation
T61609	ribosomal protein sa	metabolic process, cellular process, gene expression, biological adhesion
T48804	ribosomal protein s24	metabolic process, cellular process, gene expression
T57619	ribosomal protein s6	metabolic process, cellular process, gene expression, biological regulation
M26697	nucleophosmin (nucleolar phosphoprotein b23, numatrin)	metabolic process, cellular process, gene expression, developmental process, response to stimulus, localization, establishment of localization, biological regulation
T58861	ribosomal protein l30	metabolic process, cellular process, gene expression
T52185	ribosomal protein s19	immune system process, metabolic process, cellular process gene expression, multicellular organismal process, developmental process, locomotion, response to stimulus, localization, estabshment of localization, biological regulation

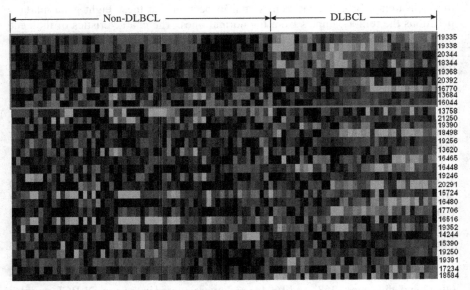

FIGURE 12.5 Heatmap of the expression levels top 30 gene markers distinguishing the tumor and normal samples of colon cancer data in terms of SNR statistic. Dark/light gray represent up–down regulation relative to black. The selected nine markers are put in the first nine rows.

TABLE 12.5 The Description and Associated GO Terms for the Nine Gene Markers Identified in Lymphoma Data

Gene_ID	Gene Description	Gene Function (GO Terms)
19335	rab23, member ras oncogene family	Nucleotide binding, binding, GTP binding, purine nucleotide binding, guanyl nucleotide binding, ribonucleotide binding, purine ribonucleotide binding, guanyl ribonucleotide binding
19338	rab33b, member of ras oncogene family	Nucleotide binding, binding, GTP binding, purine nucleotide binding, guanyl nucleotide binding, ribonucleotide binding, purine ribonucleotide binding, guanyl ribonucleotide binding
20344	Selectin, platelet	Glycoprotein binding, binding, protein binding, sugar binding, carbohydrate binding, sialic acid binding, monosaccharide binding, calcium-dependent protein binding
18344	Olfactory receptor 45	Rhodopsin-like receptor activity, signal transducer activity, receptor activity, transmembrane receptor activity, G-protein coupled receptor activity, olfactory receptor activity, molecular transducer activity
19368	Retinoic acid early transcript 1, alpha	Receptor binding, binding, protein binding, phospholipid binding, lipid binding, phosphoinositide binding, natural killer cell lectin-like receptor binding, GPI anchor binding
20392	Sarcoglycan, epsilon	Binding, calcium ion binding, protein binding, ion binding, cation binding, metal ion binding,
16770	Lactalbumin, alpha	Catalytic activity, lactose synthase activity, binding, calcium ion binding, UDP-glycosyltransferase activity, galactosyltransferase activity, transferase activity, transferase activity, transferring glycosyl groups, transferase activity, transferring hexosyl groups, UDP-galactosyltransferase activity, ion binding, cation binding, metal ion binding,
13684	Eukaryotic translation initiation factor 4e	Nucleic acid binding, RNA binding, translation initiation factor activity, binding, protein binding, translation factor activity, nucleic acid binding, translation regulator activity
16044	Immunoglobulin heavy chain sa2	Antigen binding, binding

12.7 DISCUSSION AND CONCLUSIONS

In this chapter, a cancer classification technique based on support vector machine classifier is proposed. The classification solutions yielded by different classifiers are combined through a majority voting ensemble to obtain the final solution. Further, this classification result is utilized to identify potential gene markers using SNR statistic followed by a multiobjective feature selection technique.

Results on three publicly available benchmark cancer data sets, namely, leukemia, colon cancer and lymphoma, have been demonstrated. The utility of the proposed classification ensemble technique has been demonstrated. The proposed ensemble classifier technique consistently outperformed the other kernel functions considered individually. Finally, relevant gene markers are identified using the classification result. The gene markers identified for different data sets are found to share many GO terms and molecular functions.

As a scope of further research, performance of other popular classifiers and their ensemble is to be studied. Moreover, the gene markers identified are needed to be further investigated biologically.

ACKNOWLEDGMENT

Sanghamitra Bandyopadhyay gratefully acknowledges the financial support received from the grant no. DST/SJF/ET-02/2006-07 under the Swarnajayanti Fellowship scheme of the Department of Science and Technology, Government of India.

REFERENCES

1. S. Bandyopadhyay, A. Mukhopadhyay, and U. Maulik (2007), An improved algorithm for clustering gene expression data, *Bioinformatics*, 23(21):2859–2865.

2. D. Jiang, C. Tang, and A. Zhang (2004), Cluster analysis for gene expression data: A survey, *IEEE Trans. Knowl. Data Eng.*, 16(11):1370–1386.

3. U. Maulik, A. Mukhopadhyay, and S. Bandyopadhyay (2009), Combining pareto-optimal clusters using supervised learning for identifying co-expressed genes, *BMC Bioinformatics*, 10(27).

4. W. Shannon, R. Culverhouse, and J. Duncan (2003), Analyzing microarray data using cluster analysis, *Pharmacogenomics*, 4(1):41–51.

5. R. Shyamsundar, Y. H. Kim, J. P. Higgins, K. Montgomery, M. Jorden, A. Sethuraman, M. van de Rijn, D. Botstein, P. O. Brown, and J. R. Pollack (2005), A DNA microarray survey of gene expression in normal human tissues. *Genome Biol.*, 6:R22.

6. A. A. Alizadeh, M. B. Eisen, R. Davis, C. Ma, I. Lossos, A. Rosenwald, J. Boldrick, R. Warnke, R. Levy, W. Wilson, M. Grever, J. Byrd, D. Botstein, P. O. Brown, and L. M. Straudt (2000), Distinct types of diffuse large b-cell lymphomas identified by gene expression profiling. *Nature (London)*, 403:503–511.

7. U. Alon et al. (1999), Broad patterns of gene expression revealed by clustering analysis of tumor and normal colon tissues probed by oligonucleotide arrays, *Proc. Natl. Acad. Sci.*, USA 96:6745–6750.

8. T. R. Golub, D. K. Slonim, P. Tamayo, C. Huard, M. Gassenbeek, J. P. Mesirov, H. Coller, M. L. Loh, J. R. Downing, M. A. Caligiuri, D. D. Bloomfield, and E. S. Lander (1999), Molecular classification of cancer: class discovery and class prediction by gene expression monitoring, *Science*, 286:531–537.

9. K. Y. Yeung and R. E. Bumgarner (2003), Multiclass classification of microarray data with repeated measurements: application to cancer, *Genome Biol.*, 4.

10. V. Vapnik (1998), *Statistical Learning Theory*. John Wiley & Sons, Inc., NY.

11. K. Crammer and Y. Singer (2001), On the algorithmic implementation of multiclass kernel-based vector machines. *J. Machine Learning Res.*, 2:265–292.

12. E. Alba, J. Garcia-Nieto, L. Jourdan, and E-G. Talbi (2007), Gene selection in cancer classification using PSO/SVM and GA/SVM hybrid algorithms. *Proceedings of the IEEE Congress Evolution of Computers*, IEEE Computer Society, Singapore, pp. 284–290.

13. M. P. S. Brown, W. N. Grundy, D. Lin, N. Cristianini, C. W. Sugnet, T. S. Furey, Jr, and D. Haussler (2000), Knowledge-based analysis of microarray gene expression data by using support vector machines *Proc. Natl. Acad. Sci. USA*, 97(1):262–267.

14. K. B. Duan, J. C. Rajapakse, H. Wang, and F. Azuaje (2005), Multiple SVM-RFE for gene selection in cancer classification with expression data, *IEEE Trans. Nanobiosci.*, 4(3):228–234.

15. T. S. Furey, N. Cristianini, N. Duffy, D. W. Bednarski, M. Schummer, and D. Haussler (2000), Support vector machine classification and validation of cancer tissue samples using microarray expression data, *Bioinformatics*, 16(10):906–914.

16. I. Guyon, J. Weston, S. Barnhill, and V. Vapnik (2002), Gene selection for cancer classification using support vector machines, *Machine Learning*, 46(1-3):389–422.

17. S. Li and M. Tan (2007), Gene selection and tissue classification based on support vector machine and genetic algorithm, Proceedings of the 1st International Conference on Bioformatics and Biomedical Engineering (ICBBE 2007) unhen, China pp. 192–195.

18. J. Mohr, S. Seo, and K. Obermayer (2008), Automated microarray classification based on P-SVM gene selection. *ICMLA '08: Proceedings of the 2008 Seventh International Conference on Machine Learning and Applications*, IEEE Computer Society, pp. 503–507. Washington, DC.

19. C.A. Coello Coello (2006), Evolutionary multiobjective optimization: A historical view of the field. *IEEE Comput. Intell. Mag.*, 1(1):28–36.

20. C.A. Coello Coello, D.A. Van Veldhuizen, and G.B. Lamont (2006), *Evolutionary Algorithms for Solving Multi-Objective Problems*, (Genetic and Evolutionary seves) Springer-Verlag, NY.

21. K. Deb (2001), *Multi-objective Optimization Using Evolutionary Algorithms,* John Wiley & Sons, Ltd, England.

22. N. M. Luscombe, D. Greenbaum, and M. Gerstein (2001), What is bioinformatics? A proposed definition and overview of the field. *Methods of Information & Medicine, Schatbuer*, Vol. 40(4), pp. 346–358.

23. J. Quackenbush (2001), Computational analysis of microarray data, *Nat. Rev. Genet.*, 2:418–427.

24. K. Deb, A. Pratap, S. Agrawal, and T. Meyarivan (2002), A fast and elitist multiobjective genetic algorithm: NSGA-II, *IEEE Trans. Evolut. Comput.*, 6:182–197.

13

GENE MICROARRAY DATA ANALYSIS USING PARALLEL POINT SYMMETRY-BASED CLUSTERING

UJJWAL MAULIK AND ANASUA SARKAR

13.1 INTRODUCTION

The advent of deoxyribonucleic acid (DNA) microarray technology has enabled scientists to monitor the expression levels for many thousands of genes simultaneously over different time points under multiple biological processes [1]. Since the diauxic shift [2], sporulation [3] and the cell cycle [4] in the yeast were explored, many experiments were conducted to monitor genes with similar expression patterns of various organisms, which may participate in the same signal pathway or may be coregulated.

Clustering is an unsupervised pattern classification technique, while K-means is a well-known partitional clustering approach. The present study focuses on the application of the point symmetry-based clustering method for analyzing gene-expression data sets, comprising either time-course type of data or expression levels under various environmental conditions. The most widely used clustering algorithms for microarray gene-expression analysis are hierarchical clustering [5], K-means clustering [6] and self-organizing maps (SOM) [2]. Among these conventional clustering methods, K-means is an effective partitional clustering algorithm that utilizes heuristic global optimization criteria.

Thus clustering based on K-means is closely related to the recognition of variability in compactness of different geometrical cluster shapes, whereas symmetry is considered as an inherent feature for recognition and reconstruction of shapes hidden in any clusters. In [7], Su and Chou proposed a variation of K-means algorithm with

Computational Intelligence and Pattern Analysis in Biological Informatics, Edited by Ujjwal Maulik, Sanghamitra Bandyopadhyay, and Jason T. L. Wang
Copyright © 2010 John Wiley & Sons, Inc.

a new symmetry-based distance measure (SBKM). However, it fails when symmetry lies, with respect to some intermediate point, in a cluster. To overcome it in [8], a point symmetry-based distance measure in clustering(PSBKM) has been proposed with quadratic runtime.

Gene-expression microarray data is a form of high-throughput genomics data providing relative measurements of expression levels for thousands of genes in a biological sample. Analysis of such huge data is becoming a major bottleneck. Kanungo et al. [9] defined parallel K-means to speedup timing. Following it, parallel implementation of both SBKM and PSBKM algorithms have been proposed in this chapter for microarray data sets, in a distributed master–slave environment. Its advantage lies not only in the scalability in timing, but also parallel ParPSBKM (ParPSBKM) outperforms parallel K-means (PKM) and parallel SBKM (ParSBKM) for symmetrical-shaped clusters as analyzed with four validity indices-J_m, XB, I, and $s(C)$. ParPSBKM also succeeds in correctly classifying symmetrical clusters even when PSBKM fails, and increasing the number of nodes and parallel in ParPSBKM leads to the production of better solutions.

13.2 SYMMETRY- AND POINT SYMMETRY-BASED DISTANCE MEASURES

There are several measures for proximity of clusters like Euclidean, Pearson correlation, and Spearman distances, but none of them can detect symmetry. Hence, Su and Chou in [7] defined the symmetry-based distance between any pattern $\overline{X_i}$, $i = 1, 2, \ldots, N$ and any reference centroid vector $\overline{C_k}$, $k = 1, 2, \ldots, K$ as follows:

$$d_s(\overline{X_i}, \overline{C_k}) = \min_{j=1,2,\ldots,N \text{ and } (i \neq j)} \frac{\| (\overline{X_i} - \overline{C_k}) + (\overline{X_j} - \overline{C_k}) \|}{\| (\overline{X_i} - \overline{C_k}) \| + \| (\overline{X_j} - \overline{C_k}) \|}$$

The numerator is the distance between a point $\overline{X_i}$ and its first nearest neighbor with respect to centroid $\overline{C_k}$. In [8], Saha and Bandyopadhyay proposed a point symmetry(ps)-based distance measure as follows:

$$d_{ps}(\overline{X_i}, \overline{C_k}) = \frac{(d_1 + d_2)}{2} \times d_e(\overline{X_i}, \overline{C_k})$$

where $d_{ps}(\overline{X_i}, \overline{C_k})$ is the PS distance and $d_e(\overline{X_i}, \overline{C_k})$ denotes Euclidean distance between $\overline{X_i}$ and $\overline{C_k}$. If $\overline{X_i^*}$ represents the symmetrical point of $\overline{X_i}$ and is computed as $\overline{X_i^*} = (2 * \overline{C_k} - \overline{X_i})$, then d_1 and d_2 represent the Euclidean distances of first and second nearest neighbors of $\overline{X_i^*}$.

13.3 PARPSBKM CLUSTERING IMPLEMENTATION

Both partitioning and clustering phases of ParSBKM and ParPSBKM algorithms have been implemented in a distributed master–slave paradigm. Among M

Comment: Only changes to the sequential MODSBKM algorithm for obtaining global cluster assignments on master node M_0 by combining parallely-computed local cluster assignments from all $M-1$ distributed slave nodes are shown.

Step 1 : Initialization on M_0 :
1.1: Total number of elements in data set = N. Total number of distributed nodes = M.
1.2: Make a horizontal partition of the universal dataset
    Distribute partitions and masking parameters from master node M_0 to $M-1$ slave nodes,
    maintaining equality in partition lengths in slave nodes with additional zero data assignments.
    Randomly assign N data elements to K clusters,
    so that at least one element has been assigned to each cluster.
    Calculate θ as the maximum nearest neighbor distance among all elements in the dataset.
1.3: Make an initial random non-empty cluster assignment of universal dataset at node m_0.
    Calculate initial J_m at master node J_m.
1.4: BROADCAST the initial cluster assignment and J_m to all $M-1$ slave nodes.
Step 2 : Parallel computation of centroids towards convergence :
2.1: Calculate centroids C_k for $k=1,2,...,K$ clusters on $M-1$ slave nodes.
2.2: Execute 1pass of K-means method on partial data of $M-1$ nodes to update K centroids.
2.3: Calculate local J_m on each of the $M-1$ slave nodes.
2.4: GATHER all local cluster assignments to the global cluster assignment in master node M_0.
2.5: REDUCE all local J_ms to global J_m at master node M_0.
2.6: If global J_m is minimizing towards convergence then go to Step 2
    else if the final metric convergence has been reached, stop calculation.
    Compute final centroids on master node M_0 and go to Step 3.
Step 3 : Fine-Tuning with PS distance :
3.1: In master node M_0,
    for each data point $\overline{x_i}, i=1,2,...,N$ and each cluster centroid $\overline{c_k}, k=1,2,...,K$
    Compute $mindps = min_{k=1,2,...,K} d_{ps}(\overline{x_i},\overline{c_k})$, where $d_{ps}(\overline{x_i},\overline{c_k}) = \frac{(d_1+d_2)}{2} \times d_e(\overline{x_i},\overline{c_k})$.
3.2: If $(mindps == d_{ps}(\overline{x_i},\overline{c_k}))$ assign $k^* = k$.
3.3: If $d_{ps}(\overline{x_i},\overline{c_k}^*) < \theta$
    If $\overline{x_i}$ is not already assigned to the k^*th cluster , then assign $\overline{x_i}$ to the k^*th cluster.
    else compute $mineds = min_{k=1,2,...,K} d_e(\overline{x_i},\overline{c_k})$,
    where d_e is the Euclidean distance between $\overline{x_i}$ and $\overline{c_k}$,stored in $distanceArray$.
3.4:   If $mineds == d_e(\overline{x_i},c_k^*)$ assign $k^* = k$.
    If $\overline{x_i}$ is not already assigned to the k^*th cluster , then assign $\overline{x_i}$ to the k^*th cluster.
Step 4 : Point Symmetry-based centroids updating :
4.1: Compute new centroids of the K clusters in master node M_0 as follows:
$$c_k = \frac{\sum_{i \in S_k} \overline{x_i}}{S_k}, k=1,2,...,K,$$
    where S_k is the set of elements assigned to the kth cluster till then.
4.2: Update the $distanceArray$ with the Euclidean distances from corrected centroids.
Step 5 : Continuation : If centroids converge or number of iterations is completed,
    then in master node M_0 compute final validity indices J_m, XB, MS and $I-index$
    and stop, else go to Step 3.

FIGURE 13.1   Steps of parallel PSBKM algorithm.

distributed nodes, M_0 acts as the master to ensure load balancing [10] and other $M-1$ nodes act as slaves. The ParPSBKM algorithm in Figure 13.1, composed of three phases - initial horizontal partitioning of universal data set, parallely computed local centroids updating using the K-means method and point symmetry-based fine-tuning with validation. Initial random cluster assignment puts N elements in K clusters. Each slave then performs centroids updating on partitioned data locally and next returns its local cluster assignment to M_0 [11]. The parameter M_0 then merges them into global cluster assignment, using the union-find data structure with an average runtime of inverse Ackermann's function. If optimization continues, M_0 continues with redistribution of corrected cluster assignment. The fine-tuning phase at M_0 utilizes the PS distance in lieu of Euclidean distance. The point is reassigned to a new cluster only if its symmetrical point resides inside the data set and the minimal PS distance between the point and the new centroid is greater than the threshold value θ. This value is set to 0.18 for ParSBKM and for ParPSBKM it is calculated as the maximum nearest-neighbor distance [8]. This leads to convergence and finally validity indices are computed over final symmetry-corrected solution.

13.3.1   Complexity Analysis

Time complexity of ParPSBKM is analyzed below:

1. *Initialization.* As there are $m = M - 1$ slave nodes, horizontally partitioned data set becomes $N/m \times C$ matrix, with N elements and C attributes. Hence, partitioning time for one-to-all *SEND/SCATTER* operation and *BROADCAST* operation of initial assignment leads to timing: $T_{\text{partition}} = O((N/m) * (C + 1)) \simeq O(N/m)$.

2. *Parallel Centroids Calculation.* If *maxrepeat* ($\ll N$) is the number of repetition to converge parallel centroid updation on m slaves, then complexity for K clusters becomes: $T_{\text{cluster}} = O(((N/m) * K + K) * maxrepeat)$.

3. *Fine-Tuning with PS Distance.* In M_0 with all N elements, time complexity is $O((N * (NK)) * maxrepeat\_symmetry)$, where *maxrepeat_symmetry* is the number of repetitions required for point symmetry-based centroid correction method to converge. $N >> maxrepeat\_symmetry$.

4. *Point Symmetry-Based Centroids Updating.* For K clusters, it also requires $O(K)$ time on M_0.

5. *Continuation.* A constant time in M_0. The time complexity of sequential PSBKM is $O(N^2 K)$. Yet timing of ParPSBKM reduces to $O((N/m)^2 K)$, which yields linear speedup. In ParPSBKM, *ALL-GATHER* and *ALL-REDUCE* operations for N/m rows from slave nodes in parallel clustering phase, incurs additional *maxrepeat* $* O(N/m + 1) \simeq O(N/m)$ delay in communication cost. So, for large M, communication overhead for collective operations undermines linear speedup [12].

13.4   PERFORMANCE ANALYSIS

The algorithms PKM, ParSBKM, and ParPSBKM are implemented using MPI (message passing interface) and C. Experiments are performed on IBM p690 Regatta Server, with 16 Power 4+ processors with a 1.3-GHz clock speed. Execution times are obtained using $MPI\_Wtime()$ function in seconds (5 benchmark data sets, 1 artificial and 4 microarray, are used).

13.4.1   Data Sets

This section demonstrates the benchmark data sets used to measure the performance of the parallel algorithms. It consists of 1 artificial data set and 4 benchmark microarray data sets. Each data set consists of 5000 to 45,000 elements.

13.4.1.1 Artificial Data Set

1. *Data 2.* This is a synthetic data set with 34, 468 points with a dimensionality of
10. This data set has *Center–Corners* distribution [13], in which one generated
hyper-rectangle is placed in the center and others in are in three different
corners of the space (origin, far corner, and one randomly selected corner).
All generated hyper-rectangles have uniform internal distributions and each
one represents a different class of data. Thus, each point is assigned to one of
four classes. This synthetic data set is produced by the program available at
http://www.cs.iit.edu/egalite/Data/GARDENHD/DataGenerator.zip.

13.4.1.2 Microarray Data Sets

1. *Yeast Sporulation.* This data set consists of 6118 genes measured across
seven time points (0, 0.5, 2, 5, 7, 9, and 11.5 h) during the sporulation process of a budding yeast [3]. The data set is publicly available at the website: http://cmgm.stanford.edu/pbrown/sporulation. Genes with no significant
change in expression levels during harvesting are eliminated during log2-
transformed normalization with 1.6 level threshold value for root mean squares.
The normalized set consists of 474 genes.

2. *Mitochondrial Genome.* This data set consists of the Telomerase expression,
which sensitizes the mitochondrial genome of mammalian cells to oxidative
stress through increased bioavailable Fe. There are 16,828 genes, each with
22 features. The data set is available at http://www.niehs.nih.gov/research /at-
niehs/core/microarrays/docs/santos.txt.

3. *Lung Inflammation.* This data set describes the modulatory role for retinoid-
related orphan receptor a (RORa) in allergen-induced lung inflammation. It
consists of 20,917 genes, each with 15 features. The data set is available
at http://www.niehs.nih.gov/research/atniehs/core/microarrays/docs/272jetten.
txt.

4. *Colon Culture.* This Interleukin-22 effect on colon cultures GEO data set
contains the analysis of C57BL/6 colon cultures treated with 10 ng/mL^{-1} (of
interleukin-22 (IL-22) for 24 h on Mus musculus. The IL-22, a member of
the IL-10 family of cytokines, can induce a marked antimicrobial response
in vitro. Results provide insight into the molecular basis of IL-22 induced
host defense mechanisms. This gene expression array-based ribonucleic acid
(RNA) type sample consists of log10 ratio values for 44,290 genes each with
six samples. The data set is publicly available at http://www.ncbi.nlm.nih.gov/
projects/geo/gds /gds_browse.cgi?gds=3226.

13.4.2 Timing Analysis

Tables 13.1–13.5 reports the execution times of the sequential, as well as parallel
versions of SBKM and PSBKM algorithms. These include the partitioning, clustering,
and fine-tuning phases of those algorithms both for the artificial and gene microarray
data sets. The speedup $S = \text{Time}(p = 1)/\text{Time}(p = P)$, is computed to show the

TABLE 13.1   Time Comparison of ParSBKM and ParPSBKM Algorithms for Data 2

			Execution Time					
Algorithms	Methods	P	Partition Time (s)	Cluster Time (s)	Fine Tuning Time (s)	Total Time (s)	S	TG (%)
SBKM	Sequential	1		6.478	4842.397	4848.881	1.00	0.00
ParSBKM	Parallel	2	1.772	6.416	2427.536	2435.724	1.99	49.77
		4	1.507	5.458	1537.885	1544.849	3.14	68.14
		8	1.484	5.043	988.973	995.500	4.87	79.47
		12	1.407	4.134	914.791	920.332	5.27	81.02
PSBKM	Sequential	1		6.335	2162.434	2168.776	1.00	0.00
ParPSBKM	Parallel	2	1.568	6.214	901.899	909.680	2.38	58.06
		4	1.473	5.152	453.626	460.251	4.71	78.78
		8	1.464	4.497	367.880	373.841	5.80	82.76
		12	1.404	4.066	305.523	310.993	6.97	85.66

scalability of parallel execution on each data set. Similarly, the percentage of time gain (%TG) is computed as $\%TG = \text{Time}(p = 1) - \text{Time}(p = P)/\text{Time}(p = P) * 100$ to show the performance time gain for increasing the number of processors in the parallel execution. The clustering and fine-tuning phases are expected to take quadratic runtimes for sequential execution. The decrease in runtime as the number of processors(P) increases from 1 to 2, happens not only for the increase in the number of processors, but also for the cache size limitation of individual nodes. Moreover, parallel runtimes of both the algorithms are reduced further with the increase in number of processors until the communication overhead arises.

TABLE 13.2   Time Comparison of ParSBKM and ParPSBKM Algorithms for Sporulation

			Execution Time					
Algorithms	Methods	P	Partition Time (s)	Cluster Time (s)	Fine Tuning Time (s)	Total Time (s)	S	TG (%)
SBKM	Sequential	1		0.060	1.491	1.551	1.00	0.00
ParSBKM	Parallel	2	0.019	0.050	0.975	1.044	1.49	32.71
		4	0.018	0.044	0.549	0.610	2.54	60.67
		8	0.010	0.040	0.457	0.506	3.06	67.37
		12	0.005	0.038	0.353	0.395	3.92	74.51
PSBKM	Sequential	1		0.052	1.399	1.451	1.00	0.00
ParPSBKM	Parallel	2	0.011	0.042	0.854	0.907	1.60	37.50
		4	0.008	0.036	0.436	0.480	3.02	66.93
		8	0.004	0.025	0.370	0.398	3.64	72.55
		12	0.001	0.024	0.307	0.332	4.37	77.13

TABLE 13.3   Time Comparison of ParSBKM and ParPSBKM Algorithms for Mitochondrial Genome

Algorithms	Methods	P	Partition Time (s)	Cluster Time (s)	Fine Tuning Time (s)	Total Time (s)	S	TG (%)
SBKM	Sequential	1		0.866	1670.036	1670.906	1.00	0.00
ParSBKM	Parallel	2	0.879	0.848	982.306	984.033	1.70	41.11
		4	0.874	0.803	721.535	723.211	2.31	56.72
		8	0.854	0.698	484.767	486.320	3.44	70.89
		12	0.837	0.642	458.354	459.833	3.63	72.48
PSBKM	Sequential	1		0.862	1185.614	1186.479	1.00	0.00
ParPSBKM	Parallel	2	0.873	0.838	438.614	440.325	2.69	62.89
		4	0.862	0.784	320.481	322.128	3.68	72.85
		8	0.837	0.672	269.480	270.990	4.38	77.16
		12	0.827	0.641	197.118	198.587	5.97	83.26

Table 13.1 (for the large artificial data set Data 2) shows the speedup ranging from 1.99 to 5.27 and 2.38 to 6.97, respectively, for the ParSBKM and ParPSBKM algorithms. Noticeably, the speedup obtained by the ParPSBKM algorithm is better than ParSBKM algorithm. For this artificial data set, the %TG for the ParSBKM algorithm is ranging from 49.77 to 81.02% and for the ParPSBKM algorithm, the range is from 58.06 to 85.66%.

Similarly, Table 13.2 provides the execution times for the sporulation microarray data set. Note that the ParSBKM and ParPSBKM algorithms are able to achieve speedup ranging from 1.49 to 3.92 and 1.60 to 4.37 respectively, when the number

TABLE 13.4   Time Comparison of ParSBKM and ParPSBKM Algorithms for Lung Inflammation

Algorithms	Methods	P	Partition Time	Cluster Time	Fine Tuning Time	Total Time	S	TG (%)
SBKM	Sequential	1	–	0.878	2722.107	2722.989	1.00	0.00
ParSBKM	Parallel	2	0.924	0.565	1552.107	1553.595	1.75	42.95
		4	0.904	0.474	1163.528	1164.906	2.34	57.22
		8	0.898	0.209	747.641	748.749	3.64	72.50
		12	0.892	0.193	728.548	729.633	3.73	73.20
PSBKM	Sequential	1	–	0.619	1543.691	1544.314	1.00	0.00
ParPSBKM	Parallel	2	0.728	0.439	558.673	559.840	2.76	63.75
		4	0.712	0.161	402.321	403.193	3.83	73.89
		8	0.708	0.148	323.678	324.534	4.76	78.99
		12	0.703	0.161	241.215	242.078	6.38	84.32

TABLE 13.5   Time Comparison of ParSBKM and ParPSBKM Algorithms for Colon Culture

			Execution Time					
Algorithms	Methods	P	Partition Time (s)	Cluster Time (s)	Fine Tuning Time (s)	Total Time (s)	S	TG (%)
SBKM	Sequential	1	–	0.688	5458.352	5459.044	1.00	0.00
ParSBKM	Parallel	2	0.925	0.658	2609.891	2611.474	2.09	52.16
		4	0.903	0.624	1651.973	1653.500	3.30	69.71
		8	0.899	0.582	1129.397	1130.878	4.83	79.28
		12	0.895	0.521	1008.047	1009.463	5.41	81.51
PSBKM	Sequential	1	–	0.673	2610.532	2611.210	1.00	0.00
ParPSBKM	Parallel	2	0.889	0.616	1002.944	1004.450	2.60	61.53
		4	0.883	0.589	519.438	520.910	5.01	80.05
		8	0.880	0.527	413.546	414.952	6.29	84.11
		12	0.873	0.460	322.523	323.856	8.06	87.60

of processors (P) increases from 2 to 12. The %TG for the sporulation data set is in the range of 32.71–74.51% for the ParSBKM algorithm, while for the ParPSBKM algorithm, it ranges from 37.50–77.13%. Similar boosting in the speedup and %TG can also be found for all other data sets.

For the largest microarray data set, colon culture with 44291 elements, the TG% of ParPSBKM algorithm for $P = 2, 4, 8,$ and 12 processors are, respectively, 61.53, 80.05, 84.11, and 87.60% and those of ParSBKM algorithms are, respectively, 52.16, 69.71, 79.28, and 81.51%. The speedup computation of the ParSBKM algorithm for this data set results in the range of 2.09–5.41 times and the range for the ParPSBKM algorithm is from 2.60–8.06 times. This finding shows an increasing order of speedup and %TG with an increase in the number of processors, which proves the necessity for parallelization of all those algorithms for even large microarray data sets.

Figures 13.2 and 13.3 show improvement in the execution times for ParSBKM and ParPSBKM algorithms, respectively, as P is increased from 2 to 12 while keeping the data size constant for four relatively large data sets, namely, mitochondrial genome, lung inflammation, data 2, and colon culture. The speedups for $P = 2, 4,$ and 8 tends to increase even for $P = 12$, undermining the interprocessor communication cost for all these large data sets. Moreover, the superiority of the ParPSBKM algorithm over the ParSBKM algorithm can be noted from Figures 13.2 and 13.3. Figures 13.4 and 13.5 show the overall performance of ParSBKM and ParPSBKM, respectively, in terms of total execution times for various problem sizes for $P = 1, 2, 4, 8,$ and 12. It is evident from the figures that the performance gain of ParPSBKM algorithm in comparison with the ParSBKM algorithm for the parallel execution times is in the range of 2.60–3.12 times for $P = 2$.

The scalability of parallel execution on each data set is shown in bar charts in Figures 13.6 and 13.7. As expected the scalability is high for large microarray data sets. The largest microarray data set, colon culture, with 44,291 elements, shows the

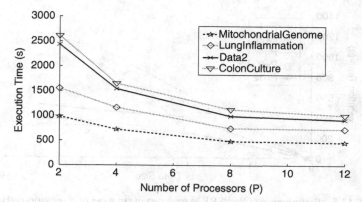

FIGURE 13.2   Performance of ParSBKM with varying data sizes and increasing number of processors.

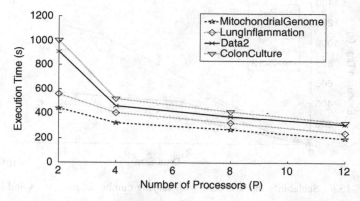

FIGURE 13.3   Performance of ParPSBKM with varying data sizes and increasing number of processors.

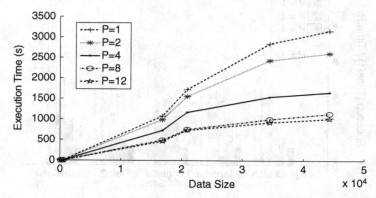

FIGURE 13.4   Performance of ParSBKM with varying number of processors and increasing data sizes.

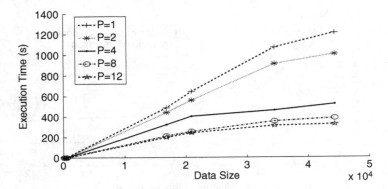

FIGURE 13.5 Performance of ParPSBKM with varying number of processors and increasing data sizes.

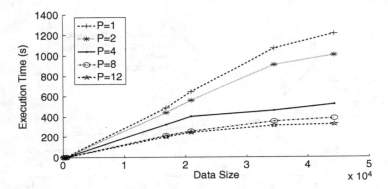

FIGURE 13.6 Scalability of ParSBKM with varying number of processors and increasing data sizes.

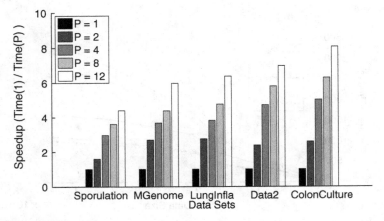

FIGURE 13.7 Scalability of ParPSBKM with varying number of processors and increasing data sizes.

TABLE 13.6   Performance Comparisons of PKM and ParSBKM Algorithms on Data Sets

		Algorithms							
		PKM				ParSBKM			
	Data Sets	J_m	XB	I	$s(C)$	J_m	XB	I	$s(C)$
Artificial	Data 2	5,364.58	1.77E+6	2.42	0.49	5,229.58	1.71E+6	3.24	0.50
Microarray	Sporulation	144.33	1329.44	7.53	0.69	143.59	1296.71	8.25	0.73
	Mitochondrial Genome	7,510.91	5.79E+6	3.62	0.53	7,483.55	4.52E+6	4.12	0.62
	Lung Inflammation	3.65E+7	287.56	1.49E+9	0.96	3.54E+7	220.41	1.91E+9	0.97
	Colon Culture	14,233.68	2.87E+5	0.82	0.66	12,987.14	1.99E+5	0.98	0.73

highest scalability of 8.06 times for the ParPSBKM algorithm with $P = 12$, forming a linear curve of speedup with other data sets. However, the ParSBKM algorithm provides a scalability of 5.41 times for the colon culture data set. Similar results are also observed for other data sets, which show that the ParPSBKM algorithm outperforms the ParSBKM algorithm even in the scalability of parallel execution times.

13.4.3   Validity Analysis

The clustering results have been evaluated objectively by measuring four validity measures J_m, XB, I index, and *silhouette index* $s(C)$, as defined in [14–17], respectively, for PKM, ParSBKM, and ParPSBKM algorithms on each data set to measure the goodness of the clustering solutions. The results are reported in Tables 13.6 and 13.7.

Note that for the microarray data set sporulation, ParPSBKM produces the best minimized J_m index as 143.512, while ParSBKM and PKM produces J_m values

TABLE 13.7   Performance Comparisons of PKM and ParPSBKM Algorithms on Data Sets

		Algorithms							
		PKM				ParSBKM			
	Data Sets	J_m	XB	I	$s(C)$	J_m	XB	I	$s(C)$
Artificial	Data 2	5,364.58	1.77E+6	2.42	0.49	3,574.89	1.63E+6	5.86	0.50
Microarray	Sporulation	144.33	1329.44	7.53	0.69	143.51	1127.26	9.68	0.74
	Mitochondrial Genome	7510.91	5.79E+6	3.62	0.53	7,206.19	4.34E+6	4.69	0.63
	Lung Inflammation	3.65E+7	287.56	1.49E+9	0.96	3.54E+7	209.87	2.10E+9	0.99
	Colon Culture	14,233.68	2.87E+5	0.82	0.66	11,834.42	1.04E+5	0.99	0.74

as 143.591 and 144.332, respectively. The ParPSBKM algorithm also provides the best XB index value of 1127.258, compared to 1296.71 and 1329.44 produced by ParSBKM and PKM, respectively. The I index values produced by ParPSBKM, ParSBKM, and PKM algorithms are, respectively, 9.681, 8.249, and 7.539, which also shows the superiority of the ParPSBKM algorithm over the other two. Similarly, the silhouette index $s(C)$ produced by the ParPSBKM algorithm [maximizing $s(C)$] is 0.739, but ParSBKM and PKM implementations provide smaller $s(C)$ values of 0.733 and 0.693, respectively. Similar results are also found for other data sets.

13.5 TEST FOR STATISTICAL SIGNIFICANCE

A nonparametric statistical significance test called *Wilcoxon's rank sum* for independent samples has been conducted at the 5% significance level [13]. Three groups corresponding to three algorithms PKM, ParSBKM, and ParPSBKM, have been created for each data set. Each group consists of the performance scores $s(C)$ produced by 10 consecutive runs of corresponding algorithm on each data set. From the median values of each group for all data sets, as shown in Table 13.8, it is observed that ParPSBKM provides better median values than both PKM and ParSBKM.

Table 13.9 shows the P- and H-values produced by Wilcoxon's rank sum test for comparison of two groups (one for ParPSBKM and another for some other algorithm, either PKM or ParSBKM) at a time. As a null hypothesis, it is assumed that there are no significant differences between the median values of the two groups. If $H = 0$, one cannot reject the null hypothesis, while $H = 1$ means the null hypothesis can be rejected at the 5% level. A larger value of P means the null hypothesis is more significant. All the P-values reported in the table are < 0.005.

We see from Table 13.9, that for microarray data set sporulation, the comparative P-value of rank sum test between PKM and ParPSBKM is $1.74E - 4$, which is very small. This indicates that the performance metrics produced by ParPSBKM is statistically significant and has not occurred by chance. Similarly for that microarray data set, $H = 1$ and $P = 1.67E - 4$ values between ParPSBKM and ParSBKM

TABLE 13.8 Median Values of Performance Parameters [$s(C)$ for Microarray Data Sets] over 10 Consecutive Runs on Different Algorithms

Data Sets		Median Values		
		PKM	ParSBKM	ParPSBKM
Artificial	Data 2	0.4924	0.4969	0.4999
Microarray	Sporulation	0.5538	0.6140	0.7331
	Mitochondrial Genome	0.4314	0.5318	0.6220
	Lung Inflammation	0.9479	0.9673	0.9829
	Colon Culture	0.6975	0.7258	0.7424

TABLE 13.9   _P_-Values Produced by Rank Sum While Comparing ParPSBKM with Other Algorithms

		P-Values			
		PKM		ParSBKM	
	Data Sets	H	P	H	P
Artificial	Data 2	1	8.17E-5	1	1.09E-4
Microarray	Sporulation	1	1.72E-4	1	1.67E-4
	Mitochondrial Genome	1	1.55E-4	1	5.59E-5
	Lung Inflammation	1	1.13E-4	1	4.55E-5
	Colon Culture	1	1.59E-5	1	4.73E-5

algorithms means that the result is not casting of the null hypothesis. Similar results are obtained for both PKM and ParSBKM algorithms over all other data sets. Hence, all results established the significant superiority of ParPSBKM algorithm over ParSBKM and PKM algorithms.

13.6   CONCLUSIONS

Gene-expression microarray is one of the latest breakthroughs in experimental molecular biology. It provides a powerful tool by which the expression patterns for thousands of genes across multiple conditions can be monitored simultaneously producing large throughput data. Although the magnitudes may not be close, the patterns they exhibit may be alike and symmetrical. The point-symmetry distance measure, as presented in this chapter, proves the closure and difference symmetry properties even on those intra and intercluster symmetrical patterns, as demonstarted with examples. The contribution of this chapter lies in faster and more efficient discovery of such symmetrical clusters of genes in large microarray data sets by the reformulation of the SBKM and PSBKM to the time-efficient scalable high-performance parallel symmetry-based clustering algorithms, namely, ParSBKM and ParPSBKM.

The primary contributions are as follows: to reduce the space requirement from linear to be factored by the number of distributed nodes, to generate global centroids updation without using an all-to-all communication pattern, and to reduce execution time by a factor of quadratic value of number of slave nodes. Generally, it was found that ParPSBKM outperforms PKM and ParSBKM not only in timing, but also succeeds in detecting symmetrical-shaped clusters in gene microarray data analysis.

REFERENCES

1. R. Sharan (2003), CLICK and EXPANDER: a system for clustering and visualizing gene expression data, _Bioinformatics_, 19:1787–1799.
2. J. DeRisi, V. Iyer, and P. Brown (1997), Exploring the metabolic and genetic control of gene expression on a genome scale, _Science_, 282:257–264.

3. S. Chu (1998), The transcriptional program of sporulation in budding yeast, *Science*, 202:699–705.

4. R. J. Cho (1998), A genome-wide transcriptional analysis of the mitotic cell cycle, *Mol. Cell*, 2:65–73.

5. M. Eisen, P. Spellman, P. Brown, and D. Botstein (1998), Cluster analysis and display of genome-wide expression patterns, *Proc. Natl Acad. Sci. USA*, 95:14863–14868.

6. S. Tavazoie, J. Hughes, M. Campbell, R.J. Cho, and G.M. Church (2001), Ssystematic determination of genetic network architecture, *Bioinformatics*, 17:405–414.

7. M.-C.Su and C.-H.Chou (2001), A modified version of the k-means algorithm with a distance based on cluster symmetry, *IEEE Trans. Pattern Mach. Intell.*, 23(6):674–680.

8. S. Saha and S. Bandyopadhyay, (2003), GAPS: A clustering method using a new point symmetry-based distance measure, *Pattern Recognition*, 10(12):3430–3451.

9. T. Kanungo, D. Mount, N.S. Netanyahu, C. Piatko, R. Silverman, and A. Wu (2002), An efficient k-means clustering algorithm: analysis and implementation, *IEEE Trans. Pattern Mach. Intell.*, 24(7):881–892.

10. A. Kalyanaraman, S. Aluru, and V. Brendel (2003), Space and time efficient parallel algorithms and software for est clustering. *IEEE Trans. Parallel Distributed Systems*, 14(12):1209–1221.

11. A. Kalyanaraman, S. Aluru, S. Kothari, and V. Brendel (2003), Efficient clustering of large est data sets on parallel computers, *Nucleic Acids Res.*, 31(11):2963–2974.

12. W. Ahmad and A. Khokhar. SPHire:Scallable High Performance Biclustering using Weighted Bigraph Crossing Minimization. *UIC ECE Tech Report TR-MSL0787*.

13. M. Hollander and D.A. Wolfe (1999), *Nonparametric statistical methods*, 2 ed., John Wiely & Sons, Inc., NY.

14. J. C. Bezdek (1981), *Pastern recognition with fuzzy objective function algorithms*, Plenum, NY.

15. X. L. Xie and G. Beni (1991), A validity measure for fuzzy clustering, *IEEE Trans. Pattern Anal. Mach. Intell.*, 13:841–847.

16. U. Maulik and S. Bandyopadhyay (2002), Pperformance evaluation of some clustering algorithms and validity indices, *IEEE Trans. Pattern Anal. Machine Intelligence*, 24(12):1650–1654.

17. P. Rousseeuw (1987), Silhouettes: a graphical aid to the interpretation and validation of cluster analysis, *J. Comput. Appl. Math.*, 20:53–65.

PART V

SYSTEMS BIOLOGY

14

TECHNIQUES FOR PRIORITIZATION OF CANDIDATE DISEASE GENES

JIEUN JEONG AND JAKE Y. CHEN

14.1 INTRODUCTION

Gene prioritization is a new approach for extending our knowledge about diseases and phenotypic information each gene encodes. We will review computational methods that have been described to date and attempt to identify which are most successful and what are the remaining challenges. The motivations and applications of this topic been well described in [1]. Therefore, we focus on how to enable a biologist to select the best existing method for a given application context. At the same time, we would like to identify remaining open research problems for practitioners in bioinformatics.

The general notion of gene prioritization assumes that one has a set of candidates and he wants to order the candidates from the most promising to the least promising one. A primary motivation for prioritization of candidate disease genes comes from the analysis of linkage regions that contain genetic elements of diseases. In this setting, the notion of a disease gene is unambiguous: a genetic element that confers disease susceptibility if its variants is present in the genome. For a particular disease phenotype, researchers often have a list of candidate genes usually genes located in a linkage interval associated with the disease. Finding the actual gene and candidate can be a subject of expensive experimental validations; however, once identified as real, these disease-associated genes or their protein products can be considered as a therapeutic target or a diagnostic biomarker. Online Mendelian Inheritance in Man (OMIM) is a representative database that links phenotypes, genomic regions, and genes. Here, we refer to a "phenotype" as a disease phenotype. To make effective

Computational Intelligence and Pattern Analysis in Biological Informatics, Edited by Ujjwal Maulik, Sanghamitra Bandyopadhyay, and Jason T. L. Wang
Copyright © 2010 John Wiley & Sons, Inc.

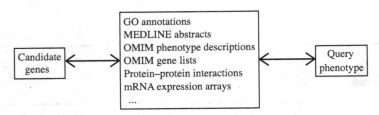

FIGURE 14.1   Different types of biological data provides the context for gene prioritizations.

use of biological resources, computational gene prioritization allows researchers to choose the best candidate genes for subsequent experimental validations.

The ultimate goal of gene prioritization is to find therapeutic targets and diagnostic biomarkers, the notion of a disease-related gene can be more general, i.e., a gene or a protein involved in the disease process either directly or indirectly. In turn, the list of candidates can originate from many data sources, e.g., genome-wide association studies serial analysis of gene expression (SAGE), massively parallel signature sequencing (MPSS) [2], or proteomic experiments. Such prioritization can be applied to either a short list of genes or the entire genome [3].

Disease gene prioritization requires researchers to take advantage of prior knowledge about both genes and phenotypes. We assume that "the truth is always there", which is embedded in large volumes of potentially relevant publications and various tabulated results from high-throughput experiments. A computational disease-gene prioritization method should be able to convert this data into insights about the relationship between candidate genes and interested disease phenotypes (see Fig. 14.1).

The first work on prioritization of candidate genes from linkage regions [4, 5] used text mining to extract phenotype descriptions and establish similarities among phenotypes and the relationships between phenotypes and genes. The underlying assumption is that a good candidate gene with a strong connection to the query phenotype, i.e., phenotype under investigation, can be identified by sifting through biomedical literature. Text mining allows more high-throughput scanning of the biomedical literature to develop credible content; therefore, it can be less costly than curation-based database development, e.g., LocusLink and RefSeq [6], GO (Gene Ontology) [7], and OMIM [8]. In Section 14.2, we will review gene prioritization methods and related databases that are developed based on biomedical text mining.

Both literature curation and text mining based approaches extract relationships between phenotypes and genes, all based on biological and biochemical processes that have been already identified. Thus, a pontential drawback is that genes that are less well characterized can be overlooked. Such "blind spot" can be targeted by complementary methods that do not rely on properties of phenotypes, e.g., lists of known disease genes or text-mined associations. One class of such complementary methods reported was to identify general properties of genomic sequences of disease genes [9–11] and relate genes from different loci (or linkage regions) of the same phenotype [12]. These methods will be reviewed in Section 14.3.

With the arrival of systems biology, several recent emerging methods have used data on biomolecular interactions among proteins and genes, most notably protein–protein interactions, biological pathways, and biomolecular interaction networks (see [13–19]). In Section 14.4, we will review different ways of gene prioritization based on interaction networks.

In Section 14.5, we describe how gene prioritization can be obtained with a unified phenotype-gene association network in which gene–gene links are taken from biomolecular interaction networks and phenotype–phenotype links are identified with results from text-mining.

One difficulty in prioritizing disease genes is the lack of data on many possible gene candidates. For example, among roughly 23,000 identified human genes, only 50–55% have GO annotations, which suggests that for the remaining genes we do not know about their biological processes, cellular components, or molecular functions. Networks of biomolecular interactions cover a similarly small percentage of genes. Gene expression data, on the other hand, can cover many genes that are otherwise uncharacterized genomic DNA. Using data of many types, especially high-throughput experimental and computational-derived data, has the potential to improve the quality of gene prioritizations that leads to new discoveries. However, the inherent "noisy" nature of high-throughput experimental data and computationally derived data raise the question how to combine different sources of data so that the integrated data improves the predictive power of gene prioritizations. We refer to this problem as the challenge of data fusion problems in gene participations and will describe different solutions in Section 14.6.

14.2 PRIORITIZATION BASED ON TEXT-MINING WITH REFERENCE TO PHENOTYPES

Perez-Iratxeta et al. [5] developed a method that uses the MEDLINE database and GO data to associate GO terms with phenotypes. Then, they ranked the candidate genes based on GO terms shared with the query phenotype. Later, they implemented this strategy as a web application [20]. The phenotype-GO term association was derived using MeSH C terms (medical subject headings from chemistry recognized in MEDLINE queries): An article stored in MEDLINE that mentions both terms creates an association pair. They measured the strengths of associations between phenotypes and MeSH C terms and between MeSH C and GO terms, and used a "max-product" rule from fuzzy logic to obtain the strength of the relationship between phenotypes and GO terms. The relationship GO term gene also has "strength" (which takes larger values for less frequent terms) and the same max-product rule can define the strength of the gene-phenotype relationship. Then, this "strength" was taken as the priority score (see Fig. 14.2). Clearly, this methods allow the aggregation of different

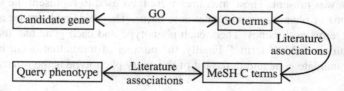

FIGURE 14.2 Chains of associations used by Perez-Iratxeta et al. in a text-mining based gene prioritization method [5].

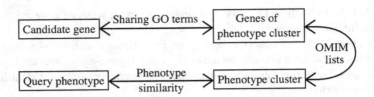

FIGURE 14.3   Chains of associations used by Freudenberg and Propping [4].

relationships between specific phenotypes and genes to identify additional information absent in biomedical texts separately. For example, one article evaluates effectiveness of a drug (MeSH C term) in the treatment of a phenotype, and another, the impact of that drug on a metabolic process (GO term). The enrichment on "artificial linkage regions" was approximately 10-fold, i.e., locating the correct candidate in the top 5% half of the time.

Freudenberg and Propping [4] used an different version of chain of associations (see Fig. 14.3). They defined between disease phenotypes a similarity score that was based on five key clinical features and clustered the phenotypes from OMIM according to the score. The OMIM also provides associations of phenotype-genetic cause, and this defines the last step in their chain. The enrichment reported in this article is similar to Perez-Iratxeta et al. [5].

van Driel et al. [21] developed a tool that could "data mine" up to nine web-based databases for candidate genes and could be used to select "the best" candidates in a linkage region. The user can specify a genomic region, which can be a linkage region, and a set of anatomic terms that describe the localization of symptoms of a Mendelian disorder provided by the user. The result gives two lists of genes from the genomic region: those that were found in at least one tissue from the set (OR list) and those that were found in all tissues from the set (AND list). The count of lists in which a gene is present can be viewed as a priority with possible values, 0, 1, or 2; in ten examples of diseases used in this chapter, they determined an average enrichment (the correct candidate was always present in the OR list). The localization of disease symptoms and the tissue localization of a disease-related protein is apparently an important part of "prior knowledge", but it is not apparent how to choose the best anatomic terms for a particular phenotype. Tiffin et al. [2] developed a method to make this decision "automatic". They used eVOC vocabulary of anatomic terms that is hierarchically organized like GO with only the "part of" relationships (e.g., retina is a part of eye). Applying text-mining, they counted MEDLINE papers that mention both the disease and the particular eVOC term. A term was counted as being present in a paper if its hypernym was present. These measures were then used to represent the strength of associations of phenotypes with anatomic terms. They obtained similar association of eVOC terms with genes. Then, each phenotype and each gene had its list of "n most significant eVOC terms." Finally, the number of terms that occur both in the list of a candidate gene and in the list of the query phenotype is the inferred priority for genes.

Both Perez-Iratxeta et al. [5] and Tiffin et al. [2] used the concept of chains of associations with different computational algorithmic flavors. Several recent papers

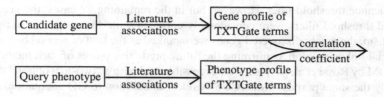

FIGURE 14.4 Using profile vectors for gene prioritizations.

used Pearson correlation of profile vectors. For example, Aerts et al. [22] used the MEDLINE database of abstracts in conjunction with the TXTGate vocabulary [23], which was developed specifically for gene analysis. A profile of "subject" X is a vector with an element for every term t and this element is the over-representation or under-representation or of occurrences of term t in articles that mention X compared with the frequency of occurrences of t in the entire database. Since both genes and phenotypes are "subjects", one can define the closeness of gene g to phenotype p as the Pearson correlation coefficient of profile(p) and profile(g) (see Fig. 14.4). This method was a component of a more complex prioritization system ENDEAVOUR that will also be discussed in Section 14.6.

14.3   PRIORITIZATION WITH NO DIRECT REFERENCE TO PHENOTYPES

Using literature to find associations between phenotypes and vocabulary terms was successful, but rarely new disease genes can be discovered using those associations. One reason is that many terms important for a given phenotype may not be discussed in articles that mention the phenotype' in addition, many new disease genes are yet to be annotated.

The POCUS method of Turner et al. [12] addressed the first problem. They applied two types of gene annotations, GO terms and InterPro domains for phenotypes that are associated with multiple genetic loci (linkage regions). The idea is that for such phenotypes one can discover important associations that were not yet reported in the literature. Within a single locus associated with phenotype p, genes with a certain term X (a type of protein domain or with a certain GO annotation) can be over-represented because of tandem duplications that place similar genes next to each other. Therefore, having term X does not identify a disease gene within that locus. However, if a gene g from another locus that is associated with p has term X, it raises the possibility that term X and gene g are significant for the query phenotype p. More precisely, gene g obtains a score because of term X if X also occurs in other loci of Phenotype p, and the score is based on the probability that two loci with a particular number of distinct terms containing the term X.

Turner et al. [12] tested POCUS on 29 phenotypes with multiple loci containing known disease genes, and on one specific disease, autism, which had two new genes discovered during the time of the research by Turner et al. In 11 cases, no disease genes could be identified using this method, due to enforcement of a stringent significance threshold filter. However, but in the remaining 18 cases, the genes that passed threshold filters were considerably enriched with disease genes. In the case of autism, the newly discovered genes were ranked as the best or second best in their artificial linkage region, confirming the future predictive power of such methods.

TOM by Rossi et al. [24] is a web-accessible tool with a "two-loci option" that has exactly the same purpose as POCUS besides. In addition to GO annotations, TOM also uses expression profile similarity.

While POCUS does not rely on prior literature to identify terms that are significant for the query phenotype, it relies on existing GO annotations that are available for approximately 60% of known human genes according to the GO annotation provided by the SwissProt database as well as available InterPro domain annotations. This motivates follow-up work that do not rely on any annotations of the candidate genes. Lopez-Bigas et al. [9] and Adie et al. [10] developed a decision tree method that is based solely DNA sequence features of the candidate gene, such as coding potential for a signal peptide, the similarity with its mouse homolog, the number of exons, and so on. The enrichment of PROSPECTR, the latter version of the approach, is close to 2-fold, i.e., the correct candidate appearing in the top 5% with a frequency of 10%. While modest, this result does not rely on any knowledge except for a DNA sequence. Further development in this direction can be promising in the context of interpretation of results from genome-wide association studies, because in those cases we know not only the DNA sequence, but also the exact type of variations.

14.4   PRIORITIZATION USING INTERACTION NETWORKS

Many methods using interactions in prioritizing candidate genes are fundamentally counting and comparing "qualified" interactions under the following underlying assumptions: 1) causative genes for a disease reside in the same biological module; 2) genes in the module have many interactions with other members within the module and relatively few interactions with nonmembers outside the module.

The observation that disease genes share interactions at a much higher rate than random gene pairs was made when protein–protein interaction (PPI) networks were assembled [25]. In this discussion, we will use some graph terms. A network is a graph composed of a set of nodes (genes as identified with their protein products) and a set of pairs of nodes called edges (that indicate the existence of interactions). If we have an edge $\{u, v\}$, we say that u and v are neighbors. For a node u, $N(u)$ is the set of its neighbors, and for a node set A, $N(A)$ is formed from A by inserting the neighbors of its elements. We will also use T to denote the set of known disease genes for the query phenotype (the training set).

George et al. [26] tested whether a PPI network could be used to propose candidates. They used the OPHID network [19] that consolidates interactions from HPRD, BIND, and MINT, curated networks of interactions that were reported in the literature, as well as results of high-throughput experiments that were performed on human proteins and proteins of four model species (baker's yeast, mouse, nematode, and fruit fly) that were mapped to their orthologous human proteins. Rather than ranking candidates, George et al. [26] were simply making predictions: any gene in

$N(T)$ that is within the investigated linkage interval is a candidate. To test the quality of these predictions, they used a set of 29 diseases with 170 genes, the same set as the set used to test the POCUS method by Turner et al. [12] . This benchmark showed very good performance: 42% of the correct candidates were identified and no incorrect candidates were identified.

The work of Oti et al. [27] drew quite different conclusions. They compared the gene prioritization results based on two networks: (1) HPRD (assembled by Gandhi et al. [25]), a curated collection of 19,000 PPIs based on the literature and (2) a network expanded with results of high-throughput experiments on human proteins and three model species. They tested the same prediction method as George et al. [26] on 1114 disease loci for 289 OMIM phenotypes that shared at least two known disease genes. This led to 432 predictions, 60% of which based on HPRD were correct as compared with 12% of which based on high-throughput data were correct. These results revealed the challenge even though biomolecular interactions may generate most trustworthy predictions, the number of such high-quality predictions is dependent on the coverage of PPI, which is still quite poor today. To make more predictions, we need to use some combination of (a) a larger network, (b) indirect interactions, and (c) methods that prioritize candidates that have these indirect connections. Otherwise, one must explore how to use prior knowledge to expand set T. In tests conducted by Oti et al. [27], the average size of T was 2, while in tests of George et al. [26], this size was more than twice as large at 4, a major motivation for the methods that we will discuss in Section 14.5.

Aerts et al. [22] used ranking based on PPI as one of the components of their ENDEAVOR program. They used the BIND PPI network developed by Bader et al. [28], which is similar to the expanded version of the network used by Oti et al. [27]. Using graph definitions, the priority score for a gene u is the count of its neighbors in $N(T)$. They subsequently order the candidate list from the largest to the smallest priority score. Here, each of the points (a–c) is addressed. However, the formula for the priority value does not take into account of very high variability of numbers of neighbors of nodes in the PPI graph, which varies between 1 and >1000. Clearly, being a neighbor of a node with degree 1 provides a much more specific hint of relatedness than being a neighbor of a node with degree 1000.

Franke et al. [29] used several data sources, but they also evaluated the use of an interaction network that had a large majority of interactions from the BIND PPI network, with a small number of coexpression-based "interactions" added (the MA+PPI data set). Their priority function is described as an empirical p-value of kernel scoring function of the shortest path distance from node u to T, but a much simpler definition defines the same ranking. If $d(u, T)$ is the distance (defined as the shortest path length) from u to T and there are k network nodes that are not further from u than $d(u, T)$, then they effectively use k as the priority value of u and they rank candidates from the smallest to the largest priority value. When they used MA+PPI only, the correct candidates appeared at the top 5 (of 100) candidates 8% of the time, hence they concluded that MA+PPI "lacks predictive performance".

The above methods are based on basic graph concepts and all are rooted in the notion of path distance in the network graph. However, measures derived from graph distance can be misleading. As we mentioned, one issue is the wide range of the numbers of neighbors that different nodes have. Moreover, disease genes are not a representative sample of all genes as they tend to have more interactions than the average. To address these issues, Aerts et al. [22] have a priority formula that is "much easier" for proteins with many interactions (network hubs) than for others, conversely, the formula of Franke et al. [29] eliminates that advantage. Which is the correct approach? Or perhaps there is a "third approach" that can avoid the pitfalls of either extreme position?

Indeed, a much more successful method was introduced recently by Köhler et al. [30]. They proposed a more elaborate network-based prioritization method based on global distance measure in the application of finding disease genes from linkage analysis. They also compared their methods with the methods based on local distance measures [26,27] and ENDEAVOUR [22] to show that their own methods performed better.

A physical example of global distance would be a resistance between two points of an electric network; computing such resistance with Kirchoff's circuit law requires us to know the entire network. We can also talk about "closeness": If we apply some positive voltage to the first point and ground to the second point, the closeness would be the resulting current. Köhler et al. [30] discussed two global distance measures, random walk with restart (RWR) and diffusion kernel. In evaluation, diffusion kernel leads to very similar results as RWR; computationally and conceptually, these methods are quite similar, so we will describe RWR only here. The general concept of these methods is to start a random walk by selecting a node in set T and use the rules of the walk to compute the stationary probability distribution of the position of the walker. A good set of rules should assure that this probability measures closeness, or relatedness, of various positions to set T, so we can rank the candidate genes based on those closeness scores.

In RWR, the random walker first decides if it should continue the walk (with probability $1 - r$) or to restart (with probability r). In the former case, it changes its position from the current node c to a randomly selected neighbor in $N(c)$; in the latter, it "jumps" to a random node in T.

To describe RWR more precisely, we will use W to denote the column-normalized adjacency matrix of the network and $\mathbf{p}^t$ to denote a vector in which the ith element holds the probability of the walker being at node i at time step t. The walker starts by moving to each disease gene (a node in T) with probability $1/|T|$, so the ith element of $\mathbf{p}^0$ is $1/|T|$ if i is in T and 0 otherwise. Then, at each time step t, the random walker has probability r to restart (i.e., to repeat the starting move) and with probability $1 - r$ the random walker chooses to follow an edge from its current node, each edge with the same probability. This defines the simple update rule of how to change the probability distribution of the location of the walker, namely, $\mathbf{p}$ changes to $r\mathbf{p}^0 + (1 - r)W\mathbf{p}$ (i.e., $\mathbf{p}^{t+1} = r\mathbf{p}^0 + (1 - r)W\mathbf{p}^t$). They repeat this update until the sum of changes of the elements of $\mathbf{p}$ becomes $<10^{-6}$, so that $\mathbf{p}$ becomes a good approximation of the steady-state distribution. The final probabilities of each node are the priority values and the ranking is from the largest to the smallest value.

For comparison with other methods, Köhler et al. [30] implemented direct interactions (DI) with other known disease-family genes and single shortest path (SP) to any known disease gene in the family. They computed results for 110 phenotypes with 783 known disease genes using a "1-out, artificial linkage region of 100" approach (the same approach as [22, 26, 29]). They tested the results on their screens of candidate genes in an artificial linkage interval, i.e., the prediction of gene g tested by removing g from T and considering a set S of 100 candidate genes that flank g in two directions on the chromosome. They also ranked genes in S with PROSPECTR, which is based on sequence-based features, and with ENDEAVOUR, which is based on several different types of data. Both mean-fold enrichment and ROC analysis showed that their methods perform much better than the other methods they were compared with.

The shortest path method, was considered by George et al. [26], but as we mentioned before, they merely tested predictions made when the shortest path has length 1, i.e., they did not test the ranking based on SP length. Correct predictions were made in 42% of the tested artificial linkage intervals where they did not observe incorrect predictions. In 61% of the cases in the tests of Köhler et al., where the approach of George et al. [26] and Oti et al. [27] yielded a correct prediction, some genes are also predicted incorrectly. An analogous situation, multiple nodes having the best priority value, is very rare for the RWR method: of the cases when the correct candidate had the top score, only 1.4% had another node within the investigated linkage interval with the same score. Moreover, RWR assigns a top score to the correct candidate more often. Thus, one of the advantages of RWR is that when SP selects several genes with the same score, RWR usually correctly picks a single good candidate. The measure for the assessing the quality of a method developed by Köhler et al., mean enrichment, can be explained as follows: if the evaluated candidate gets rank a, we score it as enrichment $50/a$, and we calculate the mean. For example, if the evaluated gene always receives a rank between 1 and 5 (out of 100 possible ranks) with equal probability, this gives mean enrichment of $(50/1 + 50/2 + 50/3 + 50/4 + 50/5)/5 = 22.8$. The mean enrichment for RWR was 26, and for SP and DI it was 18. They also tested various methods on seven recently identified disease genes and the mean enrichment for RWR and SP was 25.9 and 17.2, respectively. They also obtained ENDEAVOUR ranks for those genes and the resulting mean enrichment was 18.4. This is very intriguing because ENDEAVOUR presumably considers many data sources and obtained top evaluations in other papers. Apparently, many biases and coverage issues can confound literature or data integration based gene prioritization methods but may be addressed with the use of biomolecular interaction networks.

14.5   PRIORITIZATION BASED ON JOINT USE OF INTERACTION NETWORK AND LITERATURE-BASED SIMILARITY BETWEEN PHENOTYPES

One conclusion from the results of Köhler et al. [30] concerning the effectiveness of their RWR ranking method could be that PPI interactions alone can provide the best possible prediction of disease genes. This conclusion may be premature, because RWR was tested on phenotypes that on average had seven known disease genes.

The comparison of results of George et al. [26] and Oti et al. [27] suggests that the reliability of a method based on PPI interactions may decrease as the number of known disease genes decreases. Moreover, for roughly one-third of the phenotypes in OMIM, there are no known disease genes, and in these cases PPI methods described in Section 14.4 cannot be applied at all. However, even if no disease genes are identified for a given phenotype, we have considerable prior knowledge in the form of (1) knowledge that phenotypes are similar and (2) accumulated knowledge about the similar phenotypes.

The notion of similarity of phenotypes was used first by Freudenberg and Propping [4], who defined a measure of "closeness" for phenotypes and computed phenotype clusters as the initial stage of their prioritization method. One could simply combine that approach with, for example, RWR. Given a phenotype compute its cluster, and then use the set T that consists of all known disease genes of all members of the cluster. This requires making an arbitrary decision on whether to cluster the phenotypes or avoid clustering with the use of phenotype–phenotype similarity.

Most gene prioritization methods integrate two different types of data: literature-based data and interactome data [3, 31]. They use similarities between phenotypes based on literature curation and the interaction network, and are guided by the assumption that causative genes for the phenotypically similar diseases reside in the same biological module. In turn, a biological module corresponds to a fragment of the network that contains many interactions.

To justify that assumption, Lage et al. [31] described a situation when a protein complex is vital to some biological process, while mutations of genes of the proteins that participate in that complex have a negative impact on that process leading to diseases with different, but related symptoms. Therefore, connections in PPI network between the constituents of the complex are reflected in similarities between phenotypes that are related to their genes. Alternatively, there can be biological pathways with similar consequences: disease proteins have many interactions among themselves, which make up the basic assumption for all network-based prioritization methods. Lage et al. [31] identified so-called "disease complexes" for each candidate gene and each such disease complex can be seen as a small module (and a disease pathway would be a larger module). They made a unified network of genes and phenotypes where connections between genes were from a PPI network, each with its reliability score, and disease genes were connected to their respective phenotypes while phenotype–phenotype connections were annotated with similarity scores. Then they converted the unified network into a Bayesian network by computing posterior probability for each gene. Intuitively, those probabilities measure the strength of the following tendency: If one moves from the network node of the candidate gene to its network neighbors and then to the phenotypes (if any) associated with those neighbors, he can arrive at a phenotype that is similar to the query phenotype. Consequently, the posterior probabilities of genes define their priority values.

Following this work, Wu et al. [3] also proposed the prioritization method based on the same assumption as Lage et al. [31], but much simpler. In addition to the general assumption of all network-based prioritization methods, they made the following assumption for their method called "CIPHER," in which members of a disease module have positive correlation of gene–gene relatedness and phenotype–phenotype similarity while nonmembers lack such correlation. They also tested the levels of these correlations to predict module members. Their method can be described as the sequence of the following steps:

First, for the query phenotype p, collect similarity scores (described at the end of this section) to all other phenotypes in the phenotype–gene network. This forms a vector profile(p).

Second, for a pair of candidate gene g and phenotype q, define closeness(g, q) as the number of neighbors of g that are disease genes of q. By collecting these values for all q's we obtain a vector profile(g).

Third, the priority value of g is the Pearson correlation coefficient of profile(g) and profile(p). The gene with the highest value receives the rank of the top candidate.

They compared this method with other methods including those by Freudenberg and Propping [4], Gaulton et al. [32], and ENDEAVOR. They determined that their methods perform much better than the first two methods and have comparable performance with ENDEAVOR. A direct comparison of CIPHER with RWR of Köhler et al. [30] is not simple because Wu et al. use a different set of test cases and a different definition of enrichment. In both methods, when applied to artificial linkage intervals of size 100 (109 for CIPHER) in "leave-one-out" manner, the correct candidate had the top rank roughly 50% of the time. The additional strength of CIPHER is revealed using "leave-all-out" tests in which we remove the knowledge of all gene-disease associations for the query phenotype. The performance in those tests was only somewhat weaker than in "leave-one-out" tests. The explanation is that CIPHER uses the associations of genes with the remaining phenotypes and similarities of those phenotypes with the query phenotype. A weakness of CIPHER is its inability to prioritize genes with no known interactions with disease genes or where there is no single connected interaction network. A modification of CIPHER called CIPHER(SP) alleviated the limitation because it computes closeness(g, q) using profiles of disease genes of q and the shortest path distances from g to those genes. However, CIPHER(SP) performs worse than CIPHER. This is not surprising given the results of Köhler et al. [30], in which the shortest path distance should probably be replaced with some version of global distance. Therefore, one can expect that a "fusion" of RWR and CIPHER would have wider applicability and superior performance to either of these methods.

Of special note is the concept of phenotype similarity, which was widely used [3, 4, 31, 33]. Freudenberg and Popping [4] measured the similarity between disease phenotypes from the OMIM database using five indices, i.e., episodic, etiology, tissue, onset, and inheritance. They gave simple similarity scores for the pairs of diseases by comparing the individual indices. van Driel et al. [33] developed a text analysis technique to extract phenotypic features from OMIM to quantify the overlap of their OMIM descriptions. They defined a vector of phenotypic features in OMIM descriptions of phenotype p by mining terms from the MeSH vocabulary and for each term they counted its occurrences (including its hypernyms) in the text. Thus each term has a value in the feature vector and the similarity between two phenotypes is computed as the cosine of the feature vectors of two phenotypes. Note that this type of feature vector of phenotype p is similar to the profile(p) used by Aerts et al. [22] described in Section 14.2. This method was adapted and refined in Wu et al. [3] and Lage et al. [31].

14.6   FUSION OF DATA FROM MULTIPLE SOURCES

Each prioritization method uses several data sources that allow us to define associations that connect genes, phenotypes and other objects, on which we can compute a priority score. Adding more data sources might yield more reliable results. In particular, each source represents only a partial knowledge and potentially can complement each other to piece together a global view of the knowledge context.

This creates two challenges. First, each data source has to be incorporated in a coherent prioritization framework. Second, one need to develop an integrated formula. Typically, a single prioritization formula uses several but rarely all of these data sources, e.g., associations between genes and phenotypes from OMIM, associations between phenotypes and scientific terms from text mining in MEDLINE abstracts, and associations between genes or proteins from molecular interaction network. However, when one add new data source and associations with another type of data the problem of incorporating mixed data types looms large.

Rossi et al. [24] proposed solving this problem by defining "filters" for the candidate genes. They considered a set of candidate genes and another set of genes as the training set T (as defined in Section 14.4). Genes in T are presumed to be related to the query phenotype either by being explicitly provided by a database like OMIM or obtained in the same way as in the POCUS method, which we discussed in Section 14.3. Then, they use a data source to compute the distance of candidate genes to T. If the data source is GO, they measure the statistical significance of sharing GO terms with the training set. If the data source is the transcriptome data from public repositories, each gene has a vector of expression values, and a candidate gene has a statistical significance of the closeness of its vector to the vectors of genes in T. In this fashion, each candidate gene has two priority scores. Finally, they selected candidates for which both priority values exceed a certain threshold, and they describe them as genes that passed through two filters. This certainly raises the concern that a candidate could be identified by one data source and disqualified by the other due to the incompleteness of the data. This problem is solved by allowing the user of the system to select which filters they want to apply. Clearly, this would be inadequate if we would consider a large number of data sources.

Aerts et al. [22] designed a modular prioritization system, ENDEAVOUR, which uses a large number of data sources and produces a "synthetic" rank. They defined 10 priority scores based on a variety of data sources. Their prioritization process consisted of four steps: (1) compute priority values according to each data source, (2) convert these priorities to ratio ranks, (3) use vectors of 10 ratio ranks to compute values of a summarizing statistic, and (4) use the values of the summarizing statistic as the final priority score.

Several different methods are used in step (1). As we described in Section 14.2, they used "literature" data to represent each gene as a "profile vector" of strengths of associations of a gene with scientific terms, and Pearson correlation coefficient to measure the closeness of a candidate gene to the training set of genes. This vector methodology was used with two other data sources. One type of vector gives expression levels of a gene in 79 human tissues a the gene expression data set. Another type gives for each position a weight matrix of a transcription factor from the TRANSFAC database the best score recorded for that matrix in the cis-regulatory region of the gene.

Four data sources were treated as attributes and in those cases they compute p-values of sharing attributes with the training set in a similar manner to Rossi et al. [24]. Some of the attributes were straightforward, including GO terms, InterPro protein domains, and membership in KEGG pathways. Expression levels of a gene in human tissues can also be treated as attributes because in a dbEST library of a particular tissue, a gene is categorized as present or absent (based on the levels of its ESTs).

Two data sources define priority scores rather directly. One is the minimum e-value of a BLAST alignment of a candidate gene with the genes of the training set. The second is based on the scores of positional weight matrices of transcription factors in the cis-regulatory region of a candidate gene; however, rather than creating the profile for all transcription factors, in this variant, five most significantly ranked transcription factors are established for the training set and the total score that these five give for a candidate gene are simply added up.

The third data source is the graph of a PPI network, which we described already in Section 14.4.

Each candidate gene obtains a vector of 10 priority scores. In step (1), each priority score is replaced with its ratio rank. If there are n candidate genes being evaluated and a gene g has a bth best value, the ratio rank is b/n.

The summarizing statistic computed in step (3) is Q statistic proposed in the biological context by Stuart et al. [34]. Finally, the genes are ranked–ordered according to their values of Q statistic.

A nonstatistician can be puzzled why the Q statistic of n ranks is superior to a sum or a product of those ranks but the evaluation of the method is quite revealing. It is difficult to translate the sensitivity–specificity curves of Aerts et al. to enrichment measures described earlier, but Wu et al. [3] reported ENDEAVOUR to be the "best other method", based on their evaluations of CIPHER and a similar comparison made by Köhler et al. [30]. Among all the data sources included in ENDEAVOUR, literature profiles were most useful when tested on the OMIM phenotypes and GO annotations were most useful when tested on KEGG pathways, but the results were not significantly worse when the most useful data source was excluded. This suggests that the data fusion based on the Q statistic is effective in combining relatively noisy and incomplete data into reliable prediction.

Most compelling evaluation results were derived from the tests on 10 newly discovered disease genes. In three cases, a very good rank (1 or 3) was obtained using literature profiles alone and slightly worse (2, 3, and 4) using a synthetic rank. In both cases, the synthetic rank was drastically better, 1 and 3 and in the remaining cases the synthetic rank was also significantly better.

One can expect that ENDEAVOUR, being modular, will be improved in the future. Its protein–protein interaction component was not reported by the authors as particularly successful and it can be replaced with a better network method like RWR from Köhler et al. [30]. The application of expression data is limited to expression in healthy human tissues and provides two priority scores. The main challenge is to combine data fusion with the phenotype similarity because it would require larger changes in the modular design; one possibility would be to have a fuzzy training set where the disease genes of similar phenotypes would be available with different degrees.

14.7 CONCLUSIONS AND OPEN PROBLEMS

Gene prioritization problems benefited from the development of systems biology. As comprehensive online databases emerged, researchers used them to develop computational tools that offer practical advice to biologists. Apparently, any candidates for genes responsible for a given phenotype or involved in a biological process should be incorporated as prior knowledge (biological context). There has been significant progress in the selection of the most relevant sources of data, in the development of algorithms applied to various types of data, and finally, in the application of methods to combine results derived from different data sources. Many of the resulting methods are readily available to users either as standalone programs or as web services online.

This "success story" is clearly not yet complete. First, it is still an open question what the best way is to handle different data sources. For example, literature data can be text-mined with different controlled vocabularies. Second, one can try to give better weights to different vocabulary terms or to different types of publications. Using data on protein–gene interaction also raises a different set of questions. "What are the best interaction networks to use"? "What are the best algorithms"? "Does the answer depend on application"?

For other types of biological data, these questions are even more relevant for gene prioritizations. How should we use data on transcription regulation? Aerts et al. [22] did not comment how to practically pick "the best one". While one debates how to develop more effective methods in the future, there are plenty of questions to address even today. How to use information about protein structure? How can we use gene expression data and proteomics data? The list goes on. One thing for sure is that this area will be a subject of many new developments in the near future.

14.8 ACKNOWLEDGMENT

We thank Michael Grobe for reviewing this chapter and giving invaluable comments.

REFERENCES

1. C. Giallourakis, C. Henson, M. Reich, X. Xie, and V. K. Mootha (2005), Disease gene discovery through integrative genomics, *Annu. Rev. Genomics Hum. Genet.*, **ED-6**: 381.

2. N. Tiffin, J. F. Kelso, A. R. Powell, H. Pan, V. B. Bajic, and W. A. Hide (2005), Integration of text- and data-mining using ontologies successfully selects disease gene candidates, *Nucleic Acids Res.*, **EDL-33**(5): 1544.

3. X. Wu, R. Jiang, M. Q. Zhang, and S. Li (2008), Network-based global inference of human disease genes, *Mol. Syst. Biol.*, **ED-4**: 189.

4. J. Freudenberg and P. Propping (2002), A similarity-based method for genome-wide prediction of disease-relevant human genes, *Bioinformatics*, **EDL-18**(Suppl. 2): S110.

5. C. Perez-Iratxeta, P. Bork, and M. A. Andrade (2002), Association of genes to genetically inherited diseases using data mining, *Nat. Genet.*, **EDL-31**(3): 316.

6. K. D. Pruitt, K. S. Katz, H. Sicotte, and D. R. Maglott (2000), Introducing RefSeq and LocusLink: curated human genome resources at the NCBI, *Trends Genet.*, **EDL-16**(1): 44.

7. M. Ashburner, C. A. Ball, J. A. Blake, D. Botstein, H. Butler, J. M. Cherry, A. P. Davis, K. Dolinski, S. S. Dwight, J. T. Eppig, M. A. Harris, D. P. Hill, L. Issel-Tarver, A. Kasarskis, S. Lewis, J. C. Matese, J. E. Richardson, M. Ringwald, G. M. Rubin, and G. Sherlock (2000), Gene ontology: tool for the unification of biology. The Gene Ontology Consortium, *Nat. Genet.*, **EDL-25**(1): 25.

8. A. Hamosh, A. F. Scott, J. Amberger, D. Valle, and V. A. Mckusick (2000), Online Mendelian Inheritance in Man (OMIM), *Hum. Mutat.*, **EDL-15**(1): 57.

9. N. Lopez-Bigas and C. A. Ouzounis (2004), Genome-wide identification of genes likely to be involved in human genetic disease, *Nucleic Acids Res.*, **EDL-32**(10): 3108.

10. E. A. Adie, R. R. Adams, K. L. Evans, D. J. Porteous, and B. S. Pickard (2005), Speeding disease gene discovery by sequence based candidate prioritization, *BMC Bioinformatics*, **ED-6**: 55.

11. E.A. Adie, R.R. Adams, K.L. Evans, D.J. Porteous, and B.S. Pickard (2006), SUSPECTS: enabling fast and effective prioritization of positional candidates, *Bioinformatics*, **EDL-22**(6): 773.

12. F. S. Turner, D. R. Clutterbuck, and C. A. Semple (2003), POCUS: mining genomic sequence annotation to predict disease genes, *Genome Biol.*, **EDL-4**(11): R75.

13. S. Peri, et al. (2004), Human protein reference database as a discovery resource for proteomics, *Nucl. Acids Res.*, **EDL-32**(Database issue): D497.

14. C. Alfarano et al. (2005), The Biomolecular Interaction Network Database and related tools 2005 update, *Nucleic, Acids Res.*, **EDL-33**(Database issue): D418.

15. C. Stark, B. J. Breitkreutz, T. Reguly, L. Boucher, A. Breitkreutz, and M. Tyers (2006), BioGRID: a general repository for interaction datasets, *Nucleic Acids Res.*, **EDL-34** (Database issue): D535.

16. S. Kerrien, et al. (2007), IntAct–open source resource for molecular interaction data, *Nucleic Acids Res.*, **EDL-35**(Database issue): D561.

17. L. Salwinski, C. S. Miller, A. J. Smith, F. K. Pettit, J. U. Bowie, and D. Eisenberg (2004), The Database of Interacting Proteins: 2004 update, *Nucleic Acids Res.*, **EDL-32**(Database issue): D449.

18. C. von Mering, L. J. Jensen, M. Kuhn, S. Chaffron, T. Doerks, B. Kruger, B. Snel, and P. Bork (2007), STRING 7–recent developments in the integration and prediction of protein interactions, *Nucleic Acids Res.*, **EDL-35**(Database issue): D358.

19. K. R. Brown and I. Jurisica (2005), Online predicted human interaction database, *Bioinformatics*, **EDL-21**(9): 2076.

20. C. Perez-Iratxeta, M. Wjst, P. Bork, and M. A. Andrade (2005), G2D: a tool for mining genes associated with disease, *BMC Genet.,* **ED-6**: 45.

21. M. A. van Driel, K. Cuelenaere, P. P. Kemmeren, J. A. Leunissen, and H. G. Brunner (2003), A new web-based data mining tool for the identification of candidate genes for human genetic disorders, *Eur. J. Hum. Genet.,* **EDL-11**(1): 57.

22. S. Aerts, D. Lambrechts, S. Maity, P. Van Loo, B. Coessens, F. De Smet, L. C. Tranchevent, B. De moor, P. Marynen, B. Hassan, P. Carmeliet, and Y. Moreau (2006), Gene prioritization through genomic data fusion, *Nat. Biotechnol.,* **EDL-24**(5): 537.

23. P. Glenisson, B. Coessens, S. Van Vooren, J. Mathys, Y. Moreau, and B. De Moor (2004), TXTGate: profiling gene groups with text-based information, *Genome Biol.,* **EDL-5**(6): R43.

24. S. Rossi, D. Masotti, C. Nardini, E. Bonora, G. Romeo, E. Macii, L. Benini, and S. Volinia (2006), TOM: a web-based integrated approach for identification of candidate disease genes, *Nucleic Acids Res.,* **EDL-34**(Web Server issue): W285.

25. T. K. Gandhi, et al. (2006), Analysis of the human protein interactome and comparison with yeast, worm and fly interaction datasets, *Nat. Genet.,* **EDL-38**(3): 285.

26. R. A. George, J. Y. Liu, L. L. Feng, R. J. Bryson-Richardson, D. Fatkin, and M. A. Wouters (2006), Analysis of protein sequence and interaction data for candidate disease gene prediction, *Nucleic Acids Res.,* **EDL-34**(19): e130.

27. M. Oti, B. Snel, M. A. Huynen, and H. G. Brunner (2006), Predicting disease genes using protein-protein interactions, *J. Med. Genet.,* **EDL-43**(8): 691.

28. G. D. Bader, D. Betel, and C. W. Hogue (2003), BIND: the Biomolecular Interaction Network Database, *Nucleic Acids Res.,* **EDL-31**(1): 248.

29. L. Franke, H. van Bakel, L. Fokkens, E. D. de Jong, M. Egmont-Petersen, and C. Wijmenga (2006), Reconstruction of a functional human gene network, with an application for prioritizing positional candidate genes, *Am. J. Hum.,* **EDL-78**(6): 1011.

30. S. Köhler, S. Bauer, D. Horn, and P. N. Robinson (2008), Walking the interactome for prioritization of candidate disease genes, *Am. J. Hum. Genet.,* **EDL-82**(4): 949.

31. K. Lage, E. I. Karlberg, Z. M. Storling, P. I. Olason, A. G. Pedersen, O. Rigina, A. M. Hinsby, Z. Turner, F. Pociot, N. Tommerup, Y. Moreau, and S. Brunak (2007), A human phenome-interactome network of protein complexes implicated in genetic disorders, *Nat. Biotechnol.,* **EDL-25**(3): 309.

32. K. J. Gaulton, K. L. Mohlke, and T. J. Vision (2007), A computational system to select candidate genes for complex human traits, *Bioinformatics,* **EDL-23**(9): 1132.

33. M. A. van Driel, K. Cuelenaere, P. P. Kemmersen, J. A. Leunissen, and H. G. Brunner (2006), A text-mining analysis of the human phenome, *Eur. J. Hum. Genet.,* **EDL-14**(5): 535.

34. J. M. Stuart, E. Segal, D. Koller, and S. K. Kim (2003), A gene-coexpression network for global discovery of conserved genetic modules, *Science,* **EDL-302**(5643): 249.

15

PREDICTION OF PROTEIN–PROTEIN INTERACTIONS

15.1 INTRODUCTION

Protein–protein interactions (PPI) play a major role in many biological processes e.g., hormone receptor binding, protease inhibition, antigen–antibody interactions, signal transduction, chaperone activity, enzyme allostery, to name a few [1–8]. The associations of proteins may be transient or permanent. The interfaces of the interacting proteins have specific different characteristics. The identification of the interface residues may shed light on many important aspects, like drug development, elucidation of molecular pathways, generation of protein mimetics, and understanding of disease mechanisms, as well as development of docking methodologies to build structural models of protein complexes. Before going into the details of the various PPI prediction methodologies, a few basic definitions, which are frequently used in the analysis of PPIs, need to be introduced.

15.2 BASIC DEFINITIONS [9, 10]

Monomer. A single unit of an assembly.

Polymer. An assembly of single monomeric units [i.e., Polymer = (Monomer)$_n$].

If $n = 2$, the polymer is called a dimer

If $n = 3$, the polymer is called trimer, and so on.

Protomer. The monomeric constituent units of a protein having two or more monomeric protein chains.

Computational Intelligence and Pattern Analysis in Biological Informatics, Edited by Ujjwal Maulik, Sanghamitra Bandyopadhyay, and Jason T. L. Wang
Copyright © 2010 John Wiley & Sons, Inc.

Homomer. A protein with same monomeric constituents.

Heteromer. A protein with different monomeric constituents.

Obligate and Nonobligate Protein–Protein Complexes. A protein–protein complex where the individual partners (protomers) are not stable by themselves (e.g., the Arc repressor dimer). If the individual protomers can exist on their own, the complex is then referred to as nonobligate. For example, antibody–antigen complexes are nonobligate ones.

Transient and Permanent Complexes. If the associations between the protomers in a protein–protein complex is weak and are in a dynamic equilibrium in solution where it is broken and formed continuously, the complex is called a transient complex (e.g., the nonobligate homodimer of sperm lysine).

On the other hand, if the associations between the protomers require molecular switch to break, the complex is called a permanent complex. The heterotrimeric G protein forms a permanent complex in the presence of GDP.

Note that PPIs cannot be distinctly classified as transient and permanent, rather a continuum exists between them. The stabilities of all these complexes depend on physiological conditions and cellular environments.

Accessible Surface Area. Accessible surface area (ASA) is the fraction of the total van der Waal's surface of an atom that can come in contact with other atoms, specifically water. In the case of proteins, the accessible surface area is calculated for each atom of each amino acid residue.

Interface Patch. The interface is the contact area of the proteins. It involves those residues of the proteins that have the ASA of their side chains decreased by $>1 \text{ Å}^2$ on complex formation.

Relative Accessible Surface Area. Relative accessible surface area (RSA) is defined as the ratio of ASA to the maximal accessibility of each amino acid.

Gap Volume and Gap Index. The gap volume is defined as the volume enclosed between any two protein molecules delimiting the boundary by defining a maximum allowed distance from both the interfaces. The Gap index is calculated as *Gap index = gap volume / interface ASA*

Surface Patch. Surface residues are the amino acid residues of a protein with a relative accessible surface area of $>5\%$. A surface patch is the central surface accessible residue and *n* nearest surface accessible neighbors, where *n* is the size of the patch in terms of the number of residues. A mean relative ASA for each patch is calculated as

Patch ASA (Å^2) = sum of the RSAs of the amino acid residues in the patch / number of amino acid residues in the patch

Solvation Potential. This is the measure of the propensity of an amino acid to get solvated. It is used to quantify the tendency of a patch to be exposed to solvent or buried in the interface of a protein–protein complex.

Residue Interface Propensities. Residue interface propensities (RIPs) represent the tendency of the amino acid residues of a protein to be on the interface of the protein–protein complex. The patch interface propensity (PIP) is calculated as

PIP = Sum of the natural logarithms of the RIPs of the amino acid residues in the patch / number of amino acid residues in the patch

Hydrophobicity. The surface patch hydrophobicities are defined as

Patch hydrophobicity = Hydrophobicity value of the amino acid residues in a patch / number of amino acid residues in the patch

Planarity. This quantity of the surface patch is evaluated by calculating the root-mean-square (rms) deviation of all the atoms present on the surface patch from the least-square plane that passes through the atoms.

Protrusion Index. The protrusion index (PI) is a quantity that gives an idea of how much a residue sticks out from the surface of a protein. The patch PI is calculated as

Patch PI = Sum of the PIs of the amino acid residues in the patch/number of amino acid residues in the patch

15.3   CLASSIFICATION OF PPI

According to Ofran and Rost (2003), the PPIs [11] can be grouped into six different categories on the basis of their sequence features. They are

Intradomain. It represents the interfaces within one structural domain.

Domain–domain. It is the interface between different domains within one chain of a protein.

Homo-obligomer. It is defined as the interface between permanently interacting identical chains (having the same amino acid compositions) of proteins.

Hetero-obligomer. It is the interface between permanently interacting different chains (having different amino acid compositions) of proteins.

Homo-complex. It is defined as the interface between transiently interacting identical chains (having the same amino acid compositions) of proteins.

Hetero-complex. It is the interface between transiently interacting different chains (having different amino acid compositions) of proteins.

15.4   CHARACTERISTICS OF PPIs

The different PPIs have different characteristic features as determined by various research groups. There are a number of databases having features of PPIs. A list of web links of some important servers is given in Appendix I. A brief description of the mechanism of the functionality of the servers is presented in Appendix II.

As a whole, the following features hold good for most of the PPI.

Sequence Conservation. The PPIs have more or less conserved amino acid sequence patterns as compared to the noninterface regions of the proteins. This may be due to functional or structural reasons [9–20].

Nature of the Interface. Generally, the PPIs are flat compared to the other surface regions on the proteins. Enzymes are found to possess the largest cavities on the surfaces to which the particular substrate with a complimentary surface binds [9–20].

Distribution of Amino Acids. The PPI generally consists of hydrophobic amino acid residues, but the number of conserved residues in interfaces is a function of the interface size. Large interfaces have polar amino acids surrounded by hydrophobic rings. Generally, the PPI are rich in aromatic amino acid residues, Tyr, Trp, and to some extent Phe, as well as Arg and Met. However, in large interfaces there are a preponderance of polar amino acid residues like His, Asn, Gln, Thr, and Ser, which remain surrounded by hydrophobic shells [12,15,16].

Secondary Structure. β-Strands are the ones that are mostly found in the interfaces while α-helices are disfavored. The interfaces are also found to contain long loops.

Solvent Accessibility. The solvent accessibilities of the interfaces depend on the interface type. In general, the interfaces of obligomers are less solvent accessible than those of transient complexes. The reason is because of the ability of the protomers of the transient complexes to exist on their own by getting solvated in the cellular environments.

Conformational Entropy of Side Chains. To minimize the entropic cost upon complex formation, the interface residues are found to have less side-chain rotamers.

Interface Area. In general, the majority of the protein heterodimer interfaces are $> 600 \text{ Å}^2$.

- The interfaces of homo-obligomers are larger and more hydrophobic than their nonobligate counterparts. The individual monomers of the homo-obligomeric complexes cannot exist on their own in cellular environments. Thus they are able to form large, intertwined hydrophobic interfaces. On the other hand, the monomeric components of hetero-obligomers are able to exist individually in cells. This may be the cause of their having polar interfaces to meet the requirements of individual existence and solubility.
- Protein–protein complexes with interfaces larger than $\sim 1000 \text{ Å}^2$ may undergo conformational changes upon complexation [9,10,12].
- The complexation ability of proteins, which form transient complexes, is dependent on the cellular environments that trigger the biochemical processes [12].
- The binding free energy ΔG between the protomers is not correlated with the interface parameters (e.g., the size, polarity, and so on) [12].

- Most proteins are very specific in choosing their partners. However, multi-specific binding between protein families is also observed, such as in proteins involved in regulatory pathways (e.g., RhoA-RhoGAP) [9–20].

15.5   DRIVING FORCES FOR THE FORMATION OF PPIs

The mechanism(s) by which a protein binds another protein is poorly understood. However, a few aspects of the interactions may be generalized from the analyses of the different protein–protein complexes.

The association of the proteins relies on an encounter of the interacting surfaces. It requires colocalization and/or coexpression within a compartment. For encounter from different locations, diffusion or vascular transport of the proteins is necessary [10–20].

Local concentrations of the interacting proteins also play important roles in their binding. For example, the anchoring of proteins in a membrane helps in transmembrane protein oligomerization [10–20].

The mutual affinity of components of a protein complex may be altered by the presence of an effector molecule (e.g., adenosine triphosphate, ATP), a change in the physicochemical conditions (e.g., changes in pH, concentrations of ions, and so on), or by the covalent modifications of the proteins (e.g., phosphorylation [10–20]).

The binding interactions that hold the protein molecules together are mainly noncovalent interactions such as

- The clustering of hydrophobic residues in the interface.
- Hydrogen bonding and salt bridges between polar amino acids in the interface.
- Interactions involving the π electron cloud of aromatic rings.
- Cation-π interactions between the guanidinium ring of Arg with the aromatic π electron cloud of the amino acids (e.g., Tyr, Trp, and Phe) [12,15,16].

The only covalent interaction observed in PPIs is the disulfide bridges between Cys residues of the two interacting protomers [12,15,16].

Hydrophobic–hydrophilic interactions are the dominant ones in intradomain, domain–domain, and heterocomplex interfaces. Disulfide bridges are observed in all types of interfaces with the exception of homocomplexes, which exhibit a general preference for interactions between identical amino acid residues. Hydrophobic interactions are found to be the more frequent in permanent protein–protein associations than in transient ones.

In general, a necessary condition for high affinity interactions is the exclusion of bulk solvent from the interacting interface residues. This is generally achieved by the presence of hydrophobic amino acids in the interfaces, which causes a lowering of the effective dielectric in and around the interface, thereby favoring hydrogen bonding and ion pair formation between the interacting amino acid residues in the interface region. Thus, the effective interactions, which lead to the formation of PPIs, are both polar and hydrophobic in nature. This justifies the abundance of Trp, Tyr, and Arg in the interface regions, as these amino acids are capable of forming multiple types of interactions. Both Trp and Tyr can contribute aromatic π interactions, hydrogen bonding, and hydrophobic interactions. In addition Arg undergoes hydrogen bonding, salt bridges, and cation–π interactions (with the help of its guanidinium ring). The methylene carbon atoms of Arg contribute significant hydrophobicities [9–12,15,16,20,21].

15.6   PREDICTION OF PPIs

The PPI prediction methodologies can be broadly classified into two categories, viz, the experimental determination and the computational techniques. In most cases, the two types of methods are combined to complement each other.

15.6.1   Experimental PPI Prediction Methodologies

The prediction of PPIs requires the determination of the quaternary structures of the proteins. This needs the knowledge of the subunit composition of the system. The subunit composition of the proteins may be determined by introducing chemical cross-links between the polypeptide chains. This may also be done by comparing the molecular weights of the native protein and the constituent chains. The subunit molecular weights are obtained using denaturing gel electrophoresis.

The most accurate and important method of PPI prediction is X-ray crystallography. There are several other techniques such as, NMR spectroscopy, fluorescence resonance energy transfer, yeast two-hybrid, affinity purification–mass spectrometry, and protein chips to name a few.

X-ray crystallography [1–7 and references cited therein] is a method to determine the arrangement of atoms within a crystal (Fig. 15.1). In this method, a beam of X-rays strikes a crystal. Then, it scatters into many different directions. The electron density map of the molecule can be generated from the angles and intensities of these scattered beams to build a three-dimensional (3D) picture of the distribution of electrons within the crystal. This leads to the determinations of the mean positions of the atoms in the crystal, as well as their chemical bonds, the disorder, and various other structural properties. A fully grown crystal is mounted on an apparatus called a goniometer. After that, the crystal is gradually rotated and X-rays are passed through it, which produce a diffraction pattern of spots regularly spaced in two dimensions (2D). These are known as reflections. A 3D electron density model of the whole crystal is then created from the images of the crystal that are taken by rotating it at different orientations with the help of Fourier transforms (FT), as well as with previous chemical data for the crystallized sample. Small crystals or deformities in crystal packing lead to erroneous results. X-ray crystallography is related to several

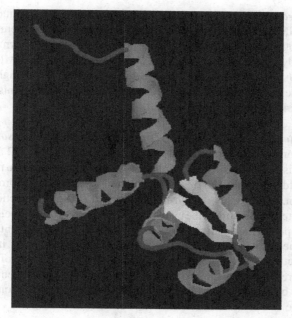

FIGURE 15.1   An example of a crystal structure. Helices are shown as ribbons and sheets are presented as arrows. The rests are coils.

other methods for determining atomic structures. Similar diffraction patterns can be produced by scattering electrons or neutrons, which are likewise interpreted as a FT.

The structure of hexamethylenetetramine was solved in 1923, and this happened to be the structure of the first organic molecule. After that, structures of a number of important bioorganic molecules (e.g., porphyrin, corrin, and chlorophyll) were solved.

X-ray crystallography of biological molecules took off with Dorothy Crowfoot Hodgkin, who solved the structures of cholesterol (1937), vitamin B12 (1945), and penicillin (1954). In 1969, she succeeded in solving the structure of insulin.

15.6.1.1 Protein Crystallography.   Crystal structures of proteins, which are irregular, began to be solved in the late 1950s. The first protein structure that was solved by X-ray crystallography was that of sperm whale myoglobin by Max Perutz and Sir John Cowdery Kendrew. Since then, X-ray crystal structures of proteins, nucleic acids, and other biological molecules have been determined. X-ray crystallography has a widespread use in the elucidation of protein structure function relationship, mutational analysis and drug design. The challenge lies in the prediction of structures of membrane proteins (e.g., ion channels and receptors) as it is difficult to find appropriate systems for them to crystallize. The reason is these proteins are integral parts of the cell membranes and it is hard to get the protein part out from the membrane component.

15.6.1.2 Nuclear Magnetic Resonance Methodologies. Proton nuclear magnetic resonance (HNMR) spectroscopy [1–6, 8 and References cited Therein] is a field of structural biology in which NMR spectroscopy is used to obtain information about the structure and dynamics of proteins. Structure determination by NMR spectroscopy usually consists of several phases, each using a separate set of highly specialized techniques. The sample is prepared, resonances are assigned, restraints are generated, and a structure is calculated and validated.

15.6.1.3 Förster Resonance Energy Transfer–Fluorescence Resonance Energy Transfer. Fluorescence resonance energy transfer (FRET) [1–7, 22 and References cited Therein] is a mechanism describing energy transfer between two molecules, both of which should be sensitive to light. This method is used to study protein dynamics, protein–protein, and protein–deoxyribonucleic acid (DNA) interactions. For FRET analysis of protein interactions, the cyan fluorescent protein (CFP)–yellow fluorescent protein (YFP) pair, which is the color variants of the green fluorescent protein (GFP), is currently the most useful protein pair that is being employed in biology. The interactions between the proteins are determined by the amount of energy that is being transferred between the proteins, thereby creating a large emission peak of YFP obtained by the overlaps of the individual fluorescent emission peaks of CFP and YPF as the two proteins are near to each other.

15.6.1.4 Yeast Two-Hybrid System. One of the important methods to analyze the physical interactions between proteins or proteins with DNA is the yeast two-hybrid screening [1–6, 23–26]. The basic principle behind the process stems from the fact that the close proximity and modularity of the activating and the binding domains of most of the eukaryotic transcription factors lead to the interactions between themselves albeit indirectly. This system often utilizes a genetically engineered strain of yeast that does not possess the biosynthetic machinery required for the biosynthesis of amino acids or nucleic acids. Yeast cells do not survive on the media lacking these nutrients. In order to detect the interactions between the proteins, the transcription factor is divided into two domains called the binding (BD) and the activator domain (AD). Genetically engineered plasmids are made to produce a protein product with the DNA binding domain attached onto a protein. Another such plasmid codes for a protein product having the AD tagged to another protein. The protein fused to the BD may be referred to as the bait protein and is typically a known protein that is used to identify the new binding partners. The protein fused to the AD may be referred to as the prey protein and can either be a single known protein or a collection of known or unknown proteins. The transcription of the reporter gene(s) occurs if and only if the AD and BD of the transcription factors are connected bringing the AD close to the transcription start site of the reporter gene, which justifies the presence of physical interactions between the bait and the prey proteins. Thus, a fruitful interaction between the proteins fused together determines the phenotypic change of the cell.

15.6.1.5 Affinity Purification. This technique studies PPIs [1–6]. It involves creating a fusion protein with a designed piece, the tag, on the end. The protein of interest with the tag first binds to beads coated with IgG. Then, the tag is broken apart by an enzyme. Finally, a different part of the tag binds reversibly to beads of a different type. After the protein of interest has been washed through two affinity columns, it can be examined for binding partners.

15.6.1.6 Rotein Chips–Protein Microarray.
This method is also sometimes referred to as protein binding microarray [1–6]. It provides a multiplex approach to identify PPIs, to identify transcription factor protein–activation, or to identify the targets of biologically active small molecules. On a piece of glass, different protein molecules or DNA-binding sequences of proteins are affixed orderly at different locations forming a microscopic array. A commonly used microarray is obtained by affixing antibodies that bind antigen molecules from cell lysate solutions. These antibodies can easily be spotted with appropriate dyes.

The aforementioned experimental tools are routinely used in laboratories to detect PPIs. However, these methods are not devoid of shortcomings. They are labor- and time-intensive expensive, and often give poor results. Moreover, the PPI data obtained using these techniques include false positives, which necessitates the use of other methods in order to verify the results. All these led to the development of computational methods that are capable of PPI prediction with sufficient accuracies.

15.6.2 Computational PPI Prediction Methodologies

Computational PPI prediction methodologies can be classified broadly as numerical value-based and probabilistic. Both of them involve training over a data set containing protein structural and sequence information [27–75]. Numerical methods use a function of the form $F = f(p_i, p_j \in n_i, x)$, where, p_i = input data for the residue i under consideration, p_j = the corresponding properties of the spatially neighboring residues and $j \in n_i$ and x = the collection of coefficients to be determined by training. The value of F determines the characteristics of residue i under consideration. It can either be I for interface or N for noninterface. If F is above a certain threshold, i is considered to be in I state otherwise it is in N state.

The value-based methods are classified as follows:

Linear Regression. This method [27, 31, 38, 67, 72, and References cited Therein] predicts the values of the unknown variable from a set of known variables. It also tests the relationship among the variables. In the case of PPI prediction methods, solvent accessibilities of the amino acid residues of the proteins are taken as inputs. The different amino acid residues have different solvent accessibility values depending on whether they are exposed or buried. Based on a collection of such values of known proteins, linear regression methods may be used to predict the nature of amino acids in unknown proteins.

Scoring Function. This is a general knowledge-based approach [31, 36, 41, 47, 48, 67, 72, and References cited Therein]. Scoring functions are based on empirical energy functions having contributions from various data. In this approach, information is generated from know protein–protein complexes present in the protein databank (PDB). This approach takes into account various physicochemical parameters of the protein complexes, (e.g., solvation potential, solvent accessibilities, interaction free energies, and entropies). These data are used to generate the scoring functions for the individual atoms of the amino acids constituting the protein complexes. The functions can then be used in case of unknown proteins to predict its mode of binding. The typical form of a scoring function is as follows:

$$U_{total} = U_{bond} + U_{angle} + U_{dihedral} + U_{nonbonded}$$

There are several methods available that use these. The significances of the individual terms are listed below:

U_{total} = Total energy of the system

U_{bond} = Bond energy of the molecules under considerations. In this case, the molecules are protein molecules.

$$U_{bond} = \sum K_b(r - r_{eq})^2$$

K_b = Force constant associated with the bond in question

r = Actual bond distance in the molecule

r_{eq} = Equilibrium bond distance

U_{angle} = Energy associated with change in bond angles from their usual values

$$U_{angle} = \sum K_\theta(\theta - \theta_{eq})^2$$

K_θ = Force constant associated with the bond angle in question

θ = Actual bond angle in the molecule

θ_{eq} = Equilibrium bond angle

$U_{dihedral}$ = Energy associated with change in dihedral angles from their usual values.

$$U_{dihedral} = \sum A_n(1 + \cos(n\phi - \delta))$$

ϕ = dihedral angle

n = multiplicity (which gives the number of minimum points in the function as the torsion angle changes from 0 to 2π)

δ = phase angle

A_n = force constant.

$U_{nonbonded}$ = Energy associated with various nonbonded interactions (e.g., H-bonding, etc.). It consists of an electrostatic and a Lennard-Jones term.

$$U_{nonbonded} = \sum \sum [(q_i q_j / 4\pi \varepsilon_0 r_{ij}) + 4\varepsilon_{ij}\{(\sigma_{ij}/r_{ij})^{12} - (\sigma_{ij}/r_{ij})^6\}]$$

The q terms are the partial atomic charges ε_{ij} and σ_{ij} are the Lennard-Jones well-depth energy and collision-diameter parameters ε_0 is the permittivity of free space and r_{ij} is the interatomic distance.

Support Vector Machines. Support vector machines (SVM) [17, 27, 30, 44, 54–59, and References cited Therein] is a supervised learning method for classification, function approximation, signal processing, and regression analysis. In this method, the input data are divided into two different sets, normaly, the interface (I) and noninterface (N) states. The SVM will create a separating hyperplane that maximizes the margin between the two different types of data. The basic principle of SVM is to first train it with a set of known data, which would create a classifier. The classifier is then used to predict whether a residue is on a PPI site or not by giving it a score. The SVM training is done by using a training file consisting of feature vectors generated using various information about the PPI complex. The typical information used for this purpose follow: hydrophobicities, accessible surface areas, electrical charges, sequence similarity and sequence conservation scores of amino acids and so on. This information is combined into feature vectors and used as input to train the SVM.

In terms of mathematics, the problem is defined as follows:

$$D = \{(X_i, C_i) | X_i \in R^p, C_i \in \{-1, 1\}\}_{i=1}^n$$

where C_i is a class representing $+1$ or -1 to which the datapoints X_i (which are nothing but some real vectors) belong. The datapoints are used to train a SVM that creates the maximum-margin hyperplane dividing the points based on the class label. Any hyperplane can be written on the basis of the datapoints (X_i) as

$$F.X - a = 0$$

where, "." is the dot product, $F =$ normal vector perpendicular to the hyperplane, $a/||F|| =$ offset of the hyperplane from the origin along the normal vector F, a and F are chosen in such a way as to maximize the distance between the parallel hyperplanes to enhance the chance of separation of the data.

The representations of the hyperplanes can be done using the equations:

$$F.X - a = 1 \quad \text{and} \quad F.X - a = -1$$

The training data are generally linearly separable, which enables us to select the two hyperplanes of the margin in a way that there are no points between them. Then we try to maximize their distance. Geometrically, the distance between the two hyperplanes is $2 / ||F||$, so $||F||$ has to be minimized. In order to prevent datapoints falling into the margin, the following constraints are added:

For each i either, $F.X_i$-a > 1 for X_i of the first class with label $+1$ and for the second class (having a label of -1) $F. X_i - a < 1$. Thus, $C_i (F.X_i - a) \le 1$, for all

$1 \leq i \leq n$. Combining everything the optimization problem looks like Minimization of $||F||$ (in F, a), when (for any $i = 1, \ldots, n$) C_i (F. $X_i - a) \geq 1$. In order to simplify, the above mentioned problem is converted to a quadratic one and the problem looks like Minimization of $||F||^2 / 2$ (in F, a), when (for any $i = 1, \ldots, n$)

$$C_i(F.X_i - a) \geq 1 \qquad (15.1)$$

Standard quadratic programming techniques can now be used to solve the problem.

The classification rule can be written in its unconstrained dual form. The dual of the SVM can be shown to be the following optimization problem: Maximization of $\Sigma w_i - 0.5 \Sigma a_i a_j \ C_i C_j X_i^T x_j$ (in a_i), when (for any $i = 1, \ldots, n$) $a_i \geq 0$ and $\Sigma w_i C_i = 0$.

The w terms are a dual representation for the weight vector in terms of the training set:

$$F = \Sigma w_i C_i X_i$$

For simplicity, sometimes the hyperplane is made to pass through the origin of the coordinate system. Such hyperplanes are called unbiased. General hyperplanes that are not passing through the origin are called biased. An unbiased hyperplane can be made by $a = 0$ in Eq. (15.1). In that case the expression of the dual remains almost the same without the equality.

$$\Sigma w_i C_i = 0$$

Another approach of SVM is called transductive support vector machines. This is an extension of the aforementioned process in such a way that it can incorporate structural properties (e.g., structural correlations) of the test data set for which the classification needs to be done. In this case, the support vector machine is fed a test data set with the test examples that are to be classified, in addition to the training set T,

$$T^* = \{X_i^* | X_i^* \in R^p\}_{i=1}^k$$

A transductive support vector machine is defined as follows: Minimization of $||F||^2 / 2$ (in F, a, C^*), when (for any $i = 1, \ldots, n$ and any $j = 1, \ldots, m$)

$$C_i(F.X_i - a) \geq 1, \ C_j^*(F.X_i^* - a) \geq 1 \text{ and } C_j^* \in \{-1, +1\}$$

Neural Network. The neural network [60, 61, 67, 72, and References cited Therein] is an interconnected group of artificial neurons (in biological perspective, neurons are connectors that transmit information via chemical signaling between cells), which are basically an adaptive system. There are hidden layers whose output is fed into a final output node. Protein information like the solvent accessibilities, free energy of interactions, and so on, are fed into the hidden layers to train them. Next, the trained model can be used to produce the output from a set of unknown data.

Random Forests. Random forests [40, 42, 63–66, 72, and References cited Therein] are a combination of tree predictors. Each of the trees is dependent on the respective values of a random vector that is sampled independently following the same distribution for all the trees in the whole forest. The more the number of trees the less is the error. Due to the law of *large numbers* there are no overfitting problems.

The steps of the algorithm can be summarized as follows: Let X = Number of samples in the training data set, Y = Total number of features or variables of the training samples, and y = The number of input variables that are to be employed to come to a decision at a node of the decision tree given that, $y << Y$.

A training set is therefore chosen for the tree to be generated and it is done by picking up the samples X times from the training data set with replacement. The remaining samples are used as a test data set to estimate the error of the tree, on the basis of the type of classes assigned to them by the classifier to be built on the training data set. The decision at each node is determined by randomly picking up y variables at that particular node and the best combination of the variables is preserved.

Random forest has a number of advantages like:

1. The method can tackle a very large number of input variables in the data sets.
2. It gives an idea of the variable importance to determine classification.
3. It gives an unbiased estimate of error.
4. If there are missing values for a particular variable, the random forests can employ a method for estimating missing data to maintain accuracy.
5. The method can give an idea about the interactions between variables.
6. It does not over fit.

The probabilistic methods are employed to find the conditional probability $p(s|x_1, \ldots, x_k)$, where s is either I or N for the range of input data $x_1, \ldots, x_k$ for a residue under consideration. Interface is predicted if the value of p(s| $x_1, \ldots, x_k$) becomes greater than a threshold value. This method can be categorized as follows:

Naïve Bayesian. Naïve Bayesian [67, 72, and References cited Therein] is a supervised learning method. It takes input data, which are assumed to be independent. Naïve Bayes is a well-known machine learning tool. This classifier assumes no dependencies between the variables to predict the class of the object under study. The mathematical formulation of the method is as follows:

$$P(H|X) = P(X|H)P(H)/P(X)$$

This equation calculates the probability of predicting the class of an object X, the observed data based on some hypothesis H. The parameter $P(H|X)$ is the posterior probability of H on X, $P(X)$ is the prior probability of X, $P(H)$ is the *a priori* probability of H that X belongs to the class C, and $P(X|H)$ is the posterior probability of X on H. In this case, the training data is used to build the decision rule. Selection of the most probable class is the rule:

$$\text{classify}(f1, f1, \ldots) = \text{argmax}\, P(C = cj)P(Fi = fi|Ci = cj)$$

The class is therefore given the maximum probability based on the rules created by training with known data. Protein sequence information can be used to generate rules for the classification. The window selects a central target residue and uses the neighboring residue information to train and predict the residues involved in interactions.

Bayesian Network. In this case [45, 67, 69, 70, 72, and References cited Therein], the input data are dependent on each other. So a joint probability is calculated. For two dependent input data, x_1 and x_2, their joint probability $P(S|x_1, x_2)$ is calculated as $P(x_1, x_2|S)$.

$P(S)$ = fraction of state S in the training dataset. In case of PPIs S represents whether an amino acid residue of the protein under study is in the interface or not.

$P(x_i)$ = probability density of input data x_i in the whole data set.

$P(x_i|S)$ = probability density of input data in the subset with a given state S.

Hidden Markov Model. Hidden Markov models (HMMs) [46, 67, 71, 72, and References cited Therein] are directed graphical models that define a factored probability distribution of $p(x, y)$. The mathematical formulation of the model is

$$p(x, y) = \prod p(x_i|y_i)p(y_i|y_{i-1})$$

This is often referred to as a generative model. The term $p(x_i|y_i)$ can be considered to be the probability that the observed result x_i is generated from the feature y_i. The second term, $p(y_i|y_{i-1})$, is actually the first-order Markov assumption term. It represents the probability of a label variable y_i that is not related to the other label variables y_{i-1} used in the study.

In case of prediction of PPIs, this method takes into account a multiple sequence alignment (MSA) of known proteins. The amino acid residues that are found to be conserved in the MSA are used to construct a profile that is used to predict the nature of the amino acids from the protein of interest.

Conditional Random Field. Conditional random field [67, 71–73, and References cited Therein] is a comparatively new method for the prediction of PPIs. In this method, each position along the protein chain is assigned to either a I or N label depending on some feature functions. This method is quite similar to

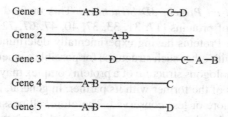

Gene 1 ——————A–B——————————C–D

Gene 2 ——————————A–B——————————

Gene 3 ——————————D——————————C–A–B

Gene 4 ——————A–B——————————C

Gene 5 ——————A–B——————————D

FIGURE 15.2 Prediction of PPIs based on the whole genome analysis.

HMM, but as opposed to HMM during prediction, the conditional probability of $p(x|y)$ is calculated.

From a biological point of view, the PPI predictive methodologies may be categorized in somewhat different ways.

Evaluation Based on Whole Genome Analysis. It has been observed that protein-coding genes that are in close proximities in different genomes are known to be interacting with each other [24–26, 67, 72, 74]. Sometimes two proteins fuse together to form a new protein in another organism. They are also considered to be interacting partners. Though the method seems interesting, but in reality it fails to predict interactions between proteins encoded by genes located far in the genome. This approach is not suitable for eukaryotes.

In Figure 15.2, the genes produce proteins A, B, C, and D. Since the distance between the proteins A and B is very small in all the genes, they may be considered to be interacting.

Evaluation Based on Evolutionary Relationships. This method is based on the phylogenetic profiles of the proteins under observations [47, 67, 72, 74, and References cited Therein]. Proteins with similar profiles exhibit functional relationships. Incorporation of evolutionary relationships furthers the prediction method.

The genome in Table 15.1 codes for Genes 1–5 with proteins A to E. Proteins A, B, and E share the same phylogenetic profiles. Therefore we may conclude that A, B, and E are interacting among themselves.

TABLE 15.1 Prediction of PPIs Based on Evolutionary Relationships

Genome	Proteins				
	A	B	C	D	E
Gene 1	1	1	0	0	1
Gene 2	1	1	1	0	1
Gene 3	0	0	1	0	0
Gene 4	0	0	0	1	0
Gene 5	1	1	0	1	1

Evaluation Based on Protein 3D Structures. This method relies on the solved 3D structures of proteins [17, 31, 33, 37, 40, 47, 67, 72, 74, and References cited Therein]. Proteins having experimentally determined 3D structures can be compared with other such structures for possible sequence identities. A suitable close homologous structure of a protein complex may indicate the possible binding modes of the former with its partner. In general, interface residues are known to be more or less conserved. Therefore, all possible protein pairs between those under observations can be predicted. In other words, the structures of the interacting protein partners are analyzed to find the best possible mode of binding and they are then compared to the existing protein complexes. The possible structures are ranked based on their energy content or some other statistical parameters. This method can also be used to find the putative binding partner from a set of 3D structures of interest.

Evaluation Based on Protein Domains. This method relies on the presence of similar domains in proteins [17, 31, 33, 37, 40, 46, 47, 67, 71, 72, and References cited Therein]. A database of protein families based on protein domains, Pfam, gives an idea about the domain structures in proteins. If the proteins of interest have similar arrangements of domains as those of some other interacting protein pairs, then these former proteins are also considered to have a similar kind interaction pattern as the latter.

Evaluation Based on Primary Structure of Proteins. This method is based on the assumption that PPIs are mediated through a specific number of short sequence motifs [61, 64, 69, 70, 72, 74, and References cited Therein]. Protein sequence information like a position specific scoring matrix (PSSM), combined with other experimental evidences (known interactions, physicochemical properties of amino acids, and so on) can be used as descriptors to train some machine-learning programs (support vector machines, random forest, etc.). The result would predict the probabilities of interactions between protein pairs.

The different methods are applied for different types of input data sets. The combinations of results for the different predictive methodologies may be used to have a comprehensive result. Protein–protein binding modes are also used to predict interfaces. The different computational methods are applied to different data sets with varying degrees of success. The results depend on the type of data used. Some methods are suitable for some specific kinds of data sets. The SVM gives fairly good results if the data set is small and balanced, whereas random forest can handle large data sets. Sometimes SVM can overfit the data, but random forest never does. However, there are a number of challenging problems that need be taken into account. They are

PPIs Associated with Large-Scale Conformational Changes. Large-scale conformational changes, (e.g., those involving domain–domain rearrangements) are difficult to analyze in terms of computation. In such cases, it might be possible for the protein-binding residues in their native complex form to get scattered when they are uncomplexed. This may lead to their elimination in the process of clustering.

One Protein, Many Partners. There are a number of proteins that have multiple partners where the interactions are mediated through the different parts of the surface. In such cases, it is possible that the different binding modes are predicted, but they have to be validated by biochemical data to identify which is for which partner protein.

15.7 DISCUSSION AND CONCLUSION

The PPIs are the central players in many of the vital biochemical processes. Cellular metabolism is guided by the PPIs be it a bacterium, an archea, or complex multicellular organisms. This made the prediction of PPIs so vital. Knowledge of PPI is useful in all aspects of biology. Many of the diseases including cancer are results of improper PPIs. Therefore prediction of PPIs has become important targets for therapy. There are different approaches for the predictions and analyses of protein–protein interactions. This chapter has made an attempt to review the different PPI prediction methodologies that are available. The experimental approaches are more accurate and would give more comprehensive and reliable results; but they are time consuming and labor intensive besides being expensive. As alternatives to the experimental approaches, computational methods have been developed. They are comparatively less accurate, but often give an overall idea of the whole process. There are various computational approaches with somewhat varying accuracies. The most important aspect is that computational approaches are cost effective, and requires less time. A word of caution is that none of the methods are cent percent accurate. To properly predict a PPI, much information is needed. The best way to perform an experiment is first to use the computational algorithms to find a PPI, and then test that via experimental means.

APPENDIX I

This appendix refers to the web links of some of the important servers used in the study of protein–protein interaction. This is not an exhaustive list and the list keeps on growing day by day. This is given for an easy reference of the computational tools available to study protein interactions.

http://protein3d.ncifcrf.gov/~keskino
http://dockground.bioinformatics.ku.edu/
http://www.ces.clemson.edu/compbio/protcom/
http://mips.gsf.de/proj/ppi/
http://mips.gsf.de/proj/yeast/CYGD/interaction/
http://dip.doe-mbi.ucla.edu/dip/Main.cgi
http://www.thebiogrid.org/
http://www.ncbi.nlm.nih.gov/RefSeq/HIVInteractions/
http://www.hprd.org/

http://wilab.inha.ac.kr/hpid/
http://www.ihop-net.org/UniPub/iHOP
http://insilico.csie.ntu.edu.tw:9999/point/
http://point.bioinformatics.tw/
http://www.compbio.dundee.ac.uk/www-pips
http://www.jcvi.org/mpidb/about.php
http://www.molecularconnections.com/home/en/home/products/NetPro
http://www.proteinlounge.com/inter_home.asp
http://itolab.cb.k.u-tokyo.ac.jp/Y2H/
http://mips.gsf.de/genre/proj/mpact/index.html

APPENDIX II

There are a number of techniques that culminate in the generation of numerous software tools for the analysis of PPIs. Of which some of them are mentioned here

PATCHDOCK (http://bioinfo3d.cs.tau.ac.il/PatchDock/). PatchDock algorithm is inspired by object recognition and image segmentation techniques used in Computer Vision. Docking can be compared to assembling a jigsaw puzzle. When solving the puzzle two pieces are matched by picking one piece and searching for the complementary one.

ELM server (http://elm.eu.org/about.html). It is based on the recognition of short linear sequence motifs on proteins (SLiM), which are considered to be the binding regions.

ISEARCH [75]. This method uses known domain–domain interfaces stored in an interface library to screen unbound proteins for structurally similar interaction sites.

GRAMM   (http://vakser.bioinformatics.ku.edu/resources/gramm/grammx/). GRAMM is a program for protein docking. To predict the structure of a complex, it requires only the atomic coordinates of the two molecules (no information about the binding sites is needed). The program performs an exhaustive six-dimensional search through the relative translations and rotations of the molecules.

GWIDD (http://gwidd.bioinformatics.ku.edu/). GWIDD is a comprehensive resource for genomewide structural modeling of protein–protein interactions. It contains interaction information for multiple organisms. The structures of the participating proteins are modeled or crystallographic coordinates are retrieved, if available, and docked by GRAMM-X. The resource is not restricted to interactions in the GWIDD database. Other sequences or structures may be entered at various stages.

Dockground (http://dockground.bioinformatics.ku.edu/). Integrated system of databases for protein recognition studies. The core Dockground data set consists of cocrystallized protein–protein structures. The data set is regularly updated and annotated.

I-2-I Site engine (http://bioinfo3d.cs.tau.ac.il/I2I-SiteEngine). Interface-to-Interface (I2I)-SiteEngine, is based on the structural alignment between two protein–protein interfaces. The method simultaneously aligns two pairs of binding sites that constitute an interface. The method is based on recognition of similarity of physico-chemical properties and shapes. It assumes no similarity of sequences or folds of the proteins that comprise the interfaces.

INTERVIEWER (http://interviewer.inha.ac.kr/). Protein–protein interaction networks often consist of thousands of nodes or more, which severely limit the usefulness of many graph drawing tools because they become too slow for interactive analysis of the networks and because they produce cluttered drawings with many edge crossings. Interviewer is based on a layout algorithm for visualizing large-scale protein interaction networks. InterViewer3 (1) first finds a layout of connected components of an entire network, (2) finds a global layout of nodes with respect to pivot nodes within a connected component, and (3) refines the local layout of each connected component by first relocating midnodes with respect to their cutvertices and direct neighbors of the cutvertices and then by relocating all nodes with respect to their neighbors within distance 2.

APID (http://bioinfow.dep.usal.es/apid/index.htm). APID is an interactive bioinformatic webtool that has been developed to allow exploration and analysis of main currently known information about PPIs integrated and unified in a common and comparative platform.

INTEGRATOR (http://bioverse.compbio.washington.edu/integrator/). Integrator is a tool for graphically searching PPI networks across several genomes. The database contains experimentally determined PPIs from various public repositories (including the DIP, GRID, and PDB) and predicts PPIs based on these collections.

PIPSA (http://projects.villa-bosch.de/mcmsoft/pipsa/3.0/index.html). PIPSA may be used to compute and analyze the pairwise similarity of 3D interaction property fields for a set of proteins.

con-PPISP (http://pipe.scs.fsu.edu/ppisp.html). It uses PSI BLAST sequence profile and solvent accessibility as input to a neural network.

PROMATE (http://bioportal.weizmann.ac.il/promate). It is based on a Naïve Bayesian method, which takes secondary structure, amino acid grouping, sequence conservation, and atom distribution as input.

PINUP (http://sparks.informatics.iupui.edu?PINUP/). It is based on an empirical scoring function that involves side chain energy terms, solvent accessible area, and sequence conservation.

PPI-Pred (http://bioinformatics.leeds.ac.uk/ppi-pred). It is based on SVM that considers six parameters.

SPPIDER (http://sppider.cchmc.org/). A neural network based technique. It takes solvent accessibilities as inputs.

SHARP[2] (http://www.bioinformatics.sussex.ac.uk/SHARP2). It calculates solvation potential, hydrophobicity, accessible surface area, residue interface propensity, and planarity and protrusion. Each parameter is combined for each surface patch and the patch with the highest value is given as the output.

This is not an exhaustive list. The list is growing day by day.

REFERENCES

1. T. E. Creighton (1996), *Proteins: Structures and Molecular Properties*, 2nd ed., W. H. Freeman, NY.

2. J. Kyte (1995), *Structure in Protein Chemistry*, 2nd ed., Garland Publishing Inc., NY.

3. C. Branden and J. Tooze (1999), *Introduction to Protein Structure*, 2nd ed., Garland Publishing Inc., NY.

4. G. A. Petsko and Dagmar Ringe (2003), *Protein Structure and Function (Primers in Biology)*, 1st ed., New Science Press Ltd., London.

5. D. Voet and J. G. Voet (1995), *Biochemistry*, 2nd ed., John Wiley & Sons, Inc., NY.

6. A. Fresht (1998), *Structure and Mechanism in Protein Science: A Guide to Enzyme Catalysis and Protein Folding*, 1st ed., W. H. Freeman, NY.

7. J. Drenth (1994), *Principles of protein x-ray crystallography*, 2nd ed., Springer, NY.

8. J. Cavanagh, W. J. Fairbrother, A. G. Palmer, III, N. J. Skelton, M. Rance (2006), *Protein NMR Spectroscopy: Principles and Practice,* 2nd ed., Academic Press, NY.

9. S. Jones and J. M. Thornton (1977), Analysis of protein–protein interaction sites using surface patches, *J. Mol. Biol.*, 272(1), 121–132.

10. S. Jones and J. M. Thornton (1997), Prediction of protein–protein interaction sites using patch analysis, *J. Mol. Biol.*, 272(1), 133–143.

11. Y. Ofran and Burkhard Rost (2003), Analysing six types of protein–protein interfaces, *J. Mol. Biol.*, 325(2), 377–387.

12. A. A. Bogan, and K. S. Thorn (1998), Anatomy of hot spots in protein interfaces, *J. Mol. Biol.*, 280(1), 1–9.

13. Y. Ofran and B. Rost (2007), ISIS: interaction sites identified from sequence, *Bioinformatics*, 23(20), e13–e16.

14. Y. Ofran and B. Rost (2003), Predicted protein–protein interaction sites from local sequence information, *FEBS Lett.*, 544(1), 236–239.

15. B. Ma, T. Elkayam, H. Wolfson, and R. Nussinov (2003), Protein–protein interactions: Structurally conserved residues distinguish between binding sites and exposed protein surfaces, *Proc. Natl. Acad. Sci. USA*, 100(10), 5772–5777.

16. Y. Ofran and B. Rost (2007), Protein–protein interaction hotspots carved into sequences, *PLoS Compu. Biol.*, 3(7), e119.

17. Jo-Lan Chung, W. Wang, and P. E. Bourne (2006), Exploiting sequence and structure homologs to identify protein–protein binding sites, *Proteins: Struct. Function Bioinformatics*, 62(3), 630–640.

18. D. Reichmann, O. Rahat, S. Albeck, R. Meged, O. Dym, and G. Schreiber (2005), The modular architecture of protein-protein binding interfaces, *Proc. Natl. Acad. Sci. USA*, 102(1), 57–62.

19. O. Keskin, B. Ma, and R. Nussinov (2005), Hot regions in protein–protein interactions: The organization and contribution of structurally conserved hot spot residues, *J. Mol. Biol.*, 345(5), 1281–1294.

20. S. Jones and J. M. Thornton (1996), Principles of protein–protein interactions, *Proc. Natl. Acad. Sci. USA*, 93(1), 13–20.

21. W. L. DeLano (2002), Unraveling hot spots in binding interfaces: progress and challenges, *Curr. Opin. Struct. Biol.*, 12(1), 14–20.

22. A. A. Deniz, T. A. Laurence, G. S. Beligere, M. Dahan, A. B. Martin, D. S. Chemla, P. E. Dawson, P. G. Schultz, S. Weiss (2000), Single-molecule protein folding: Diffusion fluorescence resonance energy transfer studies of the denaturation of chymotrypsin inhibitor 2, *Proc. Natl. Acad. Sci. USA*, 97(10), 5179–5184.

23. J. A. Wells (1991), Systematic mutational analyses of protein–protein interfaces, *Methods Enzymol.*, 202, 390–411.

24. P. Uetz et al. (2000), A comprehensive analysis of protein–protein interactions in *Saccharomyces cerevisiae*, *Nature (London)*, 403(6770), 623–627.

25. Y. Ho et al. (2002), Systematic identification of protein complexes in *Saccharomyces cerevisiae* by mass spectrometry, *Nature (London)*, 415(6868), 180–183.

26. J. Wang et al. (2009), Uncovering the rules for protein-protein interactions from yeast genomic data, *Proc. Natl. Acad. Sci.*, 106(10), 3752–3757.

27. I. Ezkurdia et al. (2009), Progress and challenges in predicting protein-protein interaction sites, *Briefings Bioinforamtics*, 10(3), 233–246.

28. K. L. Morrison and G. A. Weiss (2001), Combinatorial alanine-scanning, *Curr. Opin. Chem. Biol.*, 5(3), 302–307.

29. A. A. Bogan and K. S. Thorn (2001), ASEdb: a database of alanine mutations and their effects on the free energy of binding in protein interactions, *Bioinformatics*, 17(3), 284–287.

30. A. Koike and T. Takagi (2004), Prediction of protein–protein interaction sites using support vector machines, *Protein Eng. Des. Sel.* 17(2), 165–173.

31. H. Neuvirth, R. Raz, and G. Schreiber (2004), ProMate: A Structure Based Prediction Program to Identify the Location of Protein–Protein Binding Sites, *J. Mol. Biol.*, 338(1), 181–199.

32. F. Pazos and A. Valencia (2002), *In silico* two-hybrid system for the selection of physically interacting protein pairs, *Proteins: Struct., Function Bioinformatics*, 47(2), 219–227.

33. I. Re, I. Mihalek, and O. Lichtarge (2005), An evolution based classifier for prediction of protein interfaces without using protein structures, *Bioinformatics*, 21(10), 2496–2501.

34. N. Zaki et al. (2009), Protein–protein interaction based on pairwise similarity, *BMC Bioinformatics*, 10(150), 150–162.

35. B. Wang et al. (2005), Predicting protein interaction sites from residue spatial sequence profile and evolution rate, *FEBS Lett.*, 580, 380–384.

36. J. Fernández-Recio, M. Totrov, and R. Abagyan, Identification of Protein–Protein Interaction Sites from Docking Energy Landscapes, *J. Mol. Biol.*, 335(3), 843–865.

37. A. Garg, H. Kaur, and G.P. Raghava (2005), Real value prediction of solvent accessibility in proteins using multiple sequence alignment and secondary structure, *Proteins*, 61(2), 318–324.

38. M. Wagner, R. Adamczak, A. Porollo, and J. Meller (2005), Linear regression models for solvent accessibility prediction in proteins, *J Comput. Biol.*, 12(3), 355–369.

39. Z. Yuan and B. Huang (2004), Prediction of protein accessible surface areas by support vector regression, *Proteins*, 57(3), 558–564.

40. M. Šikić, S. Tomić, and K. Vlahoviček, Prediction of Protein–Protein Interaction Sites in Sequences and 3D Structures by Random Forests, *PLoS Comput. Biol.*, 5(1).

41. S. J Wodak and R. Méndez (2004), Prediction of protein–protein interactions: the CAPRI experiment, its evaluation and implications, *Curr. Opin. Struct. Biol.*, 14(2), 242–249.

42. X-W. Chen and M. Liu (2005), Prediction of protein–protein interactions using random decision forest framework, *Bioinformatics*, 21(24), 4394–4400.

43. L. Banci, I. Bertini, V. Calderone, N. Della-Malva, I. C. Felli, S. Neri, A. Pavelkova, and A. Rosato (2009), Copper(I)-mediated protein–protein interactions result from suboptimal interaction surfaces, *Biochem. J.*, 10, 37–42.

44. J. R. Bradford and D. R. Westhead, Improved prediction of protein–protein binding sites using a support vector machines approach, *Bioinformatics*, 21(8), 1487–1494.

45. J. R. Bradford, C. J. Needham, A. J. Bulpitt, and D. R. Westhead (2006), Insights into Protein–Protein Interfaces using a Bayesian Network Prediction Method, *J. Mol. Biol.*, 362(2), 365–387.

46. T. Friedrich, B. Pils, T. Dandekar, J. Schultz, and T. Müller (2006), Modelling interaction sites in protein domains with interaction profile hidden Markov models. *Bioinformatics*, 22(23), 2851–2857.

47. M. Landau et al., (2005), ConSurf 2005: the projection of evolutionary conservation scores of residues on protein structures, *Nucleic Acids Res.*, 33(Web Server Issue), w299–w302.

48. N. J. Burgoyne and R. M. Jackson (2006), Predicting protein interaction sites: binding hot-spots in protein–protein and protein-ligand interfaces, *Bioinformatics*, 22(11), 1335–1342.

49. A. Koike and T. Takagi (2004), Prediction of protein–protein interaction sites using support vector machines, *Protein Eng. Des. Sel.*, 17(2).

50. C. H. Yan, et al. (2004), Identification of interface residues in protease-inhibitor and antigen-antibody complexes: a support vector machine approach, *Neural Comput. Appl.*, 13, 123–129.

51. D. Meyer, F. Leisch, and K. Hornik (2003), The support vector machine under test, Neurocomputing, 55(1–2), 169–186.

52. C. Cortes and V. Vapnik (1995), Support-Vector Networks, *Machine Learning*, 20.

53. M. Aizerman, E. Braverman, and L. Rozonoer (1964), Theoretical foundations of the potential function method in pattern recognition learning, *Automation Remote Control*, 25, 821–837.

54. B. E. Boser, I. M. Guyon, and V. N. Vapnik (1992), A training algorithm for optimal margin classifiers, D. Haussler (ed.), 5th Annual ACM Workshop on COLT, ACM Press, Pittsburgh, PA, pp. 144–152

55. H. Drucker, C. J. C. Burges, L. Kaufman, A. Smola, and V. Vapnik (1996), Support Vector Regression Machines. Advances in Neural Information Processing Systems 9 NIPS MIT Press, MA pp. 155–161.

56. M. Ferris and T. Munson (2002), Interior-point methods for massive support vector machines, *SIAM J. Optimization* 13, 783–804.

57. V. Vapnik (1995), The Nature of Statistical Learning Theory, Springer-Verlag, NY.

58. V. Vapnik and S. Kotz (2006), Estimation of Dependences Based on Empirical Data. Springer, NY, 291–400.

59. O. Ivanciuc (2007), Applications of Support Vector Machines in Chemistry, *Rev. Comput. Chem.*, 23.

60. H. Chen and H-X Zhou (2005), Prediction of interface residues in protein–protein complexes by a consensus neural network method: test against NMR data, *Proteins*, 61(1), 21–35.

61. P. Fariselli et al. (2002), Prediction of protein–protein interaction sites in heterocomplexes with neural networks, *Eur. J. Biochem.*, 269(5), 1356–1361.

62. A Porollo and J Meller (2007), Prediction-based fingerprints of protein–protein interactions, *Proteins*, 66(3), 630–645.

63. Y. Qi, J. Klein-Seetharama, and Z. Bar-Joseph (2005), Random forest similarity for protein-protein interaction prediction from multiple sources, *Pac. Symp. Biocomput.*, 10, 531–542.

64. M. Šikić, S. Tomić, and K. Vlahoviček (2009), Prediction of Protein Protein Interaction Sites in Sequences and 3D Structures by Random Forests, *Plos Computa. Biol.*, W. H. Freeman, NY.

65. L. Breiman (2002), Looking inside the black box, Wald Lecture II. Available at www.stat.berkley.edu/-brelman/wald 2002–2 pdf.

66. L. Breiman (2001), Random Forests, *Machine Learning*, 45.

67. L. Skrabanek, H. K Saini, G. D Bader, and A. J Enright (2008), Computational prediction of protein–protein interactions, *Mole. Biotechnol.* 38(1), 1–17.

68. C. Wang, J. Cheng, S. Su, and D. X (2008), Identification of Interface Residues Involved in Protein–Protein Interactions Using Naïve Bayes Classifier, *Lecture Notes in Artificial Intelligence* 5139.

69. J. R. Bradford, C. J. Needham, A. J. Bulpitt, and D. R. Westhead (2006), Insights into protein–protein interfaces using a Bayesian network prediction method, *J. Mol. Biol.*, 362 (2).

70. R. Jansen et al. (2003), A Bayesian Networks Approach for Predicting Protein–Protein Interactions from Genomic Data, *Science*, 302 (5644), 449–453.

71. T. Friedrich et al. (2006), Modelling interaction sites in protein domains with interaction profile hidden Markov models, *Bioinformatics*, 22 (23), 2851–2852.

72. H.-X. Zhou and S. Qin (2007), Interaction-site prediction for protein complexes: a critical assessment, *Bioinformatics*, 23(17), 2203–2209.

73. M.-H. Li, L. Lin, X.-L. Wang, and T. Liu (2007), Protein–protein interaction site prediction based on conditional random fields, *Bioinformatics*, 23(5), 597–604.

74. S. Pitre, Md. Alamgir, J. R Green, M. Dumontier, F. Dehne, and A. Golshani (2008), Computational methods for predicting protein–protein interactions, *Adv. Biochem. Eng. Biotechnol.* 110.

75. S. Günther, P. May, A. Hoppe A, C. Frömmel, and R. Preissner (2007), Docking without docking: ISEARCH–prediction of interactions using known interfaces, *Proteins*, 69(4), 839–844.

16

ANALYZING TOPOLOGICAL PROPERTIES OF PROTEIN–PROTEIN INTERACTION NETWORKS: A PERSPECTIVE TOWARD SYSTEMS BIOLOGY

MALAY BHATTACHARYYA AND SANGHAMITRA BANDYOPADHYAY

16.1 INTRODUCTION

Biological systems are too complex to be represented with a stand-alone computational model [1, 2]. The intricacies involved in the genomic or proteomic level of an organism, even in one of the simplest (e.g., amoeba), is hard to replicate. In spite of the complexities involved in the biological systems, they abide by a set of protocols [3]. The systematic study of such complex protocols in biological systems is the main concern in systems biology. In an analytical view, systems biology cares about the emergence of phenotypic characteristics from the genotypes and figures out the protocols behind the response to alterations of these characteristics in the environment or in the system components.

Many high-throughput technologies evolved in recent decades have enabled the analysis of various properties of the transcriptome and proteome of several organisms. These properties are occasionally mapped to an interaction network structure [4]. The identification of significant modules of genes and proteins, which have a high degree of association with each other in these networks, can add potentials to this direction of research. Individual or combined mining of gene and protein cointeraction networks is a nascent area of research that has seen promise through such module-specific studies

Computational Intelligence and Pattern Analysis in Biological Informatics, Edited by Ujjwal Maulik,
Sanghamitra Bandyopadhyay, and Jason T. L. Wang
Copyright © 2010 John Wiley & Sons, Inc.

349

[5–7]. A set of genes has a high chance of participating in a common biological pathway if they form a module in both the gene–gene and protein–protein interaction networks (PPINs). Sometimes, these networks are constructed by combining multiple sources of information by way of investigating associations between them [8–10]. Thus, we can obtain a robust and integrated view of the underlying biology. However, one of the most notable properties of these biological networks explored very recently is the whimsical dynamic behavior they exhibit corresponding to the network parameters [11]. Surprisingly, the dynamics produced by these networks are in some way more reliant on the network topology. Therefore, biological network analysis at the topological level is undeniably an important direction of research in systems biology.

In the perspective of systems biology, a biological organization has several levels of abstraction, namely, genomic, proteomic, and cellular level, and so on. Unveiling the interdependencies and intradependencies of the components in these levels is a major challenge in systems biology. Of these levels of abstraction in a biological system, the proteomic level acts as the dominant functional bridge between the others. Proteins are essential components in a living being. What a protein does and how it works defines the comprehensive activity within an organism. With the availability of a large volume of protein level interaction information of various organisms from multiple sources, a new challenge has been brought into the postgenomic era of elucidating the cellular level protein functions. Unveiling the comprehensive protein interactome of an organism provides a framework for understanding biology as an integrated system [12]. Protein–protein interaction (PPI) information provides a local as well as a global view of the interaction modules of proteins participating in significant similar activities. Essentially, such PPI information can be obtained via biological studies (X-ray crystallography, yeast two-hybrid, mass spectrometry, etc.) [13] or can be predicted *in silico* (hidden Marcov model, neural network, random forest, etc.) [14]. This chapter focuses exclusively on the topological properties of interaction networks of proteins and their significance in the systems level. Instead of pursuing a piecemeal study of the single components, we pay attention to the more global analyzes of the structure, function, and dynamics of the networks in which macromolecules work [12].

This chapter is organized as follows: In Section 16.2, we discuss various topological properties and structures of interaction networks. In Section 16.3, the details on state-of-the-art knowledge on the topology-based analysis of PPINs are provided. The problem is presented formally with necessary precursory details are in Section 16.4. Sections 16.5–16.6 include the algorithmic approach to the problem and its theoretical background. In Section 16.7, the empirical analysis along with the concern of system level study is provided on the structures explored from the studied PPIN. Finally, Section 16.8 concludes this chapter.

16.2 TOPOLOGY OF PPI NETWORKS

A network $N = (V, A)$ is defined with a set of nodes $V = \{v_1, v_2, \ldots, v_{|V|}\}$ and a set of arcs $A : (v_i, v_j)$ ($v_i \neq v_j, \forall v_i, v_j \in V$) connecting these nodes. Generally, we discard self-loops or parallel arcs from a simple network and consider it to be undirected. Whenever a network is called directed, we distinguish between the two arcs (v_i, v_j) and (v_j, v_i) ($\forall v_i, v_j \in V$). A subnetwork $N' = (V', A')$ is a part of the network $N = (V, A)$, such that $V' \in V$ and $A' \in A$. Again, by the term induced subnetwork we restrict A' to include only the comprehensive set of arcs existing within the nodes of V' in N. A weighted network, $N = (V, A, W)$, is defined with a set of nodes V, a set of arcs A, and a weight function W defined over the set of arcs, such that $W : A \rightarrow \mathbb{R}_0^+$.

A PPIN is a symbolization of PPIs in the form of a network. A PPIN is defined by a doublet $\mathcal{P} = (P, I)$, where P denotes the set of proteins $\{p_1, p_2, \ldots, p_{|P|}\}$ and $I \subseteq P \times P - \bigcup_{i=1}^{|P|}(p_i, p_i)$ denotes the set of interactions. So, the set P is equivalent to V, and I is equivalent to A. Frequently, a PPIN is generalized using a triplet representation $\mathcal{P} = (P, I, W)$, where $W : I \rightarrow \mathbb{R}_0^+$ is a weight function mapping each interaction to a positive real value. These weights are used to rank the significance of the interactions between protein pairs [9]. A PPIN is called weighted or unweighted (sometimes termed as binary), depending on the inclusion or exclusion of the weight function W. In the course of study presented in this chapter, undirected and weighted PPINs will be studied throughout. Let us suppose that $|S|$ represents the cardinality of a set S and the other notations are customary, unless specified otherwise.

The physical or logical organization of the components (nodes, arcs, etc.) in a network is known to be its topology. Topology of a particular type of network is preserved through the contraction or expansion in its size. This section describes some of the important topological properties and structures useful for the study of biological interaction networks.

16.2.1 Topological Properties

Definition 16.2.1 (Degree [15]): *The degree of a node defines the cardinality of its first-order neighborhood set (i.e., the number of arcs connected to it).*

In a directed network, the degree of a node can be separated into two distinct categories, namely, the *in* and the *out degrees*. The *in* and *out degrees* of a node defines the number of arcs directed to and directed from the node itself, respectively. For such networks, the total degree of a node equals the sum of its *in* and *out degrees*.

Definition 16.2.2 (Degree distribution [16]): *Given a network $N = (V, A)$, its degree distribution is defined as the probability distribution of the degree values of its nodes.*

For a directed network, there could be two types of degree distributions, namely, the *in degree* and the *out degree distributions*.

Definition 16.2.3 (Clustering coefficient [17]): *Given a network $N = (V, A)$, the clustering coefficient of a node in N is defined as the frequency of arcs within the subnetwork induced by its first-order neighborhood.*

By the term *frequency*, we mean the fraction of the existing number arcs to that of the maximum possible number of arcs. The clustering coefficient can also be defined for a subnetwork as the frequency of arcs within the subnetwork itself. The clustering coefficient of a subnetwork is sometimes defined as its density.

Definition 16.2.4 (Core clustering coefficient [18]): *Given a network $N = (V, A)$ and a parameter k, the core clustering coefficient of a node in N is defined as the clustering coefficient of the largest subnetwork of its first-order neighborhood with minimal degree k.*

The core clustering coefficient, in contrast to the standard clustering coefficient, increases the weights of highly dense subnetworks while giving less weights to the small degree nodes [18].

Definition 16.2.5 (Betweenness centrality [19]): *Given a network $N = (V, A)$, the betweenness centrality of a node in N is defined by the fraction of all-pair shortest paths in N that includes the specific node.*

Definition 16.2.6 (Czekanowski–Dice (CD) distance [20]): *In a network $N = (V, A)$, the CD distance between two nodes $u, v \in V$, is computed as*

$$CD(u, v) = \frac{|N(u) \cup \overline{N(v)}| + |\overline{N(u)} \cup N(v)|}{|N(u) \cup N(v)| + |N(u) \cap N(v)|} \tag{16.1}$$

where $N(u)$ denotes the first-order neighbors of u and $\overline{N(u)}$ denotes the non-neighbors of u.

The set of CD distances of all the node pairs provide important topological information about the distribution of sharing of neighborhood within a network.

Definition 16.2.7 (Scale-free property [16]): *A network $N = (V, A)$ is said to follow the scale-free property if its nodes follow a power law degree distribution [i.e., the probability $P(k)$ that a node in N is adjacent to k other nodes, decays as a power law following $P(k) \sim k^{-\gamma}$ ($\gamma > 0$)].*

Now, we describe some of the topological structures used commonly in biological network analysis in Section 16.2.2.

16.2.2   Topological Structures

Definition 16.2.8 (Clique [21]): *Given a network $N = (V, A)$, a clique is defined as a complete subnetwork of N [i.e., $K \in V$ is said to be a clique if the degree of all the nodes in the subnetwork induced by K from N is $(K - 1)$].*

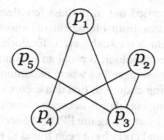

FIGURE 16.1   A $\frac{2}{3}$-quasi-clique induced by the set of proteins $\{p_1, p_2, p_3, p_4\}$ in a $\frac{1}{4}$-quasi-complete network.

Clique is one of the most exercised topological structures of a biological network. It essentially represents the all-to-all association of the nodes within it, and thus, is very useful to characterize cofunctional modules. Sometimes, the stringent all-to-all association of a clique does not prove to be useful for real-life analyzes. Thus, the concept of quasi-completeness has emerged in network analysis.

Definition 16.2.9 (γ-quasi-complete network [6]): *A network $N = (V, A)$ is a γ-quasi-complete network $(0 < \gamma \leq 1)$ if every node in the network has at least degree $\lceil \gamma.(|V| - 1) \rceil$.*

Definition 16.2.10 (γ-quasi-clique [6]): *In a network $N = (V, A)$, a subset of nodes $V' \in V$ forms a γ-quasi-clique $(0 < \gamma \leq 1)$ if the subnetwork induced by V' is a γ-quasi-complete network.*

Figure 16.1 shows a $\frac{2}{3}$–quasi-clique in a $\frac{1}{4}$-quasi-complete network. The node corresponding to the protein p_5 attains the minimum degree value 1 in the network, whereas the maximum degree value was possible up to 4. So, the complete network is only $\frac{1}{4}$-quasi-complete. But in the subnetwork induced by the proteins $\{p_1, p_2, p_3, p_4\}$, the minimum degree value is 2 (as the degree value is the same for all the nodes), and therefore, it is $\frac{2}{3}$-quasicomplete. Certainly, a 1-quasi-complete network is a complete network, whereas a 1-quasi-clique is a clique.

Definition 16.2.11 (γ-quasi-biclique [22]): *In a network $N = (V, A)$, a bipartite subnetwork $N' = (V1, V2, A)$ is said to be a γ-quasi-biclique $(0 < \gamma \leq 1)$ if the subnetwork induced by these two sets of nodes contains at least $\lceil \gamma.|V1|.|V2| \rceil$ number of arcs.*

16.3   LITERATURE SURVEY

Proteomic research is one of the early initiatives in the domains of molecular and systems biology. To date, it is one of the extensively studied domain of research.

Many studies have been carried out in the last few decades on the exploration of various topological structures from biological networks with various motivations (function prediction, system level study, etc.). Exploring cliques from interaction networks is the most studied topological problem in computational biology [21, 23]. Currently, we can find promising studies where maximum cliques have been merged with overlapping neighboring cliques to find dense cores in the PPIN of *Escherichia coli* [24]. In this study, strong correlation between cliques and essentiality of proteins have also been established by studying the PPIN of *Saccharomyces cerevisiae*. Such observed structure of essential cores have been found to take part in significant roles in the protein networks.

Due to the noise-prone behavior of biologically evolved data, clique finding in biological networks is a restrictive approach. Quasi-cliques are often suitable descriptors of a coherent module in biological networks. A number of studies are in the literature to explore quasi-cliques from networks. An earlier study presented a greedy randomized adaptive search procedure (GRASP) for finding the set of large quasi-cliques (for a given γ) in large networks of order $>10^5$ [25]. Here, the definition of a quasi-clique is somehow equivalent to the definition of density. However, the works carried out at that time neither found the complete set of quasi-cliques, nor addressed how to mine the largest quasi-clique. A current study proposes an efficient mining algorithm (Crochet) to explore the complete set of quasi-cliques [7]. Recently, the original algorithm has been improved (Crochet$^+$) keeping a similar motivation of joint mining of gene and protein interaction networks [6]. Such studies are indeed significant. However, the limitation of these approaches is that they provide the complete set of maximal quasi-cliques. So, it is computationally hard to sort out the largest quasi-clique using such an approach. In a recent study, an algorithm for finding approximately largest quasi-cliques from the human PPIN has been proposed [5].

Earlier, it was shown that quasi-cliques and quasi-bicliques are able to symbolize groups of proteins associated with coherent biological activities in *S. cerevisiae* [26]. In several biological applications, quasi-cliques have been used to represent coherent modules, whereas, the quasi-bicliques have been used to depict the cofunctionality or coregulating nature between module pairs. Mining quasi-bicliques in such networks provides an important direction toward the study of biological pathways, protein complexes, and protein function. In [26], several quasi-cliques and quasi-bicliques were identified from the PPIN of *S. cerevisiae* using spectral analysis and validated using the annotation information. Again, in a later study quasi-bicliques were explored using a branch and bound method based on second-order neighborhood information [27]. In a recent study, maximum quasi-bicliques have been searched out from PPIN of *S. cerevisiae* using a divide and conquer approach [28]. This approach has the limitation of dependency on the selection of start splitting node, which restricts it often in reaching the global optimum.

There are several network-based prediction methods of protein functions [15]. Several works have focused solely on the functional module identification from PPI data. We describe some approaches that are based on the decomposition of the PPIN into subnetworks based on some topological properties. The molecular complex detection algorithm (MCODE) [18] is one such approach. It consists of the consecutive stages of node weighting, complex prediction, and an optional postprocessing step. This approach has motivated several successive improvements [29]. In a relatively recent study, expression similarity information (obtained from microarray data) has been integrated with topological information (obtained from high-throughput interaction data) to explore significantly connected subnetworks [4] jointly active connected subnetworks (JACS). A subnetwork is significant if it is highly connected in the interaction data, and in addition, has high average internal coherence in the corresponding gene coexpression network. These subnetworks are termed as jointly active connected subnetworks JACS. The algorithm proposed in this work, MATISSE [4], explores JACS by the successive steps of initializing dense subnetworks (seed) by enumeration, expansion of the seed, and filtering based on their significance. Again, the limitation of this approach lies in the prerequisite of network connectivity that is influenced by the high rate of false-negative interactions.

Literature studies strongly emphasize that the locally dense regions (cliques–quasi-cliques–subnetworks) of an interaction network represent protein complexes. However, defining density in the locality of PPINs is itself a dynamic concept. Several possible interpretations of dense regions are in existence and they mostly differ from the motivation with which they are used. A k-core is a maximal subnetwork such that each node in the subnetwork has at least degree k. A k-plex is a subnetwork such that each node in the subnetwork has at least degree $(O(N) - k)$, where $O(N)$ is the order of the subnetwork. A k-block is a maximal subnetwork such that each pair of nodes in the subnetwork is connected by k node-disjoint paths. An n-clan is a subnetwork such that the distance between any two nodes is less than or equal to n for paths within the subnetwork. These are some of the different representations of dense regions (protein complexes) that are currently emerging in use for interaction network analysis [30]. Here, we propose a heuristic algorithm to find the largest dense k-subnetwork in large scale-free networks that are sparse. We construct a PPIN, by integrating multiple topological properties, that is both sparse and scale-free. Finally, we explore our defined dense protein modules (dense k-subnetworks) by mining the network. The way we define a dense region in a weighted human PPIN is promising. Again, this kind of approach is novel in the perspective of systems biology.

16.4 PROBLEM DISCUSSION

Suppose, a set of proteins and their corresponding PPIN is provided. Here, we address the problem of searching the largest PPI modules that have a high degree of association therein. First, the problem is given formally accompanying the necessary precursory details. Then, the method of mining is presented in the later sections.

Definition 16.4.1 (k-subnetwork of a weighted network): *A k-subnetwork of any arbitrary weighted network, $N = (V, A, W)$, denoted by V^k, is defined as an induced subnetwork of N of order $k \in [1, |V|]$.*

Definition 16.4.2 (Association density of a node): *Given a weighted network* $N = (V, A, W)$, *the association density of a node* $v_i \in V$ *with respect to a k-subnetwork* V^k ($v_i \notin V^k$), μ_{v_i/V^k}, *is defined as the ratio of the sum of the arc weights between* v_i *and each of the nodes belonging to* V^k, *and the cardinality of the set* V^k. *The association density of a node* v_i *with respect to the k-subnetwork* V^k *is computed as*

$$\mu_{v_i/V^k} = \frac{\sum_{v_j \in V^k} W_{v_i v_j}}{k} \qquad (16.2)$$

where $W_{v_i v_j}$ *denotes the weight of the arc* (v_i, v_j).

Definition 16.4.3 (Dense node): *We call a node* v_i *within a k-subnetwork* V^k, *dense with respect to an association density threshold* δ, *if* $\mu_{v_i/V^k} \geq \delta$.

Definition 16.4.4 (Association density of a k-subnetwork): *The association density of a k-subnetwork,* V^k, *is defined as the minimum of the association densities of all the nodes in it with respect to the remaining* $(k-1)$-*subnetworks. So, the association density of a k-subnetwork* V^k *is given by*

$$\mu_{V^k} = \min_{\forall v_i \in V^k} \left(\mu_{v_i/V^k - \{v_i\}} \right) \qquad (16.3)$$

Definition 16.4.5 (Dense k-subnetwork): *We call a k-subnetwork,* V^k, *dense with respect to an association density threshold* δ *if* $\mu_{V^k} \geq \delta$.

As mentioned in Section 16.2, the density of a network–subnetwork is defined as the ratio of the total number of arcs existing in and the maximum number of arcs that could possibly appear within them. Thus, it may so happen that a k-subnetwork becomes dense although it contains some low degree values. In the network shown in Figure 16.2, the density of the k-subnetwork $\{p_1, p_2, p_3, p_5\}$, in the conventional sense, is 4.5/6. However, it is evident that the association of the node p_5 is poor as it has very low connectivity with the other nodes. A dense association should not only satisfy a high overall density, but also a high participation density of each member. Earlier studies also suggest that the computation of dense clusters should include some minimum density threshold for each node [31]. So, the concept of minimum association density threshold (a cutoff participation factor) has been included in Definition (16.4.4). Now, we present the problem of finding the largest dense k-subnetwork in a PPIN formally.

Problem Statement Given a weighted PPIN, $\mathcal{P} = (P, I, W)$, and an association density threshold of a k-subnetwork δ, locate a dense k-subnetwork $P^{k_{max}}$ in $\mathcal{P}$ that has the maximum cardinality, that is, $k_{max} \geq k : \forall \mu_{P^k} \geq \delta, \forall k = \{1, 2, \ldots, |P|\}$.

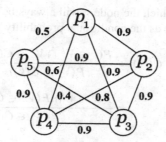

FIGURE 16.2   A dense subnetwork within a PPIN of order 5.

16.5   THEORETICAL ANALYSIS

As in this chapter, we are focusing on PPINs and they are generally found to follow the scale-free property [5]. We will concentrate on this special type of network to explore the largest dense k-subnetworks. In this regard, some theoretical analysis has been covered to devise the final algorithm.

Suppose $N = (V, A)$ is an arbitrary undirected and connected scale-free network with decay constant γ ($\gamma > 0$). Thus, the probability $P(k)$ that a node in N is adjacent to k ($\max(k) = |V| - 1$) other nodes, decays as a power law following $P(k) \sim k^{-\gamma}$. Evidently, this probability distribution of the discrete degree function adjoins the additional constraint $\sum_{k=1}^{|V|-1} P(k) = 1$. In this case $P(0) = 0$, as we have assumed the network N to be connected. Let the probability with which the arcs occur in N be $p(N)$ and the probability with which an arbitrary node v attaches with the other nodes be $p(v)$. Then, we have the following theorem:

Theorem 16.5.1   *Given, $p(N)$ and $p(v)$ for any arbitrary network N and for a node v within it, the probability with which v will appear in a clique selected randomly from N is given as*

$$P(v \in V^k | V^k \in C(k)) = \frac{k}{|V|}\left[1 + \frac{\Delta p(v)}{p(N)}\right]^{(k-1)}$$

Proof   Suppose, $C(k)$ denotes the set of all the cliques in N of size k. Then, the probability that a k-subnetwork (a subnetwork with k nodes), V^k, selected randomly from N will be in $C(k)$, if it contains v, is given by

$$P(V^k \in C(k) | v \in V^k) = p(v)^{(k-1)} p(N)^{\frac{(k-1)(k-2)}{2}} \tag{16.4}$$

The probability with which the node v will always belong to the set $C(k)$ can be computed using Eq. (16.4) as the conditional probability

$$P(v \in V^k | V^k \in C(k)) = \frac{P(v \in V^k \cap V^k \in C(k))}{P(V^k \in C(k))}$$

$$= \frac{P(v \in V^k).P(V^k \in C(k)|v \in V^k)}{P(V^k \in C(k))}$$

$$= \frac{\frac{\binom{|V|-1}{k-1}}{\binom{|V|}{k}} . p(v)^{(k-1)} p(N) \frac{(k-1)(k-2)}{2}}{p(N) \frac{k(k-1)}{2}}$$

$$= \frac{k}{|V|} \left[\frac{p(v)}{p(N)} \right]^{(k-1)}$$

$$= \frac{k}{|V|} \left[1 + \frac{\Delta p(v)}{p(N)} \right]^{(k-1)} . \qquad \square$$

Let, $v_{\max}$ be the node having the highest degree value in N, and consequently, $p(v_{\max})$ be the probability with which it connects the other nodes. Then, we have

$$P(v_{\max} \in V^k | V^k \in C(k)) = \frac{k}{|V|} \left[\frac{p(v_{\max})}{p(N)} \right]^{(k-1)}$$

$$= \frac{k}{|V|} \left[1 + \frac{\Delta p(v_{\max})}{p(N)} \right]^{(k-1)} \qquad (16.5)$$

Evidently, the probability value produced in Eq. (16.5) becomes higher with the increasing value of $\Delta p(v_{\max}) (= p(v_{\max}) - p(N))$. In the case of scale-free networks, the probability with which the arcs occur ($p(N)$) rests at a very low value due to the scale-free degree distribution. Thus, the nodes having comparatively higher degree values have a higher probability to be selected in the largest dense k-subnetwork. Therefore, selecting the nodes with higher association density values and merging them heuristically might produce better approximation in the final result. Being inspired from the aforementioned probabilistic intuition, we now discuss the solution methodology in Section 16.6.

16.6 ALGORITHMIC APPROACH

The problem addressed here belongs to the NP complexity class. For this reason, it cannot be solved deterministically in polynomial time, unless P = NP [32].

Considering this, a heuristic solution method for providing an approximate solution of the problem has been presented in the following algorithm:

Algorithm A heuristic solution approach for the problem

Input: A weighted PPIN $\mathcal{P} = (P, I, W)$ and an association density threshold δ.
Output: The largest k-subnetwork $P^{k_{\max}}$ in $\mathcal{P}$ satisfying the association density threshold δ.
Steps of the algorithm:

1. For each protein $p_i \in P$, arrange the proteins in $(P - \{p_i\})$ in the form of a list, $NList(p_i)$, such that any two entries p_1, p_2 satisfies $W_{p_i p_1} \geq W_{p_i p_2}$, if p_1 appears before p_2 within $NList(p_i)$.
2. Suppose, $NList(p_i, j)$ denotes the jth entry in the list $NList(p_i)$. Select an arbitrary protein $p_{\max}$ from the set of proteins for which $\sum_{n=1}^{k} W_{p_{\max} NList(p_{\max}, n)} < \delta k$ is satisfied for the maximum k.
3. Initialize $P^{k_{\max}}$ with $p_{\max}$
4. Let $Connector(n) = NList(p_{\max}, n), \forall n \in \{1, 2, \ldots, |P| - 1\}$
5. **while** $k_{\max} \leq |P|$ and $\mu_{p^{k_{\max}}} \geq \delta$ **do**
6. $P^{k_{\max}} \leftarrow P^{k_{\max}} \bigcup \{Connector(1)\}$
7. $Order(p_i) = Index(Connector(n), p_i)(k_{\max} - 1) + Index(NList(Connector(1), n), v_i), \forall p_i \in P$
   /* $Index(P, p_i)$ denotes the position of the element p_i in set P */
8. $Connector(n) \leftarrow p_t$, where $p_t \in P - P^{k_{\max}}$, such that $Order(Connector(i)) \leq Order(Connector(j))$, for each $i < j$
9. **end while**

We reproduce the algorithm proposed in [33] with nominal modification. In the beginning (step 1), a linked list is prepared for each protein $p_i \in P$, which contains all the remaining proteins, in the order of their descending weights with respect to the corresponding protein p_i. This is basically a neighboring list of proteins in the order of closeness. After this (step 2), the protein that can associate the largest number of proteins with it satisfying the association density threshold is determined. In case of a tie, it is selected randomly, and finally is used to initialize the largest k-subnetwork, $P^{k_{\max}}$ (step 3). Construction of the largest k-subnetwork then proceeds following steps 4–9. To start with, a connector list is prepared from the list of neighboring proteins of $p_{\max}$, taken from the $NList(p_{\max})$ (step 4). Then, the first member of the connector list is attached with the current dense k-subnetwork, $P^{k_{\max}}$ (step 6). This is in fact the closest neighbor of $p_{\max}$ and thus most similar in terms of the interaction weight. Thereafter, the connector list of $P^{k_{\max}}$ is updated by taking a weighted aggregation of the current connector list of $P^{k_{\max}}$, contained in $Connector$ and $NList(Connector(1))$, the corresponding $NList$ entry of $Connector(1)$ (step 8). The weights in this aggregation depends on the cardinalities of the two sets $P^{k_{max}}$ [before the attachment of the protein in *Connector*(1)] and *Connector*(1) itself. Certainly, the former one is of size ($k_{max} - 1$), whereas the later one is a singleton set. The iterative process continues (steps 5–9) till either all the proteins are included in $P^{k_{max}}$ or it falls short of the association density threshold δ.

16.7   EMPIRICAL ANALYSIS

We have carried out the experimental analysis both in the directions of mining the interaction networks and verifying the significance of the protein sets explored (within the largest k-subnetworks) through a biological perspective. In order to prepare the basic interaction network, PPI information of *Homo Sapiens* has been collected from the Human Protein Reference Database (HPRD) [34]. The version of interaction data we have collected reports 37, 107 interactions between 25, 661 human proteins. The clustering coefficient of the entire network is $\sim 1.13E - 4$ [5]. So, the network is prominently a sparse one. To visualize the degree distribution in this network, we have plotted the probability of attachment of the nodes against their degree values, that is, $P(k)$ denotes the probability of any arbitrary node of having a degree value of k. Scale-free degree distribution is observed in the PPIN employed in this study [16]. This is shown in Figure 16.3.

We have incorporated a novel method of integration in this topological study. Two kinds of topological information, the interaction between protein pairs and the sharing

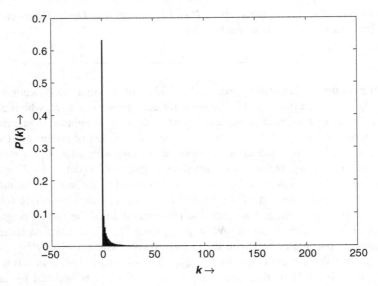

FIGURE 16.3   The degree of distribution in the human PPIN constructed from the HPRD interaction resource.

of first-order neighborhood between protein pairs, have been employed to build up a unified framework for the topological structure analysis. First, a PPIN $\mathcal{P} = (P, I, W)$ has been constructed from the up-to-date data collected from HPRD resource. Second, the sharing of first-order neighborhood information of every protein pair has been computed using the Sim_{CD} measure (inspired from the CD distance) to construct a separate network $\mathcal{P}_{CD} = (P, I_{CD}, W_{CD})$. Recently, some existing approaches have established the usefulness of accounting the common interacting partners between two proteins as an estimate of their functional similarity [20]. This Sim_{CD} is said to be the CD similarity and is computed between two proteins $p_1, p_2 \in P$ using the following final equation:

$$Sim_{CD}(p_1, p_2) = 1 - CD(p_1, p_2)$$

$$= 1 - \frac{|N(p_1) \cup \overline{N(p_2)}| + |\overline{N(p_1)} \cup N(p_2)|}{|N(p_1) \cup N(p_2)| + |N(p_1) \cap N(p_2)|}$$

$$= \frac{2.|N(p_1) \cap N(p_2)|}{|N(p_1) \cup N(p_2)| + |N(p_1) \cap N(p_2)|} \qquad (16.6)$$

Certainly, we have $W_{CD_{p_1 p_2}} = Sim_{CD}(p_1, p_2) \in [0, 1]$. Therefore, $\mathcal{P}_{CD}$ is a weighted network, whereas in the former one, constructed from the HPRD data, $\mathcal{P}$, is a binary network. Finally, these two networks are combined to produce an integrated network $\mathcal{P}^+ = (P, I^+, W^+)$, where the weight function is defined as $W^+ = 0.5 * (W + W_{CD})$. For those interactions absent in I in the network $\mathcal{P}$, we assume a weight of zero. Thus, $\mathcal{P}^+$ becomes a weighted and complete undirected network.

On constructing the integrated network $\mathcal{P}^+$ for the topological study, we have applied the algorithm described in Section 16.6 to investigate the largest dense k-subnetworks. We have set the association density threshold to $\delta = 0.55$. Fixation of δ to this value has been done to ensure that for any protein pair p_1, p_2, $(W_{p_1 p_2} + W_{CD_{p_1 p_2}})$ is at least 1.1. Because both of the weight functions W and W_{CD} have an upper bound of 1, the tuning of δ to 0.55 will confirm that none of these are individually zero for any protein pair. Thus, we can make it certain that the protein pairs selected within the dense k-subnetwork have prior interaction support, and as well, prior support of sharing a common neighborhood.

By applying the algorithm on the final network, we have obtained the largest dense k-subnetwork (with respect to $\delta = 0.55$) to contain 11 proteins. The biological analysis of this protein module is provided in the following sections. We have validated the functional significance of the protein set using the resource of HPRD [34] and a functional enrichment tool FatiGO [35].

16.7.1   Gene Ontology Studies from HPRD

The information regarding the biological process, molecular function, and molecular class (cellular component) of the genes (corresponding to the proteins found in the

TABLE 16.1 Biological Involvement of the Proteins Found in the Largest *k*-Subnetwork as Annotated from the Biological Process Information

Protein Name	Biological Process
ALDH1A1	Aldehyde metabolism
CHRNA1	Transport
APEH	Metabolism, Energy pathways
ADD2	Cell growth and/or maintenance
ADORA2A	Cell communication, Signal transduction
ARF3	Cell communication, Signal transduction
FDX1	Metabolism, Energy pathways
ADM	Regulation of physiological process
ALDOA	Metabolism, Energy pathways
SAA1	Lipid transport, Inflammatory response
CD59	Immune response

k-subnetwork) collected from the HPRD provides an insight into the system level participation of these proteins. We have accumulated the participation of the proteins found in the largest *k*-subnetwork in these three categories of gene ontology. Complete information is listed in Tables 16.1–16.3. As seen from Table 16.1, four proteins, namely, ALDH1A1, APEH, FDX1, and ALDOA are responsible for the biological process of metabolism (and often for the energy pathways) and their corresponding molecular functions (observe in Table 16.2) are related to the activities of aldehyde dehydrogenase, hydrolase, oxidoreductase, and lyase, respectively. In fact, these four proteins are separate enzymes (see Table 16.3) associated with the common biological activity of metabolism. Enzymes act as catalysts for many of the biochemical reactions

TABLE 16.2 Biological Involvement of the Proteins Found in the Largest *k*-Subnetwork as Annotated from the Molecular Function Information

Protein Name	Molecular Function
ALDH1A1	aldehyde dehydrogenase activity
CHRNA1	Intracellular ligand-gated ion channel activity
APEH	Hydrolase activity
ADD2	Cytoskeletal anchoring activity
ADORA2A	G-protein coupled receptor activity
ARF3	GTPase activity
FDX1	Oxidoreductase activity
ADM	Peptide hormone
ALDOA	Lyase activity
SAA1	Transporter activity
CD59	Receptor activity

**TABLE 16.3 Biological Involvement of the
Proteins Found in the Largest *k*-Subnetwork
as Annotated from the Molecular Class
(Cellular Component) Information**

Protein Name	Molecular Class
ALDH1A1	Enzyme: Dehydrogenase
CHRNA1	Intracellular ligand gated channel
APEH	Enzyme: Hydrolase
ADD2	Anchor protein
ADORA2A	G protein coupled receptor
ARF3	G protein
FDX1	Enzyme: Oxidoreductase
ADM	Peptide hormone
ALDOA	Enzyme: Aldolase
SAA1	Transport/cargo protein
CD59	Cell surface receptor

organized within an organism. Usually, these enzymes are very specific to a certain biochemical reaction [36]. In this regard, the four enzymes detected by the algorithm within the module are very significant. Similarly, from Table 16.1, we can identify the two proteins ADORA2A and ARF3, both of which are associated with the common tasks of cell communication and signal transduction, and again from Table 16.3 the later one is found to be a G protein, whereas the former one is its receptor. These results, obtained by combining the information provided in the Tables 16.1–16.3 suggest that the explored dense *k*-subnetwork is indeed a strongly coherent module of proteins. In Section 16.7.2, we produce the functional enrichment result produced from the tool FatiGO [35].

16.7.2 Study of Functional Enrichment with FatiGO

We have prepared two protein sets for the analysis using FatiGO. The first is a reference set, containing the 11 proteins found in the largest dense *k*-subnetwork, and the other one is a background set, containing the 25, 650 proteins remaining after mining in the initial interaction network. We have performed a two-tailed statistical test by removing the duplicates from the protein sets using the tool FatiGO [35]. The significant terms found in the functional enrichment test are provided in Table 16.4.

As observed in Table 16.4, the three proteins (ADORA2A, SAA1, and CD59) explored in the module are associated with the activities of coagulation, regulation of body fluids, and response to external stimulus with very low *p*-values. Going into a deeper analysis, it is found that these three proteins are responsible for blood coagulation. This finding is significant in the sense that <1% of the total proteins in the human protein set are related with this kind of biological activity. The *p*-value

TABLE 16.4   Significant GO Terms Found in the Biological Process to be Associated with the Proteins Found in the Largest k-Subnetwork

Level	GO Term	Module (%)	Remain (%)	p-Value
3	Coagulation	97.55	2.45	5.40E-05
3	Regulation of body fluids	97	3	9.92E-05
3	Response to external stimulus	89.45	10.55	8.87E-04
4	Hemostasis	97.43	2.57	6.28E-05
4	Response to wounding	92.09	7.91	2.69E-04
5	Wound healing	97.05	2.95	9.10E-05
6	Blood coagulation	97.73	2.27	4.02E-05

of this observation is as low as the order of $1E - 05$. From the analysis of HPRD repositories, as shown in Table 16.2, we have identified that the activities of the two proteins SAA1 and CD59 are in the form of transporter and receptor in immune response. Thus, they are responding to the immune system by participating in the blood coagulation along with the protein ADORA2A. As a whole, we have obtained six significant GO terms in the category biological process. In all of these cases, >89% of the proteins found in the largest dense k-subnetwork are associated with the corresponding GO term. The third column in Table 16.4 refers to the percentage of proteins found in the module associated with the specific GO term (biological process, molecular function, or cellular components) and in the fourth column the percentage of match with the remaining set of proteins. In all of these cases the probability of occurrence of these enrichment are not obtained by chance, as suggested by the very poor p-values computed.

The complete set of gene ontology terms categorized into biological process, molecular function, and cellular component form a directed acyclic graph structure (DAG). We produce the DAG representation of the significant terms found the protein module in Figure 16.4. This representation depicts the relations between the significant terms at the hierarchical level. Going into the lower levels in such DAG representation signifies a function into more specific form. In this regard, we found the most specific significant biological process of this protein module to be the regulation of body fluid levels. Such specific findings are therefore very important in the perspective of systems biology.

16.8   CONCLUSIONS

This chapter includes an integrated approach of analyzing topological characteristics of PPINs. The approach used in this study for combining two topological properties can also be extended for combining multiple properties at a time. We use a heuristic mining algorithm to find out dense protein sets from the integrated interaction network. Here, the denseness of a subnetwork has been defined in a novel way by

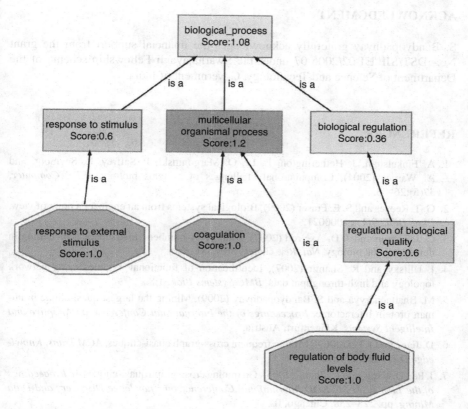

FIGURE 16.4   The gene ontology directed acyclic graph for biological process as annotated using the protein module (partial view of the significant terms).

thresholding minimum association of each node with the others in the weighted subnetwork. The analytical studies provoke a new integrative approach of studying biological systems as initiated in [4].

The success of such topological studies highly depend on the accuracy and quality of the high-throughput interaction resources. Unfortunately, the enormous volume of interaction information accumulated by various research groups worldwide principally focus on positive interactions. Researchers are generally biased to finding protein pairs that physically or functionally interact, not those having no provable interactions. There is no doubt that casting aside the negative interaction data is a major drawback of interactome analysis. Recently, it has been empirically validated that negative training data sets can add potentials to the final outcome of computational analysis on biological data [37]. Analyzing PPINs covering both validated positive and negative interaction information will thus be a promising improvement in this direction.

ACKNOWLEDGMENT

S. Bandyopadhyay gratefully acknowledges the financial support from the grant No.- DST/SJF/ET-02/2006-07 under the Swarnajayanti Fellowship scheme of the Department of Science and Technology, Government of India.

REFERENCES

1. A. Finkelstein, J. Hetherington, L. Li, O. Margoninski, P. Saffrey, R. Seymour, and A. Warner (2004), Computational challenges of systems biology, *IEEE Computer*, 37(5):26–33.

2. G. T. Reeves and S. E. Fraser (2009), Biological systems from an engineer's point of view, *PLoS Biol.*, 7(1):e1000021.

3. C. J. Tomlin and J. D. Axelrod (2007), Biology by numbers: mathematical modelling in developmental biology, *Nat. Rev. Genet.*, 8(5):331–340.

4. I. Ulitsky and R. Shamir (2007), Identification of functional modules using network topology and high-throughput data, *BMC Systems Biol.*, 1:8.

5. M. Bhattacharyya and S. Bandyopadhyay (2009), Mining the largest quasi-clique in human protein interactome. *Proceedings of the International Conference on Adaptive and Intelligent Systems*, Klagenfurt, Austria.

6. D. Jiang and J. Pei (2009), Mining frequent cross-graph quasi-cliques, *ACM Trans. Knowledge Dis. Data*, 2(4):16.

7. J. Pei, D. Jiang, and A. Zhang (2005), On mining cross-graph quasi-cliques. In *Proceedings of the 11th ACM SIGKDD International Conference on Knowledge Discovery and Data Mining*, pp. 228–238, Chicago, IL.

8. M. Bhattacharyya and S. Bandyopadhyay (2009), Integration of co-expression networks for gene clustering. *Proceedings of the 7th International Conference on Advances in Pattern Recognition*, pp. 355–358, Kolkata, India.

9. H. N. Chua, W. Hugo, G. Liu, X. Li, L. Wong, and S. K. Ng (2009), A probabilistic graph-theoretic approach to integrate multiple predictions for the protein-protein subnetwork prediction challenge. *Ann. NY Acad. Sci.*, 1158:224–233.

10. I. Lee, S. V. Date, A. T. Adai, and E. M. Marcotte (2004), A probabilistic functional network of yeast genes, *Science*, 306:1555–1558.

11. Q. A. Justman, Z. Serber, Jr. J. E. Ferrell, H. El-Samad, and K. M. Shokat (2009), Tuning the activation threshold of a kinase network by nested feedback loops, *Science*, 324(5926):509–512.

12. M. E. Cusick, N. Klitgord, M. Vidal, and D. E. Hill (2005), Interactome: gateway into systems biology, *Human Mol. Genet.*, 14(Rev. Issue 2):R171–R181.

13. S. C. Gad (2005), *Drug Discovery Handbook*. John Wiley & Sons, Inc., NY.

14. A. Panchenko and T. Przytycka (Eds.) (2008), Protein–protein interactions and networks: Identification, computer analysis, and prediction, *Computational Biology*, Vol. 9. Springer, NY.

15. R. Sharan, I. Ulitsky, and R. Shamir (2007), Network-based prediction of protein function, *Mol. Systems Biol.*, 3:88.

16. A. L. Barabási and R. Albert (1999), Emergence of scaling in random networks, *Science*, 286:509–512.

17. D. J. Watts and S. H. Strogatz (1998), Collective dynamics of 'small-world' networks, *Nature (London)*, 393:440–442.

18. G. D. Bader and C. W. Hogue (2003), An automated method for finding molecular complexes in large protein interaction networks, *BMC Bioinformatics*, 4:2.

19. O. Tastan, Y. Qi, J. G. Carbonell, and J. Klein-Seetharaman (2009), Prediction of interactions between hiv-1 and human proteins by information integration. *Proceedings of the Pacific Symposium on Biocomputing*, pp. 516–527, Hawaii.

20. C. Brun, F. Chevenet, D. Martin, J. Wojcik, A. Guenoche, and B. Jacq (2003), Functional classification of proteins for the prediction of cellular function from a protein-protein interaction network, *Genome Biol.*, 5(1):R6.

21. I. M. Bomze, M. Budinich, P. M. Pardalos, and M. Pelillo (1999), The maximum clique problem. D. Z. Du and P. M. Pardalos (Eds.), *Handbook of Combinatorial Optimization: Supplementary Volume A*, pp. 1–74. Kluwer Academic, Dordrecht, The Netherlands.

22. X. Liu, J. Li and L. Wang (2008), Quasi-bicliques: Complexity and binding pairs. *Computing and Combinatorics*, Vol. LNCS 5092, pp. 255–264, Springer, NY.

23. L. Royer, M. Reimann, B. Andreopoulos, and M. Schroeder (2008), Unraveling protein networks with power graph analysis, *PLoS Comput. Biol.*, 4(7):e1000108.

24. C. C. Lin, H. F. Juan, J. T. Hsian, Y. C. Hwang, H. Mori, and H. C. Huang (2009), Essential core of protein-protein interaction network in *Escherichia coli.*, *J. Proteome Res.*, 8(4):1925–1931.

25. J. Abello, M. G. C. Resende, and S. Sudarsky (2002), Massive quasi-clique detection, *Theoretical Informatics*, Vol. LNCS 2286, pp. 598–612. Springer, NY.

26. D. Bu, Y. Zhao, L. Cai, H. Xue, X. Zhu, H. Lu, J. Zhang, S. Sun, L. Ling, N. Zhang, G. Li, and R. Chen (2003), Topological structure analysis of the protein-protein interaction network in budding yeast. *Nucleic Acids Res.*, 31(9):2443–2450.

27. H. Liu, J. Liu, and L. Wang (2007), Searching quasi-bicliques in proteomic data. *Proceedings of the International Conference on Computational Intelligence and Security Workshops*, pp. 77–80, Washington, DC.

28. H. Liu, J. Liu, and L. Wang (2008), Searching maximum quasi-bicliques from protein-protein interaction network, *J. Biomed. Sci. Eng.*, 1:200–203.

29. J. F. Rual, K. Venkatesan, T. Hao, T. Hirozane-Kishikawa, and A. Dricot (2005), Towards a proteome-scale map of the human protein-protein interaction network, *Nature (London)*, 437:1173–1178.

30. M. Altaf-Ul-Amin, Y. Shinbo, K. Mihara, K. Kurokawa, and S. Kanaya (2006), Development and implementation of an algorithm for detection of protein complexes in large interaction networks, *BMC Bioinformatics*, 7:207.

31. X. Yan, M. R. Mehan, Y. Huang, M. S. Waterman, P. S. Yu, and X. J. Zhou (2007), A graph-based approach to systematically reconstruct human transcriptional regulatory modules, *Bioinformatics*, 23:i577–i586.

32. M. R. Garey and D. S. Johnson (1979), *Computers and Intractability: A Guide to the Theory of NP-Completeness*. Freeman & Co., NY.

33. S. Bandyopadhyay and M. Bhattacharyya (2008), Mining the largest dense n-vertexlet in a fuzzy scale-free graph. In *Technical Report No. MIU/TR-03/08*, Machine Intelligence Unit, Indian Statistical Institute, Kolkata, India.

34. T. S. K. Prasad et al. (2009), Human protein reference database—2009 update, *Nucleic Acids Res. (Database issue)*, 37:D767–D772.

35. F. Al-Shahrour, R. Díaz-Uriarte, and J. Dopazo (2004), FatiGO: a web tool for finding significant associations of gene ontology terms with groups of genes, *Bioinformatics*, 20:578–580.

36. J. Setubal and J. Meidanis (1999), *Introduction to Computational Molecular Biology*, PWS Publishing Company, Boston.

37. S. Bandyopadhyay and R. Mitra (2009), TargetMiner: MicroRNA target prediction with systematic identification of tissue specific negative examples, *Bioinformatics*, 25(20):2625–2631.

INDEX

Computational Intelligence and Pattern Analysis in Biological Informatics, Edited by Ujjwal Maulik,
Sanghamitra Bandyopadhyay, and Jason T. L. Wang
Copyright © 2010 John Wiley & Sons, Inc.

Wiley Series on

Bioinformatics: Computational Techniques and Engineering

Bioinformatics and computational biology involve the comprehensive application of mathematics, statistics, science, and computer science to the understanding of living systems. Research and development in these areas require cooperation among specialists from the fields of biology, computer science, mathematics, statistics, physics, and related sciences. The objective of this book series is to provide timely treatments of the different aspects of bioinformatics spanning theory, new and established techniques, technologies and tools, and application domains. This series emphasizes algorithmic, mathematical, statistical, and computational methods that are central in bioinformatics and computational biology.

Series Editors: **Professor Yi Pan** and **Professor Albert Y. Zomaya**
pan@cs.gsu.edu   zomaya@it.usyd.edu.au

Knowledge Discovery in Bioinformatics: Techniques, Methods, and Applications
Xiaohua Hu and Yi Pan

Grid Computing for Bioinformatics and Computational Biology
Edited by El-Ghazali Talbi and Albert Y. Zomaya

Bioinformatics Algorithms: Techniques and Applications
Ion Mandiou and Alexander Zelikovsky

Analysis of Biological Networks
Edited by Björn H. Junker and Falk Schreiber

Computational Intelligence and Pattern Analysis in Biological Informatics
Edited by Ujjwal Maulik, Sanghamitra Bandyopadhyay, and Jason T. L. Wang

Printed in the United States
By Bookmasters